D1525084

Pioneer Work with
Maladjusted Children

Maurice Bridgeland, M.A., M.Ed.
Lecturer in Special Education, University of Liverpool

Pioneer Work with Maladjusted Children

A Study of the Development of
Therapeutic Education

Staples Press London

Granada Publishing Limited
First published in Great Britain 1971 by Staples Press Ltd
3 Upper James Street London W1R 4BP

ISBN 0 286 62750 7
Printed in Great Britain by Willmer Brothers Ltd
Birkenhead Cheshire

'There are three things which last for ever:
faith, hope and love; but the greatest of
them all is love.'

To my Mother

As this book was going to press, *New Society* on 8 April 1971, published a review by A. S. Neill of Freud's 'Introductory Lectures on Psychoanalysis' (published by Allen & Unwin). In this review Neill made clear his opinion that individual psychoanalysis based on Freudian methods, and education based on the Freudian principle that 'The child must learn to control his instincts ... accordingly education must inhibit, forbid and suppress', provided no answer to the problems of a neurotic society. The solution he proffers is Reichian prophylaxis and education based on the motto 'Thou shall not obey' a method and a motto which he says 'I am sure old Sigmund would not have accepted'. See Chapter 9.

Acknowledgements

The Author wishes to make grateful acknowledgement for permission to quote from the following works.

BADLEY, J. H. *A Schoolmaster's Testament*, Blackwell, London, 1937: BARRAN, A. T. 'Preparing a Child for Placement', *The New Era*, p. 32, 43, 1962: BARROW, A. T. 'What is Therapy – What is Training?' *Therapeutic Education*, p. 35, Autumn 1969, The Association of Workers for Maladjusted Children: BAZELEY, E. T. *Homer Lane and the Little Commonwealth*, pp. 109–114, Allen & Unwin, London, 1928: BURT, C. *The Young Delinquent*, p. 615, University of London Press, 1944: Caldecott Community; various publications: CHILD, H.A.T. *The Independent Progressive School*, p. 8, Hutchinson, London, 1962: City of Leicester Education Committee Annual Report 1932: City of Leicester Education Committee pamphlet 'The Education of Retarded and Difficult Children in the Leicester Schools', 1937: COLE, M. and PADLEY, R. The Evacuation Survey; A report to the Fabian Society, p. 42, 1940: COLEMAN, J. *Childscourt*, pp. 47–8, Macdonald, London, 1967: DOCKAR-DRYSDALE, B. *Therapy and the Child*, pp. 26–7, Longmans Green, London, 1968: FIORE, Q. and MCLUHAN, M. *The Medium is the Massage*, p. 188, Allen Lane, The Penguin Press, 1967: *The Guardian*, 23 February 1966: HARING, N. G. and PHILIPS, E. L. *Educating Emotionally Disturbed Children*, p. 11, McGraw-Hill, New York, 1962: HAVIGHURST, R. J. and PECK, R. F. *The Psychology of Character Development*, John Wiley, New York, 1960: HOLMES, EDMOND. *What is and What Might Be*, p. 195, Constable, London, 1911: H.M.S.O. The Curtis Report, Section 494, Cmnd 6922, 1946: H.M.S.O. Education Act, Section 33 (i) 1944: H.M.S.O. Seebohm Report, Section 242, Cmnd 3703, 1968: H.M.S.O. Kilbrandon Report, Section 178, Cmnd 2306, 1964: JONES, H. *Reluctant Rebels*, p. 12, pp. 72–3, Tavistock, London, 1960: LANE, HOMER. *Talks to Parents and Teachers*, pp. 12–13, Allen & Unwin, London, 1928: LENNHOFF, F. G. *Exceptional Children*, p. 34, Allen & Unwin, London, 1960: LYWARD, G. A. 'Feeling Their Way

Through', *New Era*, p. 115, 3, No. 7, 1938: LYWARD, G. A. 'In Conclusion', in Problems of Child Development, *New Era*, p. 94, 29, 1948: PEDLEY, R. *Comprehensive Education – A New Appraisal*, Victor Gollancz, London, 1956: Scottish Council for Research in Education, Publication XXii V.L.P., 1944: SHAW, OTTO L. *Maladjusted Boys*, pp. 81–6, Allen & Unwin, London, 1965: SIMEY, T. S. 'The Concept of Love in Child Care', National Children's Home, 1961: SUTCLIFFE, B. and KELLMER PRINGLE, M. L. *Remedial Education – An Experiment*, p. 29, The Caldecott Community and the Department of Child Study, University of Birmingham, 1960: *The Times Educational Supplement*, 6 January 1914: VAN MORRIS, C. *Existentialism in Education*, p. 148, Harper and Row, New York, 1966: WHITBOURN, F. *Lex: Alexander Devine, Founder of Claysmore School*, p. 91 and pp. 125–6, Longmans Green, London, 1937: WILLS, W. D. *Throw Away Thy Rod*, p. 18, Victor Gollancz, 1960: WILLS, W. D. *Homer Lane, A Biography*, pp. 12–13, p. 76 and p. 139, Allen & Unwin, London, 1964: WILLS, W. D. *The Barns Experiment*, p. 65, Allen & Unwin, London, 1945.

Contents

Foreword

I feel so much flattered by being asked to write a preface to Maurice Bridgeland's book that I hesitate to criticise it, but I will overcome my hesitancy and utter my one small criticism – the title is inadequate. It is inadequate because Maurice has written not only a most comprehensive and all-inclusive account of what has so far been done specifically for and with maladjusted children but he has also examined the ancestry and collateral branches of that work in ordinary and 'progressive' education, in the approved-school system, in psychiatry, in psychology and in legislation. He has thus provided a much needed conspectus of the whole field, which will enlighten the layman and stimulate the student. All this he is well qualified to do by virtue of his own record of experience in ordinary education, in schools for maladjusted children and in the training at university level of others who hope to do similar work. His counsel as an officer of the Association of Workers for Maladjusted Children has been greatly valued, and his imminent translation to a distinguished headship in the realm of 'normal' boarding-school education is one which causes us some little apprehension lest that counsel should henceforward be lost to us.

If I may speak as one of the pioneers to whom he has made reference, the development that gives me most satisfaction – and which is dealt with fully within these covers – is the appearance in recent years of what one may think of as the second wave. If, as Maurice suggests, people like George Lyward, Otto Shaw and myself are father figures, then the next generation are people like Barbara Dockar-Drysdale, Richard Balbernie and Arthur Barron. What I most like about them is that they possess so abundantly a capacity I have always lacked – the capacity to examine what they and others are doing within the terms of reference of scientific disciplines.

I have in my own work done what I believed (and still believe) to be right and have tried to convince others of its rightness by means of what can only be thought of as *ex parte* pleading. The new wave are altogether more rigorous and scientific in their examination and conceptualisation of what is being done, and yet they are not simply academic theorists – certainly not those I have named – because they have all been deeply involved in residential work for many years, often in most unpropitious circumstances and often with the most difficult children. They are developing what we lacked and what indeed we failed to provide for those who were to follow us – a highly professional and scientific rationale of therapeutic education and environment therapy.

This delights me, and I am glad that Maurice has given it its proper place between these covers. It is true that my delight arises in part from the self-complacent feeling that this careful scientific approach tends on the whole to confirm what we earlier people were doing which, naturally, is gratifying. What is more gratifying however is the consequence that follows from this, namely, that the new wave will not have to spend time starting afresh from new premises and concepts but are able to move forward along the road on which they have already started, to a greater understanding and to more effective endeavours in a field where there is still much to learn, and where there is enormous scope for improved methods and techniques.

Highly relevant here is the new approach to juvenile delinquency revealed in the Children and Young Persons Act 1969. No longer, if all goes according to plan, will an emotionally disturbed child receive different treatment according to whether or not he happens to have broken the law. This highly artificial distinction is, we hope, gone for good, and it is clearly the intention of the Home Office that the kind of therapeutic environment that has hitherto been available in schools for maladjusted children shall henceforward be at the disposal of all unhappy children. *Hoc erat in votis* says the Latin tag, and this indeed was in the prayers of all of us.

Hook Norton   W. DAVID WILLS

Introduction

Since the only real starting point in history is the present moment, historians are always being overtaken by events. In writing this account of one aspect of education and therapy I am conscious that impending legislation and administrative changes may make some of my conclusions redundant. If so I shall be delighted.

The maladjusted, like the poor, are always with us; so, more fortunately, are the pioneers. My justification for reviewing pioneer work from the vantage point of 1970 is that I can look backwards from this watershed to an era of individual endeavour and forward to one of national expansion, rethinking and responsibility. I have tried to review the characteristics of the former and preview those of the latter.

In considering pioneer work I have been hampered, as all historians are, by both the presence and the absence of facts. Both may distort perspective. Facts may prove a very unreliable guide to truth. One can never know all the relevant facts even about one person's life experience nor how these facts impinge on one another. There are no isolated events in a person's life. Thus one can never tell whether the facts one knows are more, or less, important than those which one does not know. One suspects less. Perhaps the nearest one can get to reality is how it is perceived by the person concerned. Something which did not happen but which is perceived as important may be much more real than something which did happen but which is not perceived as important.

My own perception of events has been immeasurably assisted by that of many of my subjects, of their colleagues and of their former pupils. Personal contact and correspondence with most of the living pioneers and with the widows of Dr Dodd, Dr Fitch and W. G. Sharman has been invaluable. To all of these I offer my admiration for their achievement and my thanks for their co-operation. To a large extent one has to consider not only what they did but also what others thought that they were doing, for part of their achievement lay in creating myth which inspired others. Indeed it is clear that if the many different techniques described were all as effective as their protagonists claim then the element common to all was faith.

This may also be true of psychotherapeutic techniques derived largely from practice and observation. The latter form the rationale of techniques differing widely in their objects and methods but which contain common elements of love, care and individual personal relationships. These constitute the 'philosophers' stone' in the alchemy, rather than the science, of education and therapy. To say that there is no scientific evidence that any psychotherapeutic technique *works* in the way in which it claims to work is not to undervalue it. Success can be measured only in terms of aim and in any sphere as complex as personality development one can never know, absolutely, that any of the variables perceived are those which are producing the effect. One can get nearer to the truth only by looking at, and comparing, the methods and theories in as much detail as is available and often, necessarily, in terms of the results perceived by those people who were involved in, or who observed, the process. In the future we may hope to get closer to reality by techniques of research which were largely unavailable to pioneers. Science may yet give that support to educational alchemy which modern medicine has sometimes given to medieval insight. The reason may have been wrong but the method right.

The whole concept of 'therapeutic education' involves a value judgement. Education presupposes a change in behaviour. Therapy posits an improvement in health. Therapeutic education therefore suggests that changes in behaviour and health are interrelated. A child whose behaviour damages his chances of normal healthy enjoyment of what society can offer him needs educational aid. A child whose emotional imbalance inhibits normal and acceptable behaviour in such a way that he cannot be happy in any society needs therapy. To help an individual both to establish himself and to exist happily in society constitute the twin aims of 'therapeutic education'.

The pioneers in this work were essentially optimistic. They knew, with Erickson, that children 'fall apart' repeatedly and, unlike Humpty Dumpty, grow together again; they also knew that 'there is little that cannot be remedied . . . there is much that can be prevented from happening at all'.* It is with this hope that pioneers did their

*Erickson, E. H.: in Schaffner B. (ed.), *Group Processes*. pp. 83 and 104. Josiah Macy Jnr. Foundation, New York, 1950.

work and in recording it I have tried to point to ways in which their insights may help us to prevent as well as to cure maladjustment.

In this endeavour I have received much help. To the pioneers themselves, to the many people who have given me information, to Miss Kate Guthrie, who was so much more than a secretary, and to those from whose valuable thoughts and writings I have quoted, I offer my thanks. To Professor J. W. L. Adams, who first gave me the opportunity to pursue my interest; to David Wills who encouraged me in it, and to my friend and colleague David Pritchard, who meticulously edited the result, I acknowledge my debt. To my family who have unfailingly supported me in this endeavour I return their love.

Liverpool University   M. BRIDGELAND

List of Abbreviations

A.W.M.C.	Association of Workers for Maladjusted Children
C.G.C.	Child Guidance Clinic (Centre or Council)
C.M.O.	Chief Medical Officer
C.S.E.	Certificate of Secondary Education
D.E.S.	Department of Education & Science
E.S.N.	Educationally sub-normal
H.M.I.	Her (or His) Majesty's Inspector
I.L.E.A.	Inner London Education Authority
L.E.A.	Local Education Authority
L.C.C.	London County Council
N.E.F.	New Education Fellowship
N.A.M.H.	National Association for Mental Health
N.F.E.R.	National Foundation for Educational Research (in England & Wales)
P.S.W.	Psychiatric Social Worker
S.C.E.A.	Scottish Campaign for Educational Advance
S.C.R.E.	Scottish Council for Research in Education
S.E.D.	Scottish Education Department
V.A.D.	Voluntary Aid Detachment
W.R.I.	Women's Rural Institute
W.V.S.	Women's Voluntary Service

PART ONE

Definitions

1

Pioneers

Radical experiments in institutions for problem children have been comparatively few, presumably because they call for more than ability and imagination. Great courage is also needed for the innovator has to be willing to take risks, as well as to face the hostility of a fearful and insecure general public. He must, in fact, be himself a person with a strong sense of inner security.[1]

It may be thought that by presenting the history of the progress of therapeutic education largely in terms of the individual pioneers involved I am putting too great an emphasis on the personal factor. In this particular study, however, this approach is I think justified. In few other spheres of work is the individual person so important, so essential, so central. Therapy through education depends on the establishment of close personal relationships between adult and child and the actual means of therapy are largely dictated, in a small community, by the interests, training, ability and personality of the central figure. Although most of the early experimenters were essentially individualistic any generalization of their techniques depended largely on their ability as conceptualizers and communicators or on that of people who studied them in action. Practice almost always preceded theory and until the Underwood Report[2] in 1955 there was little official attempt to see practice in terms of anything other than the — often unwelcome — experimenting of a number of independent individuals. This 'new' approach to the care and cure of those who were recognized as unhappy rather than as 'naughty' children was essentially individualistic. This is, perhaps, one of the characteristics of pioneering in any field. R. W. Shields, writing in 1962, said: 'Up to the present virtually all the pioneer research work in the treatment of maladjusted children has been done in private or independent schools. In these schools one outstandingly gifted individual has built around himself a therapeutic environment and a treatment team, and has been able to conceptualize and communicate what is being done.'[3]

Shields, I feel, establishes the right order of precedence. Few of the pioneers began with a concept to which they adhered in practice but rather the concept was evolved through practice. Alice Woods, in discussing experiments in education in the early 1920s, points out that they were not, on the whole, 'scientific' in the sense of being the systematic examination of phenomena isolated from all extraneous variables—a situation generally recognized as an unattainable ideal even in the psychological laboratory when the subjects are human beings—but rather an insightful probing into the unknown. 'Authority, having some definite aim before it, deliberately departs from some established usage ... overthrows some convention, or starts some entirely new plan, and then notes ... the changes that come about.'

'The experimenter may have an idea or a "plan" but it is constantly modified by experience in the same way that the explorer may have a rough map but, finding one route to his goal blocked by something which he had not, or could not have, foreseen, seeks an alternative way to his objective. The educator sets his imagination to work and pictures the ideal state of school and scholar that he wishes to bring about. He turns over in his mind such knowledge as he possesses of child nature, thinks out some plan which will under such circumstances as he can command lead, as he hopes, to the desired results, and then puts it into practice and notes the effects on the children. Should the effect appear to be satisfactory he pursues his scheme with renewed ardour; should it be unsatisfactory he bravely abandons it and either returns to the old regime or starts another working hypothesis.'[4]

This is, indeed, the pioneer approach, progressive in the sense of dynamic; pragmatic and formative in the sense of being observed, noted and conceptualized; and experimental in the sense of exploring beyond the safe bounds of the known and established.

A pioneer is not merely a lone figure early in the field. He must have the power to communicate to, and inspire, others who follow after. An explorer without this power may be merely a rash adventurer in uncharted regions. He must survive the experience and live at least to 'tell the tale'.

Apart from their willingness to experiment, to take risks and to meet opposition, these pioneers had few things in common. A few of them were teachers, others were therapists, journalists, doctors, engineers or sheep-farmers. Some, like Leila Rendel and Barbara

Dockar-Drysdale, came from secure upper-class backgrounds; others, like N. B. C. Lucas, from difficult or broken homes. Many rejected their own backgrounds and sought, like A. S. Neill and Homer Lane, to build a new order, while others endeavoured, as did Leila Rendel, to preserve the virtues of an older and more settled order of things. For many school had been, as it was for Norman MacMunn, a place of terror, or, as it was for Lane, Fitch and Neill, a stimulus to rebellion. A few were happy in school and tried to communicate their happiness to others. Religion was to David Wills, Father Owen or Edward Seel the essential foundation of their work; others like Bill Malcolm or Lucy Francis rejected it as something essentially injurious to mental health.

Personalities, too, appear to differ widely, although here, perhaps, there is more common ground. Whatever the regime through which they operated, pioneers in this difficult work needed a natural authority, a real sympathy and a strength of conviction which enabled them to overcome all obstacles. Each was, and is, 'like a prophet who has no doubts'. This faith in themselves, a strong tendency to be dogmatic and the isolation of their position frequently made them intolerant of others not numbered among their converts.

They are, on the whole, more successful in their relationships with children than with fellow adults, who might threaten their essential faith in themselves or compete to share the paternal role. Where failure has occurred it appears to have been largely the result of attempts to share authority, as at Arlesford Court; of inadequate definition of role; of inability to communicate the nature of the work to an apprehensive outside world or, as possibly in the case of Homer Lane, a flaw of personality which led to fatal over-involvement.

As Howard Jones suggests, the most important attribute is probably an 'inner security' whether it is derived from religious faith, a secure social order, an unshakable confidence in oneself or the depth of one's own self-knowledge. Without this one can hardly hope to lead the immature, insecure, anxious and disturbed child towards satisfactory self-adjustment.

I have examined the educational and social background against which the pioneers worked in order to reveal both the originality of that work and the interaction between it and the prevailing ethos. In considering individual pioneers I have endeavoured to show their work in relation to their lives, their principles and the structure of their institutions. While revealing their particular contributions I have suggested its interrelation with that of other pioneer figures in the allied spheres of education, child care and mental health, and have tried to assess their achievements and suggest ways in which their work may have a continuing effect.

2

The Maladjusted Child and His Setting

The Department . . . might bear in mind the extremely confused situation at present in which every local authority has its own definitions of the term 'maladjusted' and 'educationally sub-normal'. This lack of nationally agreed definition means that no picture exists about the current overall position of these young people and that consequently research into their problems and provision for their adequate care are hindered – Editorial, *New Education p* 21. September 1965.

The Editor's dismay, above, is echoed by all who are thus hindered. 'Maladjustment' is one of those terms which Reid and Hagan tellingly describe as a 'catch-all nosological waste-basket'.[5] Many workers and researchers would wish it consigned to the waste-basket either as undesirable, static, imprecise and pejorative[6] or as something more positively harmful in that the use of such an amorphous term may conceal the true nature of the condition.

Dr Kenneth Soddy, speaking at a National Association of Mental Health conference in 1957, said 'I do not believe that one advances the cause of understanding by regarding maladjustment as a phenomenon standing in its own right that has to be treated as if it has an independent meaning of its own'[7] and yet its very breadth and inclusiveness gives it a certain administrative convenience which assures its continuance. 'Provided that it is not used as a medical entity but as an umbrella term which is administratively convenient there seems little reason for changing a term which now covers such a wide variety of psychological conditions.'[8]

The wide variety of conditions covered are described in two useful appendices to the report of the working party on the *Ascertainment of Maladjusted Children, Scotland*, 1964, which consider both causes and symptoms—particularly those associated with the 'Scottish cultural environment' (the recognition of a cultural variable is significant).[9] Other 'umbrella' definitions and comprehensive lists of symptoms and causes may be found in most publications on the subject, such as Katherine d'Evelyn's *Meeting Children's Emotional Needs*[10] or, in more general terms, in the earlier Scottish report: *Pupils who are Maladjusted because of Social Handicap*.[11]

Since the term 'maladjusted' had no agreed or official meaning before the 1945 regulations, to talk of 'maladjusted' children before that time may be historically imprecise, in that there were officially no schools for a handicap which had no statutory existence. As David Wills points out: 'The Act of 1944 does not even mention, much less define them. The regulations of 1945 attempted a definition and the Ministry were so pleased with it—or frightened of it—that they did not tamper with it when the regulations were revised in 1953.'[12] The accepted definition was: 'Pupils who show evidence of emotional instability or psychological disturbance and require special educational treatment in order to effect their personal, social or educational re-adjustment'.[13] The Underwood Committee of 1955 finds this definition inadequate[14] and tries to define by example by giving detailed lists of symptoms[15] and causes.[16] Any tentative definitions are qualified, however, by such observations as 'Maladjustment is an individual matter on which it is hard to generalize'[17] and 'The reasons why one child succumbs rather than another seem to be deep and, at present, obscure'!

GENERAL DEFINITIONS

Maladjusted children are unhappy children. Unhappy whether their failure to 'adjust' is related to their own inner conflicts, to their families or to their wider social environment. They are unbalanced children. Unbalanced whether they are trying to reconcile their own conflicting impulses, their own physical and emotional development, their own personal needs or the conflicting demands of individual existence and the pressures of social conformity. Such a child is 'unable to live healthily in the normal context of home and school without pain to himself or disturbance to his environment.'[18]

If one accepts the proposition that a child is born neither adjusted nor maladjusted but is, nevertheless, born a person, with individual nervous responses and metabolic balance—a proposition not lacking in empirical support[19]—one can also accept that subsequent environmental pressures will have differing effects as the process of what Dr Soddy considered 'warping' continues.[20]

Some children will be emotionally fragile and will surrender their individuality too easily. Such children may become over-anxious, over-conformist, prone to psychosomatic conditions or phobic states, or may withdraw into a fantasy world within which they can defend themselves against painful reality. Others may be emotionally 'tough' and will carry on their fight to retain individuality through aggression, destruction and delinquency. Such reactions to stress will be described as 'symptoms' either neurotic or behavioural, but, as Dr Wolff points out, the symptom is a communication with no particular meaning outside the particular individual's complete life experience.[21]

In unbalanced children the critical stages of the essential 'ego' development (the successful resolution of the struggle between what we want and what we are allowed—and the eventual discovery of 'self'), will produce frustration and conflict without adjustment. For all children the traumatic experiences of birth; of identity with, and separation from, mother; of early training; of the experience of family life; of the death of, or separation from, others; of deprivation of all sorts; of adjusting to the demands of school and wider social groups—all of these experiences may be successfully or unsuccessfully met depending on their severity, the 'strength' of the child and the availability of 'the basic psychological nourishment without which the human infant does not become a human being in the full sense of that term.[22] This last, Professor Morris saw as the unconditional love of good parents for which, for the damaged child, a residential situation in which the characteristics of good family life are implicit may have to act as substitute.

We are all unhappy and unbalanced at some point in our emotional development. Most of us have at some time stolen, lied, been anxious, hysterical or depressed; we have withdrawn into fantasies, we have missed school or misbehaved in school, we have wet the bed, had nightmares, been aggressive and unco-operative. Had we not we could scarcely be considered normal.

The 'adjusted' child, however, has either produced these symptoms at an appropriate stage of development, has had help in a supportive home, or has been able to cope without help. The maladjusted child, who is usually, for a variety of reasons, emotionally immature, not only behaves in a way inappropriate to his years[23] but cannot, without help, cope with his own problems.

PIONEER DEFINITIONS

The interpretation put on such words as 'maladjusted' and 'delinquent' by those pioneer workers who offered help to the problem child (the child with problems) was, like their personalities and practices, individualistic. This is important in that the nature of their work (and the type of structure through which they chose to do it), was partly conditioned by their idiosyncratic interpretations of those expressions of maladjustment with which they found themselves dealing. Since they were largely independent of state control they were able to select the children whom they thought would respond best to the type of treatment which they offered.

For Wills the delinquent child and maladjusted child were indistinguishable 'beyond the technical point that a delinquent child has been charged and found guilty at a juvenile court and a maladjusted child has not necessarily had that experience'.[24] His approach was, in any case, equally appropriate, being essentially concerned with moral re-education. 'A maladjusted child, in my view, is one whose capacity to make relationships, and thus to identify and acquire moral standards, has failed to develop owing to early deprivation or maltreatment.'[25] Lyward is typically paradoxical in saying 'I have no hesitation in describing the delinquent as, for the most part, over-moral'[26] while Dr Fitch ignores all subtle moral distinctions and says flatly: 'All delinquent children are maladjusted.'[27]

Asked to define 'maladjusted', A. S. Neill gave a predictably dogmatic answer: 'Angry 'cos of lack of love mostly',[28] while Mrs Dodd, though stressing that Dr Dodd would probably have rejected the term, thought that if pressed he would have said:'Unable to cope with the circumstances with which faced'.[29]

Others, although not rejecting possible alternative definitions, put the emphasis on various causal factors—Homer Lane on the stupidity of society, Leila Rendel on social and emotional deprivation, Dockar-Drysdale on the absence of satisfactory 'primary experience', and Bill Malcolm—one suspects—on the insistence by psychiatrists and psychologists that such a condition exists.

Just as their theoretical definitions varied, so the pioneers made distinctions in practice between the conditions they were prepared to handle or considered susceptible to treatment. Wills, whose views are very catholic, makes only one proviso for admission, pointing out, of schools for the maladjusted, that since they are 'intended to be therapeutic institutions . . . this carries with it an important corollary; if we are expected to cure our children we cannot be expected to receive into our schools the manifestly incurable',[30] e.g. the brain-damaged or mentally defective. Beyond this he makes no stipulation other than that the child must have the need to be made whole and happy. In particular Wills rejects any criterion of intelligence, beyond educability.

Others, like Shaw and Lennhoff, are much more selective because what they have to offer is different. Shaw's 'first criterion of selection is whether a child is accessible to psycho-therapy or psycho-analysis'. He does not accept children with I.Q.s below 130—'for we are, after all, a grammar school'—nor deeply schizoid, psychopathic or psychotic children. Children who are epileptic or suspected of brain damage are rejected—'We are not a hospital'.[31]

Although few pioneer schools were selective to this extent the majority had some criteria for admission which were, in essence, an expression of the personality of their directors, as were the schools themselves. Lennhoff considered that 'the special school must be designed to fulfil the therapeutic needs of different types of maladjusted children'.[32] He begs a great many questions in discussing the differences in types of maladjustment and the treatment he considers desirable but he suggests, rightly, that what a child needs and, to some extent, what maladjustment is considered to be is partly a condition of what is available for him. He continues:

One school may be educationally more conventional—the main emphasis being on the teaching of subjects. Another may concentrate primarily on the therapeutic activities before attempting a more formal education. Others are good at dealing with children of low intelligence; they offer a strong stable background, conformity to rule, and a more rigid training throughout. Other schools are best suited to children of high intelligence, who respond to freedom, shared responsibilities, and intellectual and cultural activities. Others are, perhaps, especially interested in cure through the arts or other aesthetic values of some kind. Whatever the main motive of the school's work each had something special to give to a particular kind of child.

All of these types of treatment considered appropriate to different categories and conceptions of maladjustment were indeed represented among the pioneer schools, although it must be admitted that provision for intelligent maladjusted children tended to be out of proportion to their relative numbers and, indeed, that some workers with maladjusted children thought that the intelligent ones were the only ones capable of, or in some sense worthy of, re-education.

MALADJUSTMENT AND DELINQUENCY

Since early definitions of maladjustment tended to be in terms such as 'Maladjusted children are children in need of special educational treatment', the type of child re-educated in the early, independent 'special' school probably, to a large extent, conditioned people's understanding of the term and may have contributed much to its various eventual definitions.

As the term 'maladjustment' was not current and had no administrative meaning at the beginning of this century, an absolute distinction between delinquency and maladjustment would rule out of consideration as pioneers such major characters as Homer Lane and such minor ones as William Henry Hunt, except insofar as their work had a direct influence on later practitioners. Similarly over-fine distinctions between the 'deprived' and the 'maladjusted' would be unrealistic when considering the work of Leila Rendel.

In fact almost all early schools (and most existing ones) accepted children who were both deprived and technically delinquent, and perhaps the majority of the children were what is popularly known now as 'pre-delinquent' or 'at risk'. Almost all of Homer Lane's adolescent charges at the Little Commonwealth had come as the result of being in conflict with the law, as had those of David Wills at the Hawkspur Camp. Both Lennhoff and Shaw admit that 'about a third of our children have shown their deep underlying troubles in the form of delinquency and have appeared before the courts at one time or another'[33] and consider, as did Father Owen, that one of the most important roles which their schools play is to give the maladjusted and delinquent child a protected environment in which to act out his anti-social impulses.

Most schools accepted both the socially and emotionally disturbed without making Barbe's implied distinction between delinquency and maladjustment: 'The socially disturbed include such groups as juvenile delinquents; the emotionally disturbed include neurotic and psychotic children who may or may not behave anti-socially'.[34]

The pioneers tended to see emotional deprivation as a common factor whether this was expressed in anti-social activities or not. They were, on the whole, more concerned with care and cure than with subtle definitions of the condition and this I take to be the distinction, necessary to this survey, between workers in schools for the maladjusted and those in contemporary approved schools. Thus I shall include pioneers such as Lane, Wills and Lyward, who dealt with delinquents as if they were maladjusted, i.e. therapeutically, and exclude those early workers in approved schools and other institutions who, by a basically authoritarian attitude, maintained the distinction.[35]

If, as Wills and Fitch suggest (see above), and the Kilbrandon Report and Seebohm Report appear to accept, there is no essential distinction between maladjusted and delinquent children, then their treatment needs will be the same and pioneers in the treatment of maladjusted children will be seen, as they now are even in official quarters, as being equally pioneers in the treatment of delinquent children. The reverse also applies.

Increasingly emotional deprivation is seen to be as, or *more,* important than social deprivation in the production of the persistent law-breaker. Dockar-Drysdale's 'frozen children' and John Bowlby's 'affectionless' ones are as much the material of which delinquents are made as are Homer Lane's Cockney 'street arabs'. These last may, as Lane averred, be acting normally in an intolerable social environment which is itself in need of rehabilitation. Mays suggests that delinquency is a widespread social phenomenon which in most cases should be regarded as normal but accepts that there may be some children for whom 'the forbidden act is either a drug or a distress signal sent up to draw attention to themselves and their plight'.[36] Wertham makes an important distinction between a delinquent *act* and a maladjusted *child.* The delinquent act may be the result of inadequate social training or a reasonable protest against a bad or frustrating environment. A maladjusted child, however, commits a delinquent act as a symptom of his disturbance. This will not be an isolated deviation but will be typical of his whole distorted behaviour pattern and system of relationships; his is by far the greater problem and his the greater need for help.[37]

The most intractable and habitual law-breaker is distinguished by his inability to consider the consequences of his acts or to profit from experience. He is, therefore, fearless of, and invulnerable to, punishment. His emotional reactions are infantile, he cannot bear

B

frustration and he will express his frustration in temper tantrums and his fears in violent, unprovoked attacks. He will demand attention but be unable to give affection.[38]

In treating such an emotionally and socially undeveloped person the pioneers had in common that they saw the futility of punishment and the necessity of love. Beyond this their interpretations and practice differed widely. Dockar-Drysdale would have recognized an absence of 'primary experience' and would have responded with psychotherapeutic mothering;[39] Wills would probably have seen a more general lack of the experience of affection and would have relied on the love of man and of God and on developing, through shared experience, the sense of social responsibility,[40] while Shaw might have diagnosed an unresolved Oedipus complex and would have prescribed psychoanalysis.[41]

All, however, would have been concerned only with care and cure and not with constraint and coercion. All, also, would have considered much of their preventive and therapeutic work with this sort of child virtually impossible out of the context of the complete experience of a residential school. It was relevant to ask 'Why?'

RESIDENTIAL TREATMENT

Almost all of the pioneer schools referred to were residential. With two exceptions day schools for maladjusted children were of later growth and were the product of State rather than individual action. This was largely an historical artefact. While day schools for maladjusted children such as those of Oxford or Leicester evolved largely from remedial and observation classes for children who were perceived to be under-achieving in school, the more typical pioneer establishment derived its residential form from a variety of sources in which treatment away from home was implicit.

The work of William Henry Hunt, Leila Rendel and Father Owen, for instance, was derived from the needs of individuals many of whom would otherwise have been either potentially, or in fact, the responsibility of the poor-law or child-care authorities. Their charges were mainly the socially deprived, without families or without adequate families, for whom a residential placement was either desirable or essential. The Little Commonwealth and the Hawkspur

Camp were envisaged as therapeutic alternatives to some form of punitive detention under the aegis of the Home Office.

Some of the earliest work, such as that of Dr Dodd and Dr Fitch, arose from the recognition by early workers in child psychiatry of the need for residential placement if clinical work was not to be wasted by the unhelpful home backgrounds of their disturbed patients—an obligation which they eventually undertook themselves. Others like Shaw, Lyward and Dockar-Drysdale created a milieu within which they could develop their own individual techniques of therapy unhampered by too much official, or in some cases parental, contact. This was, in a sense, true of most other pioneers in that they created their work around themselves and would not easily have submitted to the daily interference likely in a non-residential setting.

Later establishments, like Chaigeley and the Barns Hostel schools, evolved from the need for residential placement of evacuees whose degree of disturbance prevented them from being billeted with ordinary families; while schools such as Lendrick Muir developed from private boarding schools which had, through the abilities and interests of their proprietors, evolved techniques of education and therapy which were seen to be of particular value to maladjusted children. The State also—to some extent by default—reinforced the idea of the value of residential treatment to the seriously disturbed child. Since maladjustment was not recognized as a specific handicap before 1945, any child who clearly required treatment for 'nervous debility' or other more severe psychological disorder could seldom be coped with within the existing educational framework and had to be placed in an independent—and therefore probably residential —establishment, whether for the maladjusted or for the mildly physically handicapped, if his condition were to be alleviated. It is not surprising, therefore, that not only did those engaged in dealing with maladjusted children evolve theories of treatment in which residential placement was implicit, e.g. 'Planned environmental therapy', but that many of their assumptions about the proper milieu for maladjusted children were embodied in the Underwood Report.

It is nevertheless proper to question these assumptions and to consider if there is, in fact, any form of maladjustment which responds particularly well, or badly, to residential treatment.

Balbernie, in 1966, declared with ample justification that 'Evidence as to the outcome of residential treatment of children ascertained as maladjusted is very scanty, and the criteria of success or failure, as used in penal institutions, is irrelevant. . . . There is so far no reliable evidence of results which might show when and for which children residential or day treatment was more appropriate.'[42] Nevertheless from his own considerable research and experience he concludes that short-term residential placement is valuable for children undergoing temporary emotional stress in an unsatisfactory family situation (but where there is no basic neurosis requiring specialized psychotherapeutic techniques),[43] and that placement in an institution available all the year round, and with adequate facilities for treatment, is necessary to provide the severely disturbed child not only with opportunities for aggression but also with the secure and loving family atmosphere necessary to him.[44]

As Howard Jones points out, the case for removing a maladjusted child from home deserves very careful consideration. 'The very act of removing him from home, by reducing the opportunities for conflict, reduces also the incentives that both the child and parents would otherwise have to co-operate in treatment.'[45] Jones establishes five criteria for placement in residential institutions:

1 If the child is damaging or being damaged by his own environment;
2 If lowering the tension level in the family group makes productive work possible;
3 If the problem is not such that it lies masked or dormant while the child is away from home;
4 If the group experience is likely to have a catalytic function;
5 If it is impossible for the child ever to return home.

Shields[46] suggests that the generally accepted criteria of conditions of maladjustment requiring residential treatment are emotional disturbances and behavioural disorders resulting from the child's own environment having failed him. The child may be in revolt against parental attitudes, e.g. excessive or inadequate discipline, cruelty, insecurity, incest or instability. The child may also be deprived emotionally in more general and subtle ways and his reaction may make the environment even less accepting. A new loving and permissive environment gives very many children a 'second chance' through which they are able 'to correct the earlier emotional bias towards the community'.

Such institutions must, however, offer something more than a change of environment. They must be more, also, than '... mere dumping grounds for children temporarily or permanently deprived of good enough parental care and for whom all else has failed; the final end of a long process of social scape-goating and projection of responsibilities'.[47]

What this 'something more' is, as has been pointed out by Lennhoff, above, is very variously interpreted. As late as 1955 it was possible for Dr Charles Burns to claim, with some justification although with, perhaps, too little insight into the subtle distinction between schools, that 'treatment consists in the main of the impact made upon the child by the new environment in which he finds himself'.[48]

Apart from unsatisfactory home backgrounds, which should never be the sole reason for sending a child to a residential special school since 'deprived children are not necessarily maladjusted . . . but suffering from the effect of a bad environment', the chief reason for residential treatment is the presence of those forms and symptoms of neurotic illness which make it difficult for a child to remain in the community or in an intolerant, or even unsympathetic, home.

The Association of Workers for Maladjusted Children investigating the differences between schools for the maladjusted and ordinary boarding schools[49] discovered that the most usual symptoms found in residential special schools were, in order of occurrence: enuresis, stealing, withdrawn and apathetic behaviour, depression, encopresis, abnormal sex behaviour and asthma. These are the symptoms which are likely to increase the rejecting behaviour which in many cases produces them.

I myself, in studying the reasons for referral of thirty girls and thirty boys to Lendrick Muir, found that they were, in order of frequency:

GIRLS—School attendance (20), stealing (15), incompatibility with parents (15), general behavioural disorders (9), lying (8), depression (7), anxiety (7), introversion (7), temper tantrums (6), sibling rivalry (6), enuresis (5), hysteria (4), learning difficulties (4), hyperactive behaviour (4), sex difficulties (3), encopresis (2).
BOYS—School attendance (17), stealing (17), anxiety (15), general behavioural problems (12), extraversion (8), enuresis (7), lying (6), depression (6), sibling rivalry (6), temper tantrums (5), intro-

version (5), hyperactivity (4), difficulty with parents (3), learning difficulties (2), hysteria (1), encopresis (1).

It will be obvious that almost every child has more than one symptom; some have as many as six or seven.[50]

This wide variety of symptom is matched by an even wider range of causes and it is clear that only what Wills calls 'a splendid capacious umbrella' term such as 'deviance from social norms' can cover all—a term so wide as to be useless for any other purpose. I shall, therefore, find it necessary, from time to time, to consider the particular type of maladjustment—emotional disturbance and social nonconformity—with which the individual pioneers were primarily concerned in bringing the hope of emotional balance and social acceptability to the 'maladjusted' children for whom they cared. For, at least forty years earlier than it appeared in an official report, a handful of pioneers believed that 're-adjustment is a hope to be cherished and not an idle dream'.[51]

REFERENCES

CHAPTER 1: Pioneers

1   JONES, H. *Reluctant Rebels, p* 12. Tavistock, London, 1960.
2   MINISTRY OF EDUCATION: Report of the Committee on Maladjusted Children (The Underwood Report), H.M.S.O., London, 1955.
3   SHIELDS, R. W. *A Cure of Delinquents, p* 183 Heinemann, London, 1962.
4   WOODS, A. *Educational Experiments in England, pp* 77–78. Methuen, London, 1920.

CHAPTER 2: The Maladjusted Child and his Setting

5   REID, J. H. and HAGAN, H. R. *Residential Treatment of Disturbed Children.* Child Welfare League of America Inc., New York, 1952.
6   SCOTTISH EDUCATION DEPARTMENT. *Ascertainment of Maladjusted Children, Scotland, p* 8. H.M.S.O., Edinburgh, 1964.
7   SODDY, K. Contributing Factors, in *The Maladjusted Child—the Underwood Report & After.* (Proceedings of N.A.M.H. Conference 11th–12th April, 1957).
8   CHAZAN, M. Maladjusted Pupils: Trends in Post-War Theory and Practice. *Educational Research*, VI (1) *p* 30. 1963.
9   SCOTTISH EDUCATION DEPARTMENT, op. cit.
10 D'EVELYN K. *Meeting Children's Emotional Needs.* Prentice-Hall. (Englewood-Cliffs, N.J.) 1957. Also Haring, N. O. and Phillips, E. L.: *Educating Emotionally Disturbed Children. pp* 35–36. McGraw-Hill, New York, 1962.
11 SCOTTISH EDUCATION DEPARTMENT. *Pupils who are Maladjusted because of Social Handicap. pp* 8–10, 14, 33. H.M.S.O., Edinburgh, 1952.
12 MINISTRY OF EDUCATION. *Handicapped Pupils and School Health Service Regulations.* H.M.S.O., London, Revision 1953.
13 Ibid. 1945.
14 MINISTRY OF EDUCATION. (Ref 2) *p* 22.
15 Ibid. Appendix B. *p* 156, and Sections 96–115.
16 Ibid. Sections 116–137.
17 Ibid. *p* 23.

18 SHIELDS, R. W. *A Cure of Delinquents.* p 53. Heinemann, London, 1962.
19 MUSSEN, P. H. *et al. Child Development and Personality.* pp 67–80. Harper & Row, London, 1963.
20 SODDY, K. op. cit.
21 WOLFF, S. *Children Under Stress.* p 22. Allen Lane, Penguin Press, London, 1969.
22 MORRIS, B. in *The Maladjusted Child–The Underwood Report and After.* N.A.M.H., 1957.
23 ROSWELL, F. and NATCHEZ, G. *Reading Disability.* p 12 et seq. Basic Books Inc., New York, 1964. Also Quay, H. C., Morse, W. C., Cutler, R. L., Personality Patterns of Pupils in Special Classes for the Emotionally Disturbed, in *Educating Emotionally Disturbed Children,* Dupont, H. (ed.), Holt, Rinehart and Winston, N.Y., 1969.
24 WILLS, W. D. *Throw Away Thy Rod,* Gollancz, London, 1960.
25 PERSONAL COMMUNICATION
26 BURN, M. *Mr Lyward's Answer.* p 52. Hamish Hamilton, London, 1956.
27 FITCH, A. Speech made at Bath to the National Council of Women, 28 October, 1952.
28 PERSONAL COMMUNICATION
29 PERSONAL COMMUNICATION
30 WILLS, W. D., op. cit., p 12.
31 SHAW, O. T. *Maladjusted Boys.* p 17. Allen & Unwin, London, 1965.
32 LENNHOFF, F. G. *Exceptional Children.* p 34. Allen & Unwin, London, 1960.
33 Ibid. p 141.
34 BARBE, W. B. *The Exceptional Child.* p 85. The Centre for Applied Research in Education, N.Y., 1963.
35 WILLS, W. D. op. cit., p 28.
36 MAYS, J. B. *Crime and the Social Structure.* p 17 Faber & Faber, London, 1967.
37 WERTHAM, F. *The Circle of Guilt.* Dennis Dobson, London, 1958.
38 WILLS, W. D. *Commonsense about Young Offenders.* Gollancz, London, 1962.
39 Dockar-Drysdale, B. The Residential Treatment of Frozen Children, *Br. J. of Delinq.,* 14 [2] 1958.
40 WILLS, W. D. *The Hawkspur Experiment* (2nd Edn.) Allen & Unwin, London, 1969.
41 SHAW, O. T. *Prisons of the Mind.* Allen & Unwin, London, 1969.
42 BALBERNIE, R. *Residential Work with Children.* pp 68–69. Pergamon, Oxford, 1966.
43 Ibid. p 53.
44 Ibid. p 55.

45 JONES, H. *Reluctant Rebels, p* 210. Tavistock Publications, London, 1960.
46 SHIELDS, R. W. *A Cure of Delinquents. p* 15 Heinemann, London, 1962.
47 BALBERNIE, R. op. cit., 182.
48 BURNS, C. L. C. *Maladjusted Children.* Hollis & Carter, London, 1955.
49 PRINGLE, M. L. K. Differences between Schools for the Maladjusted and Ordinary Boarding Schools. *Br. J. Ed. Psych.*, **xxvii** *pp* 29–36. 1957.
50 It is interesting to compare this list with that given in McNair, *A Survey of Children in Residential Schools for the Maladjusted in Scotland. p* 19. Moray House Publication No. 6. Oliver and Boyd. Edinburgh, 1968.
51 SCOTTISH EDUCATION DEPARTMENT. (Ref. 11) Section 6.

PART TWO

Some Nineteenth Century Precursors

3

Mental Health

Michael Maher, aged thirteen. This boy was quite unmanageable by any means within the reach of his father or friends. They knew no way to make him obey but that of force or blows. He was formerly a tolerably bright boy, but he had been in this condition for years, and was rapidly growing worse. He seemed to live in continual terror and seldom spoke a word. The first time that I heard him utter a word was one day when his father took hold of him to make him obey some command, upon which, with his knees fairly knocking and his body trembling all over, he screamed convulsively 'Will good boy – Will good boy'. This was enough to show that, whatever may have been the cause of his strange condition, the daily treatment he was receiving was gradually crushing his feeble intellect, and would tend to drive him into hopeless idiocy or insanity.... The boy, therefore, was taken into our school at once. He is still a little shy, but he has lost all the appearance of terror; he not only comes readily when called, but often goes up to those belonging to the home, and puts his arms affectionately about them, and returns their caresses. He takes his place in class, and strives to imitate all the motions of the scholars, and obey the signs of the teacher. He can select the letters of the alphabet, and understands a few words. He is obedient and docile, and tries hard to learn with the others. He is affectionate and much gratified by any mark of praise or approval. He begins to talk and is rapidly improving in every respect.... The improvement is mainly attributable to the spirit of gentleness which pervades the household. This has quieted all his terrors and soothed his spirit....[1]

This case, one of many similar cases admitted to Dr Howe's school for defectives founded in Boston in 1845, makes one wonder how far the general label 'imbecile' was applied to any child whose behaviour was in any way extreme or bizarre and whose educational progress was consequently retarded. The Misses White, who started an establishment 'for the reception and training of idiot children' in Bath in 1846, reported similar cases of remarkable recoveries in children who, admitted as being beyond help or restraint, made considerable adjustment towards normality of behaviour and educational achievement given kindly and systematic care.

H.B., aged eight at the time of his admission; was violent and unmanageable to a great degree: subject to fits of rage, during which he would throw himself on the floor, kicking and screaming until exhausted. In walking through the streets he was with difficulty restrained from rushing into the shops and seizing everything he saw in them, and has frequently attracted the notice of those passing by. He could only articulate a few broken sentences; nor could he give an answer to a question. He is now able to read and write fairly, can repeat many texts of Scripture, hymns etc., and is perfectly orderly when walking, asking questions as to what he sees passing around him. His temper is equally improved.

G.C. was nine at the time of her admission. She was so unruly at home as to be generally tied to the table, which she would drag about the room. She is now perfectly under control; reads, writes and works at her needle; assists also at household work, washing and dressing the younger children.[2]

Those working in close contact with so-called 'idiot', 'imbecile' or 'fatuous' children were not satisfied with these arbitrary labels and sought, sometimes through misleading physiological assessments, to establish causes and categories. Some realized that there was 'a large class of persons who are born with a certain capacity, and who, with proper treatment, would have manifested a moderate share of intellect, but who have been badly managed, and become idiotic, or have been misunderstood and considered idiotic . . . among these unfortunates left to grovel in the lowest idiocy, there are many who can be redeemed, and rendered comparatively intelligent, happy and useful.'[3] There was a growing consciousness of the need for observation, comparative studies and the development of special educational and therapeutic techniques.

The formation in 1847 of the London Society for the establishment and support of an asylum for idiots, directed by the Rev. Dr Andrew Reed, resulted in the foundation of two large asylums, in Highgate and Redhill, which in 1855 had 259 pupils under observation and training. Most of these pupils were probably mentally deficient or retarded for reasons other than emotional disturbance but, particularly in the light of our present limited knowledge of the condition of 'autism' and other infantile psychoses, one inevitably speculates about those who 'have been misunderstood and considered to be idiotic'. For instance:

F.W., a boy, aged fourteen years admitted May 1851; could not read, write, draw or do anything; he was said to be beyond improvement was very spirited and ran away from home several times.... For eighteen months after his entrance all efforts appeared useless, and patience was almost exhausted, as he did not know a single letter. Now he knows most of the alphabet, writes in a copy-book, is obedient and tractable, and has made several pairs of shoes and slippers. B.T., a boy, aged fifteen years ... was the sport of all the boys in the village; was afraid of strangers; would not speak to anyone, even to his friends he appeared quite hopeless. He did not speak for four months after admission ; was constantly moping. He has now found that he is with friends, and is gaining courage, and can speak well ... can read and write well; and is a basketmaker.[4]

In view of recent physiological and behaviourist approaches to the re-education of brain-damaged children[5] and of the extent to which certain types of maladjusted children, e.g. the hyperactive, are now considered to be minimally brain-damaged, it is interesting to note that the directors of the Highgate asylum, beginning from the opposite premise, evolved an approach to treatment which was in many ways similar.

The board have acted on the principle that always there is mind, and that, in itself, it is perfect; and that it has imperfect or deranged organization. The education therefore, has been primarily physical and the board have availed themselves of separation, and of classification, in conducting it. They have educated the eye, the ear, the mouth, the brain, the muscle, the limb and have thus endeavoured to reach the better portion of our nature, that it also might be trained to moral and spiritual exercises.[6]

THE PSYCHOLOGICAL APPROACH

The work of individuals and of voluntary societies with deficient, deranged and disturbed children continued to expand in the last half of the nineteenth century, but more accurate assessment and a more scientific approach to re-education and treatment was largely the product of the last few decades of the century.

When, by 1880, school attendance became compulsory, attention was inevitably focused on children who had previously not attended, or who had been excluded from, school because of their inability or disruptive behaviour. They could no longer merely be ignored as embarrassments, or jeered at as butts, by the community. The new situation pointed the problem and the new science sought for the solution.

The original investigatory approach concentrated primarily on broad categorizations and gross defects. An anthropometric survey of the British Isles, directed in 1877 by Galton, and numerous more limited surveys of physical and mental health conducted by Dr Francis Warner[7] and others, revealed the presence of large numbers of children who were quite incapable of coping with, or profiting by, board school education. Warner, a professor of anatomy and physiology, reported about 15 per cent of schoolchildren as defective physically, mentally or morally. Since, however, the basic method of assessment was by head-measuring and searching for the supposed 'stigmata' of mental defect, Warner's figures are of doubtful value. The purely physiological explanation of 'moral defect' and educational failure propounded by such eminent people as Maudsley,[8] and the medieval methodology used, had an effect, however, of great consequence. If all deviant behaviour was of organic origin detectable by physical examination, then clearly the appropriate diagnostician was the physician with his tape-measure rather than the psychologist with his educational and mental tests. Treatment too would be medical or surgical[9] rather than educational or social. What became a very damaging battle between psychiatrists and psychologists was joined.

Three things were particularly significant about the Elementary Education (Defective and Epileptic Children) Act, 1899, which followed these revealing surveys. Three new categories of handicap were recognized for which educational provision was to be made; the medical interpretation of defectiveness was accepted and school medical officers were to be responsible for assessment; and local education authorities could, if they wished, make special education compulsory until sixteen. The assumption behind this last provision was that, although a child might begin his education handicapped in some way, he might, given time and the appropriate treatment, catch up.

Such a philosophy not only developed naturally from the

environmentalist views inherited from Locke through the Utilitarians, but may have been given credence by the sort of experience, quoted above, which those working in close contact with disturbed and 'imbecile' children were beginning to observe and report. It was felt necessary, however, to provide philosophy with some firm scientific base.

Galton, however, thought in evolutionary terms of the new science of psychology, as one of inherited individual differences, and endeavoured by measurement and categorization to make clear what those differences were. He evolved that study of the behaviour of the individual child which became the educational basis of child guidance, for although his chief contribution was probably as 'the true father of the mental test'[10] it was also he who 'first advocated the scientific study of the individual pupil, expressly with a view to practical recommendations for treatment and training both at home and at school'.[11] Indeed his 'anthropometric laboratory' established at the International Health Exhibition 1884-5 (subsequently at University College, London) may be considered the first 'child guidance centre' in this country. Galton offered advice both to teachers and parents on the basis of a systematic testing of the child's mental abilities.

Galton's statistical approach attracted Cattell, who assisted him in his laboratory before becoming America's first professor of psychology. The clinic which Cattell set up preceded that of William Healy, which was eventually to have such a significant effect on the treatment of the delinquent and maladjusted, both in the United States and in England.[12]

Another eminent disciple of Galton, McDougall, became the director of that laboratory which Sully had opened in 1896, the first in Britain to be devoted exclusively to psychology and to contain an education section where students and teachers received a systematic course in child study.

Sully's emphasis, in the earlier British tradition of Alexander Bain, was on observation and practical work, and it is from him, rather than Galton, that work with the maladjusted, rather than the retarded, child primarily derived. His *Studies in Childhood* (1895) was 'the first systematic study in England of the development of children's behaviour'.[13] He distinguished three main types of deviation on which assessment of need was to be based: intellectual dullness, emotional instability, and deviations from acceptable moral conduct. Educational, neurotic and behavioural disorders and difficulties were seen as essentially interlinked in the unity of the child. It was, perhaps, unfortunate that in a search for greater accuracy and 'scientific' validity Sully's assistants and successors, such as McDougall and Spearman, should have diverted a large part of the effort to the pursuit of the Galtonic chimera of 'intelligence', although much useful work and discussion was incidentally generated, including that which concerned 'a spurious form of mental deficiency... not infrequently associated with bad home conditions'.

Sully and McDougall, moreover, had 'come more and more to the view that, if effective work was to be done among schoolchildren, it was essential that *local* centres should be established ... and that the work of the psychologist should be carried out within the education department'.[14] Such psychological work, Sully thought, should cease to be medically orientated towards abnormality, but should rather be concerned primarily with the adjustment of normal children temporarily maladjusted by circumstance. To Sully 'the normal child is one who is in adequate adjustment with his environment; the so-called abnormal child is, in the vast majority of cases, merely a maladjusted child, not a child suffering from gross pathological defect'. This appears to be the first use of the term 'maladjusted' with its modern connotation, i.e. of a child who, for whatever reason, is not in adequate adjustment to his environment. In Sully's view many such children were 'incapable of being benefited by ordinary instruction, not by reason of mental defect... but by reason of various accidental circumstances, and might, with individual study and guidance, be converted into reasonably efficient and law abiding citizens'.[15]

Sully's importance as the real originator of what might be called the 'British school' of educational psychology has recently been reassessed.[16] His approach was essentially based on the study of the normal child and on seeking educational rather than medical solutions. He saw the educational psychologist, supported by a local child guidance organization and armed with insight born of experience (as well as with psychometric tests), as the key figure. He thought it essential, also, that teachers and educational administrators should be trained to appreciate individual differences through child study and a knowledge of psychology.

The aims of the British Child Study Association, which was founded in 1893 to encourage that interest in Sully's work which was developing in schools, training colleges and universities throughout the country, provide a clear statement of his views.

The Society has for its object the scientific study of the mental and physical condition of children, and also of educational methods, with a view to gaining greater insight into child-nature and securing more sympathetic and scientific methods of training; to be attained by all or any of the following methods:

by interesting parents, medical practitioners, teachers and others in the systematic observation of children and young people; by scientific enquiry and research;

by efforts to ascertain the educational methods and conditions of the environment of children during school life, best suited to ensure their mental and physical development, including those children who are abnormal;

by supplying information and diffusing knowledge by means of publications, lectures etc. upon points connected with the mental and physical status of child; and by acting as a consulting body on questions concerning educational methods, so far as they relate to the child. . . .[17]

Branches of the association grew, university courses in child psychology developed, and psychological laboratories offering advice to teachers about their problem children were opened in Oxford (1904), Liverpool (1907) and London.

The work in Liverpool and London, and later throughout England, was inspired by Cyril Burt. Burt, a pupil of McDougall, was noted for his breadth of interest and vision. In 1903 he had devised tests of higher intelligence and 'laid the foundation of the mental measurement movement as applied to education'. In Liverpool, after 1907, he not only 'devoted his attention to research into all the practical problems of the schools and especially to an exploration of the psychology of individual differences so important for the adaptation of education to the rhythms of child growth'[18] but also developed his interest in the social causes of delinquency and educational subnormality.

In 1913, despite the opposition of representatives of the medical profession to 'lay' psychologists, Burt was appointed psychologist by the London County Council. His brief was to examine children referred by parents, medical officers, care-committee workers and magistrates and to recommend training or treatment; to assist and advise in academic selection procedures; to organize educational surveys, to advise the education committee and to disseminate psychological information.[19] He performed much more than his brief. Indeed 'Burt's various contributions to the development of psychological services in England are difficult to overestimate'. Apart from his research, his contributions to the methodology of psychology and his immensely important works *The Backward Child* and *The Young Delinquent*, 'the service which he created set a pattern of close co-operation with the schools, of investigation by rigorous scientific methods of the practical problems of education, of the treatment of individual cases and of the integration under the guidance and inspiration of the psychologist's office of the many special educational facilities of a large authority—a pattern which still dominates the best services in England'.[20]

That this pattern of an educationally and psychologically based school psychological service developed as slowly and unevenly as it did was partly the result of the interruption caused by the First World War bringing the nineteenth century to an end. This broke continuity in services and enabled the indigenous growth of British educational psychology to be sacrificed to the imported American product of the child-guidance clinic. Surviving only in the remoteness of Scotland and scattered areas of England the school psychological services shared the fate of the red squirrel.

4

Child Care

If, as Balbernie suggests,[21] it is the inadequate home, above all, which is productive of severe maladjustment, it is the provision of care for the children of such homes that one should study for much of the origin of work with disturbed children. In the nineteenth century, when social services were too primitive to protect the child from the consequences of parental poverty and crime, it seems inevitable that many deprived children should act out their disturbance through delinquent activities. It seems reasonable, therefore, that an account of the treatment or care of the deprived and delinquent should be considered relevant to a study of the treatment of maladjusted children, although, such is the resilience of childhood, that this view may apply only to a minority of children.

Any recognition of the special needs of deprived and delinquent children before this century will have to be sought outside the organizations provided by the State. By and large the State either ignored deprived children outside the workhouses or incarcerated them with, but not usually together with, their parents. For those within the workhouse the only relief from the demoralizing effect of total inactivity was normally picking oakum. The State eventually took notice of such children outside the workhouse only when they tried to preserve their independence or help their families by joining in their parents' criminal activities. They were then generally sent to prison or to the penal colonies.

The futility of these measures as means of rehabilitation and reform was widely realized, and need not be elaborated upon. There were, however, both inside and outside the system, people whose despair at this futility spurred them to philanthropic action.

In the middle of the eighteenth century, at the instigation of Sir John Fielding and Mr Fowler Walker, the Marine Society (1756) was founded 'for the redemption and reformation of young criminals' by training them for the Navy, and the former was also instrumental, two years later, in founding both the Female Orphan Asylum and the Magdalen Hospital for destitute and 'erring' girls. In 1788 the

Philanthropic Society was founded 'for the protection of poor children, and the offspring of convicted felons, and the reformation of children who have themselves been engaged in criminal practices, that they might learn the happiness and benefit of a home'. Founded originally on a 'cottage-home' system, it was subsequently reorganized into a prison school for delinquents, and two training schools for pauper children—one for girls and one for boys.[22]

The prison school, concentrating largely on sedentary employment, was found to be ineffective and in 1849 was moved to a farm site at Redhill, Surrey, where hard, creative, outdoor work was substituted. The boys came 'either as volunteers after completing their imprisonment, or at the desire of their parents, or having received a conditional pardon'. The regime, in terms of the time, was very liberal, and an 80 per cent success rate was claimed, 'thanks to the power of religious influence, to the attractive and subduing force of kindness, to the self-respect, thoughtfulness, and sense of personal responsibility created (especially in the older lads) by their free position and the confidence reposed in them, and last, not least, to the interest attaching to the varied and active occupation of agricultural life'.[23] It is interesting that the Rev. J. Turner, the resident chaplain, who gave evidence to the Committee of the Commons in 1850, should report the same phenomenon as that noted by Homer Lane and others who later dealt with the delinquent and disturbed in a free environment, i.e. that it was the least tractable delinquent who made most progress and 'as a general rule, the best prisoner makes the worst free boy, the most difficult and troublesome boy to deal with, because he has been so accustomed to depend on the mechanical arrangements about him, that he finds self-action almost impossible; such are the most reluctant to work, and the most untrustworthy; directly they are free, certain dispositions develope [sic] themselves, which under the restraint of the prison were mastered and hidden'.

Another interesting experiment in rehabilitating delinquents was that of the reformatory school at Stretton-on-Dunsmore, Warwickshire, which provided a home with 'the advantages and comfort of a well-ordered family' for about twenty boys, who were sent out to work in the neighbourhood while completing their sentences.[24]

THE PRECURSORS OF DAY SCHOOLS

If it may be considered that the schools already mentioned performed some of the functions of present-day residential schools and hostels for the delinquent and maladjusted, the precursors of day schools for the maladjusted may be found in the ragged schools, free day schools and industrial feeding schools of the nineteenth century. The maladjustment may have been largely of social origin (since these schools were essentially for the most deprived classes) and set against a social background in which, although destitution was tolerated, nonconformity was not, but early workers in such schools had no doubt that many of their charges had been seriously disturbed by their childhood experiences in the 'perishing and dangerous classes'. Indeed John Pounds, the Portsmouth cobbler whose impromptu school is usually taken to be the first 'ragged school' (other than a Sunday school), expressed a preference for 'little blackguards' when there was competition to receive instruction from him.[25] By 1851, when the Ragged School Union was founded, there were about sixty schools in existence, many with their own special characteristics—industrial training schemes, seaside camps and emigration training schemes.

In June, 1848, in Parliament Lord Shaftesbury, analysing the clientele of ragged schools, said: 'Of 1,600 children in fifteen ragged schools, 162 had been in prison, 116 had run away from home because of ill-treatment, 170 had slept in lodging houses, 253 lived by begging, 216 had no shoes or stockings, 68 were children of convicts, 101 had no bed-linen, 219 never slept in beds, 125 had step-mothers, 306 had lost one or both parents.'[26]

Although the difficulty of organizing such schools limited their effect (as many as 2,000 children passed through one London school in five years) the movement was nevertheless an important one. Young and Ashton, although 'doubtful whether the methods used in the ragged schools have anything specific to offer to the study of modern group work', perceive four valuable contributions:

The schools were sited where they were most needed—where deprivation and depravity were most to be found.

The less ordered regime of the ragged schools demanded teachers of high quality, whose standards and methods were diametrically opposed to those in normal schools.

'A third contribution was the importance the ragged-school teachers attached to the whole person of the child, physical, mental, moral, to his family and to his future. For it was the common practice among ragged-school teachers to visit what homes the children had, in the hope of creating a better understanding, and of giving help and advice if possible.'

The ragged schools' most important contribution was possibly the insight given to people who were associated with them such as Lord Shaftesbury, Mary Carpenter, Dr Barnardo, Charles Dickens and Dr Guthrie, into the needs of those children whom they were subsequently to help so much.[27]

Much the same influence might be claimed for the free day schools which, although fewer in number, had the advantage that they were in operation throughout the week, rather than on occasional evenings, and had some professional, rather than willing but untrained amateur, teachers. The clientele were the same as those of the ragged schools—children who were too poor, filthy, unruly or delinquent to be accepted in the normal day school. These schools will be exemplified more fully when the work of Mary Carpenter is considered.

The objective of industrial feeding schools (of which Mary Carpenter was a strong advocate) was to train those children whose condition was such that they could not even attend ragged schools, in the hope of enabling them to escape from their hopeless conditions. These were in particular vagrants and children who, either by begging or stealing, helped to maintain themselves and their families. It was hoped that by maintaining and educating them during the day at public expense they would not only be able to reform themselves but also their families, who were of the lowest social and criminal stratum. Although large towns such as Manchester and Liverpool founded such schools they did little to touch the problem. Children who were habitual vagrants did not respond to school discipline and failed to attend. Parents, who needed the support of their children's mendicant or delinquent activities to survive, kept them away. After the Poor Law Act, 1834, taxpayers complained at the expense of maintaining the destitute in both workhouses and schools. Above all, except in Scotland, magistrates had no power, before the Youthful Offenders Act, 1854, to insist on attendance at industrial schools, a provision which was necessary to rescue these children both from their parents and themselves. In Aberdeen, where in the 1840s, under Sheriff Watson, attendance at an industrial school was made compulsory for all children found guilty of begging or vagrancy, complete success was claimed both in rehabilitating what were, perhaps significantly, called 'quasi-delin-quents' and in freeing Aberdeen from their activities.[28]

One of the important characteristics of such schools, shared by day schools for the maladjusted today, is that children were not divorced from their backgrounds, however bad. It was considered important 'that they should feel that they had homes to which they were bound by feelings implanted by nature'. The alternative, particularly in England, for children who either begged or starved was the Union school.

The Union school—the State's alternative to prison or complete destitution—was such that 'no one can visit an ordinary Union school without the painful sentiment that here the youthful faculties and affections are crippled and stunted, and that a race of paupers are being trained up to make the Union their final home'.[29]

Many children whose families were non-existent or inadequate, and who were themselves unwilling or unable to turn to crime, were prepared to starve rather than to seek the doubtful refuge of the dreaded 'workhouse'. Workhouse schools were either too small, and too ill-provided, to do any effective work or, after the grouping together of pauper children into separate workhouse schools between 1845 and 1870, too large to provide for the education and care which these particularly deprived children needed. After an unsatisfactory report on the barrack-type school in the 1861 Royal Commission on Education there was a move towards the establishment of cottage-homes based on the Continental pattern of the Rauhe Haus or Mettrai, which had been strongly advocated by Joseph Fletcher in a paper to the Statistical Society in 1851, and subsequently urged by Mrs Nassau Senior, the first woman to be appointed inspector of workhouses and pauper schools.

In the cottage homes, between fifty and 300 children would be grouped into units of from ten to thirty under house parents, the children going from these homes to the community schools in which the emphasis was on fitting children for life. Joseph Fletcher considered that 'Labour must be the staple of the poor man's training. To live is the first necessity . . . labour on the land and industry in the workshop is the first desideratum, religious and moral training on example realized in daily life is the next, and intellectual culture . . . used rather as a relief from other occupations than as the greatest feature of a pauper school'. This more purposeful type of training, and its basis in the healthy and varied experience of family life, was an undoubted improvement in providing for the needs of these most deprived children. Towards the end of the century, however, it was realized that such communities had the disadvantage (subsequently associated with many residential schools for the maladjusted and delinquent) of being too self-contained and isolated, not only from society at large but also from the urban environments to which most of the children belonged. There was subsequently a move towards boarding out and a 'scattered home' system, which were thought to have the advantages both of family care and social integration.

For those destitute children who would not accept the workhouse in any form, or whom the workhouse would not accept, cottage-homes developed in the last half of the nineteenth century under the aegis of various philanthropic individuals or societies. The Farning-ham Home for Little Boys was founded in 1865, Princess Mary's Village Homes for Girls in 1870 and Dr Barnardo's Village Home for Orphan and Neglected Girls in 1875. Dr Barnardo's work for deprived children is too well known to require elaboration and there has, in recent years, been an increasing realization by the Dr Barnardo's Society of the extent to which deprivation and emotional disturbance are interconnected, which has led both to the evolution of homes considered to be particularly suited to the needs of the maladjusted child and to the foundation or support of schools for maladjusted children (e.g. Craigerne; see Chapter 17).

Another who was much interested in the work of the Rauhe Haus and of the Continental agricultural colonies was Dr T. B. Stephenson, who was largely instrumental in the foundation of the National Children's Homes in the 1870s and after. One of the most interesting of these homes (which endeavoured to specialize in different types of experience for different needs) was that founded on the moors at Edgworth. Here a group of the most difficult senior boys carved out from the moor a farm and village accommodating several hundred children to whom the experience gave a real sense of responsibility and maturity,[30] an experiment which, in many ways, foreshadows that of David Wills at the Hawkspur Camp (see Chapter 12).

MARY CARPENTER

Of the many nineteenth-century philanthropists concerned with the needs of deprived children, the most significant and 'pioneering' is probably Mary Carpenter. The daughter of an eminent churchman who was headmaster of a boys' school, she received a liberal education and was soon herself involved in teaching. After meeting Dr Tuckerman—a Boston philanthropist—she began her active work with pauper children in Bristol by founding the Bristol Working and Visiting Society (1835), and subsequently a 'Ministry to the Poor'. Turning her attention to the problems of education and reform, she opened, in 1846, a ragged school at Lewin's Mead in the slums of Bristol, later moving to larger premises in 'a filthy lane called St James's Back'. With this practical experience behind her, she wrote two powerful and effective books, *Reformatory Schools for the Children of the Perishing and Dangerous Classes and for Juvenile Offenders* (1851) and *Juvenile Delinquents, their Condition and Treatment* (1853), and in order to vindicate her own theories in a society which, even when sympathetic, tended to be essentially punitive, she opened her own reformatory school at Kingswood in 1852. This was originally coeducational but in 1854 she founded Red Lodge reform school for girls, which she supervised personally as far as her extremely crowded social and political life would allow her. In the year when Red Lodge was opened the Youthful Offenders Act (10 August, 1854) legalized private reform schools and made them eligible for Government grant and inspection. The passing of this Act owed much to Mary Carpenter's propagandist activities, and to the evidence which she and her supporters had submitted to the Parliamentary Enquiry into Juvenile Delinquency, which reported in May 1852. Mary Carpenter was particularly notable in never divorcing theory from practice and her next foundation—an industrial school, also in the Kingswood area—arose from her desire to stimulate work arising from the Industrial Schools Act of 1857. Many of her subsequent proposals, born of experience, were incorporated into amendments to the Act in 1861 and 1866. Indeed, in 1876, the year before her death, she at last succeeded in persuading the Government to authorize her plan for allowing school boards to establish day-feeding industrial schools. Meanwhile she had travelled extensively in Germany, the United States, Canada and India to stimulate her ideas, disseminate her principles, and extend her philanthropic activities. She died on 14 June, 1877.[31]

Her ragged day school in St James's Back was described with approval in Mr Fletcher's Report to the Committee of Council on Education in 1850.[32] Mary Carpenter attached central importance to the quality of the teacher, and after the first year, in which the pupils were gathered together by a good but untrained master well known to them as a temperance worker in the area, they were put in charge of two trained teachers. Mary Carpenter considered the new master's mode of teaching ideal. His aim was to engender mutual confidence and respect in a setting which contained 'a great deal of individual freedom in the boys, with an imperative sense of duty'.

The school was converted out of a delapidated court. 'The School room . . . is large, airy and light, well warmed and ventilated, with three similar rooms for classes; it is supplied with washing apparatus, and has a bath house adjacent. There is a playground . . . provided with swings, leaping poles etc., and a spacious airy play-room.'[33] Great emphasis was put on the need for play as a means of 'strengthening and calling out the intellectual powers', of promoting mental health and as a means by which the involved teacher could observe and influence the children. 'By mingling familiarly in their sports with them, he greatly increases this attachment to him, without in any way lessening his authority, and has a valuable opportunity of observing the free developing of their characters, and checking what is wrong more effectually than by a formal lesson.'[34]

The stated aim of the school was 'physically, intellectually, socially and spiritually, to raise the children out of their debasement, and prepare them to become better members of society'. The school was to be non-sectarian and two of the rules laid down by the committee are of particular interest:

'No corporal punishment, or holding up to public shame or ridicule, shall be made use of: but discipline must be maintained by the Master's own firmness, order and kindness';

'The master shall make himself acquainted with the parents and homes of the scholars. . . .'

The pupils received not only the formal education of the normal school but also such industrial training in sewing, shoemaking and tailoring as was thought useful to them and necessary for inculcating habits of industry.

Both godliness and cleanliness were considered necessary for moral development and suitably emphasized. Great efforts were made to celebrate festivals such as Christmas and May Day appropriately, and the children were at other times taken to museums and exhibitions.

The general effect of the school was impressive: '... from one to two hundred of the most destitute and neglected children of this large city are seen coming voluntarily and regularly to School ... acquiring habits of neatness and industry by learning to make and repair their clothes—improving rapidly in reading, writing, figures and general knowledge—manifesting increasing familiarity with the scriptures, and interest in them—and exercising, in general, sufficient self-control to behave in an orderly manner, unawed by the fear of punishment...' (report to the committee).

Effectiveness was, however, limited by the difficulty of securing regular attendance from the most delinquent, the hostility of some of the magistrates and citizens of Bristol, the impossibility of keeping children long enough to be useful as monitors and teaching assistants, the shortage of money, and above all the continuing depressing effect of home circumstances.

It was partly to counter some of these disadvantages that Mary Carpenter subsequently turned to residential reform schools of the Rauhe Haus type,[35] in which the family units provided the necessary parental care and the school's influence was not constantly counteracted by parental example or an intolerably debased urban environment.

Kingswood and Red Lodge reform schools were cottage-home communities in rural surroundings in which the emphasis was on creative work in the open air. In organizing and controlling them, Mary Carpenter endeavoured to put into practice those principles she so staunchly advocated.

First, there was the Christian basis of the enterprise, valuable not only in itself but for the respect it engendered between adults and children as equal beings in the sight of God.

'Secondly. Love must be the ruling sentiment of all who attempt to influence and guide these children. This love must indeed be wise as well as kind, but it must be so evidently the pervading feeling of the teacher to his charge, that no severity on his part shall alienate them from him.... None can tell but those who have witnessed it, the responsive love which is awakened in the heart of one of these forsaken ones by a kind look or word, or the purifying effect of the feeling, now by many experienced for the first time, that they are "loved for themselves".' Love provides the strongest basis for all law.

Long before Bowlby, and before such modern experts as D. W.

Winnicott or Dockar-Drysdale (see Chapter 15) based their therapeutic techniques on an understanding of the vital importance of
the unity of the child and the mother in 'primary experience', Mary
Carpenter understood the essential nature of the disturbance of
'affectionless' and 'frozen' children.

That faith or trust, so characteristic of childhood, which springs from
a sense of utter helplessness, from a confidence in the superior power
and wisdom of those around, and of their loving anxiety for their
welfare, scarcely exists in these children; for the instinctive clinging to
the parent, which is perhaps hardly ever utterly annihilated, has never
been elevated by a perception of what is excellent and worthy of love.
The *will* therefore of these children ... is their only guide ... they
only do what is 'right in their own eyes' unless compelled to do otherwise. Any kind of real obedience is unknown to them..,.[36]

With these children, who may fairly be called seriously maladjusted, and of whom she had abundant experience, Mary
Carpenter saw that love was the first essential above—and essentially
preceding—faith and obedience. Such a child had to be restored
'to the true position of childhood.... He must be brought to a
sense of dependence by awakening in him new and healthy desire
which he cannot himself gratify ... he must have his affections called
forth by the obvious personal interest felt in his own individual
well-being by those around him. This ... is the fundamental
principle of all true reformatory action with the young.'[37]

The family structure was therefore considered to be essential and
the 'parents' chosen 'to restore health to the mind diseased' had to
be people of the highest faith, ability, tolerance and capacity for love.

'Intellectual training should be directed rather to the awakening
and exciting of the mind itself to work on objects higher than those
of the sense, than to the mere infusing of elements of knowledge.'[38]
This was to be achieved through the practical experience of labour,
and in particular of agricultural labour—the virtues of which, as an
aid to moral and intellectual growth, had been so stressed by M.
Wichern, the director of the Rauhe Haus.[39]

Such labour must essentially be voluntary and must be balanced
by much opportunity for play in which, although the master plays
an essential part, all formality must be discarded.

Discipline must be firm in that what is expected must be made
clear by the person whom the children have learnt to love and
follow, and must not depend on rules to be learnt or savage punish-

ments to be endured. Pilfering, which Mary Carpenter found to be almost universal, is to be countered not by 'Thou shalt not steal' but by a recognition that deprived children have a great need to possess personal property, so that by being given things of their own which they value they should realize the importance of personal possessions.

Ideally, as Mr Fletcher suggested, and as was the Continental practice, the families should be coeducational, but this depended to some extent on the age and length of stay of the inhabitants. It was considered desirable that children should be admitted under twelve years of age and should stay until seventeen.

Great attention was to be paid to aftercare in placing children in suitable employment and in maintaining contact with, and interest in, them.

That there is so much which is startlingly modern about Mary Carpenter's work is, above all, a tribute to her understanding of essential child nature. She would, in most respects, have been an enthusiastic supporter of the proposals of the Curtis Report (1946), the 1969 Children's Act and the principles of *The Child, the Family and the Young Offender,* and of the Kilbrandon Report and Seebohm Report. She saw no essential distinction between delinquency and other forms of disturbance which postulated a need for child care. She regarded delinquency as activity which was created by social conditions and, to some extent, by the inequality of the law. She did not doubt that what she called 'moral delinquency' existed in all strata of society, but asserted that the children of the upper classes were protected from the consequences of their actions both by their parents and by the officers of the law.[40]

That delinquency was more frequently expressed in the most deprived classes she attributed primarily to the absence of adequate parental care and control—'the firm authority of a father, the yet more powerful check of a mother's love'.

These poor pariah children, these "moral orphans", who watches over them with tender care through their early years? The street their nursery, and elder brother or sister already well versed in crime their nurse, sometimes driven almost from their mother's breast to seek their own living, knowing a father often only by hearing his curses, or bearing his drunken brutality, defying in the earliest years a parental authority which has been used but to abuse them, they have at twelve,

perchance even at eight or nine years of age, the determined will, the
violent passions, even the knowledge, in crime, of a man.[32]

This may seem over-written except in terms of some of the
examples which Mary Carpenter quotes—many of which might still
be matched today with the backgrounds of children in approved
and special schools. The following examples are by no means the
most extreme, but are the shortest and perhaps those which
particularly point to the deprived or maladjusted child rather than
the delinquent act:

W.L.—Slept at night under the stairs or behind doors on a little straw
with a sack to cover him. . . . Father dead eight years; mother left him
in a workhouse when two years old, and does not know her; saw her
on Sunday morning going to church, did not know her then ; was told
it was his mother ... been in this condition for at least three years.'
    J.W.—No home, . . . when no money, sleeps in courts or on landing
about four nights a week. Father deserted mother fifteen years; mother
dead two years. . .
    D.F., aged about 14—Mother dead several years; father a drunkard
and deserted him about three years ago. Has lived since as best he
could; sometimes going errands, sometimes begging and thieving. Slept
in lodging houses when he had money, but very often walked the street
at night, or lay under arches or on doorsteps. . . . Sent to Giltspur-
Street prison (for stealing a pocket handkerchief); was fed on bread and
water. Instructed every day by the chaplain and schoolmaster, much
impressed by what the chaplain said; felt anxious to do better; behaved
well in prison. Was 'well flogged' the morning he left back bruised
but not quite bleeding. Was then turned into the streets ragged,
barefooted, friendless, homeless, penniless. . . . Met next day with some
expert thieves in the Minories went along with them, and continues
in a course of vagrancy and crime.[42]

It is hardly surprising that, with such backgrounds and such treatment, the most intelligent and spirited boys were often the most
notably delinquent.

C. and J. are well-educated, clever boys; they are at large, corrupting
those around them, and engaged in felonious acts; C. was lately an
accomplice with Z. in stealing lead he escaped, but is now in prison for
stabbing his mother. . . . F. is a passionate high-spirited boy, whom a
few years ago a word or a touch of kindness could soften or bend; now
he is brazen and reckless, one of the well-known juvenile gang who may
constantly be seen in Lewin's Mead, unchecked, plotting mischief in

open day. The rest are wild boys ready for any sort of evil. . . . A.S. had long been known as the worst boy in the neighbourhood . . . he has fine talents and a powerful spirit, which finds no scope but in mischief, as he is at present circumstanced.[48] And so on.

Mary Carpenter recognized that social deprivation was not the only cause of 'moral disease', and realized that the presence of parents was often more harmful than their absence. The 'morbid condition' might be 'merely accidental' or the result of vicious upbringing, or be a 'deep-rooted and hereditary malady'.

Whatever the cause and the condition her work held out more hope to the deprived, delinquent and disturbed than perhaps any other that was done in England in the nineteenth century, through its insight, its breadth and its practical effect.

Before her death Mary Carpenter had been instrumental in the passing of several important Acts of Parliament (see above), had seen the growth of reformatories (forty-five in 1858) and industrial schools (nineteen in 1861), and had been of immense importance in establishing the structure of child care for the deprived and delinquent in this country for the next century. That subsequent children's homes and approved schools did not always live up to her principles does not diminish her own work.

C

5

Education

There is little in the history of education in the nineteenth century which foreshadows the growth of special educational provision for the maladjusted. Public schools may have liberalized their curricula and, to some extent, their teaching methods, but there is little evidence that the hearty, games-playing, science-teaching new public school of the Oundle persuasion was any better milieu for the disturbed child than was the more violent but perhaps less organized pre-Arnold model. Indeed individual idiosyncracies might have found freer range in the latter and at least the maladjusted child would not have been so burdened with moral guilt as he would have been under an Arnold or a Howson.

Nor did the early progressive public schools, whatever their subsequent influence, perceive the adjustment of the maladjusted as part of their function, although the improved staff/pupil relationships in schools such as Abbotsholme and Bedales may have had this effect with some children. Abbotsholme (1889) may have substituted manual labour for team games and crafts for the classics but —with its red, white and blue colours, its autocratic structure and its school motto of 'Liberty is Obedience to Law'—it still sought to produce a masculine élite of a basically 'public school' type.

Of the new race of progressive school autocrats Alexander Devine, the founder of Clayesmore (1896), offered the greatest hope. Having, as a young court reporter for the *Manchester Guardian,* observed the condition and treatment of juvenile delinquents, he realized the futility of punitive suppression of youthful energies. His reaction was characteristically immediate and energetic. His first venture on behalf of the deprived and delinquent was the foundation of the Hulme and Chorlton-on-Medlock Lads' Club in 1886, which flourished despite the public-school structure which Devine imposed. Working with an adolescent enthusiasm (which appears to have remained with him until his death in 1930), Devine established two more clubs of a similar pattern and united them in the Manchester

Working Lads' Association. He also instigated holiday camps for his deprived boys on non-military lines, subsequently imitated by the universities and public schools.

He also founded the Gordon Boys Home in 1888, in which he housed forty-five boys rescued by him from the courts in his new role as honorary police court missionary. Under the provisions of the First Offenders Act, 1887 he accepted 255 delinquents in the first year: '117 of these were cases of destitution, 34 of simple larceny, 24 of begging, 21 of sleeping out, 18 of trespassing on railway stations, 16 of obstructing the footpath, 5 of gambling, and 4 of stealing food. In 19 cases only were boys who had been released under the provisions of the Act and helped by the Home subsequently re-convicted and sent to prison.'[44] His work was widely praised but little imitated. Florence Nightingale wrote '. . . as far as I know, yours is the only machinery in England which . . . offers the magistrate the means of carrying out the Act successfully.'[45] The general approval of what Miss Nightingale called Devine's 'social physic' did not, however, save the extravagant and egoistic Devine from his creditors and enemies. By 1890 he had been removed from the control both of the boys' clubs and the boys' home, and he decided to leave Manchester.

In defending himself to his committee he gave an interesting description of his daily routine:

From ten o'clock until half past twelve every morning I am at the police courts, trying to secure for any lad brought up the benefit of the First Offenders Act. The early part of the afternoon I devote to seeing persons at my office – destitute lads, out of work, in trouble; parents, employers of labour. From four o'cock until half past six I am busy with my correspondence. From half past six until ten I am at one of the Clubs; and once or twice a week I am out most of the night in the poorer districts of Charter Street and Angel Meadow, engaged in work among the lodging houses. In my enthusiasm I have been sacrificing all I possess, health, means and the best years of my youth, living absolutely cut off from old associations and family ties, in the middle of Ancoats. I am overworked to the limit of my endurance; yet I do not complain.[46]

The next venture to which Devine addressed his enthusiasm is, perhaps, the most relevant. In 1892, at the age of twenty-seven, he moved to London with twelve of his Gordon Home delinquents and a year later decided to profit by his experience with the disturbed to found a school for 'public school misfits and scallywags'. 'He saw himself as the pioneer of something new in English life and education, the saviour of a section of mankind which had hitherto been execrated, cast out as waste, when it might have been profitably cultivated.'[47] Had he remained true to his mission he might well have made a significant contribution to the problem which George Lyward saw, and tackled, in the 1930s.

The new school was established at Salisbury Grange, Edmonton, in 1894. His appeal to the headmasters of public schools—'Don't expel your bad boys! Send them to me and see what I can do with them!'—was eagerly responded to, and Devine moved to larger premises at Glebelands, Mitcham. He appears to have had no particular policy or theory of treatment, but relied on the effect of his own personality to produce reformation. An admirer, Dr Dearmer, wrote of him:

What then is wanted? A man who has the rare gift of understanding boys and who has cultivated that gift in the school of experience. We want several schools under such men. And we are glad to be able to say that one such establishment is already in existence, and that its existence has already been attended with such success as to justify the strongest hopes upon this subject. The founder is an English gentleman who has engaged upon the work from pure devotion to the cause. He has had a wide practical experience and has made a careful study of both the English and the Continental school systems. We are able to bear witness to his possession of remarkable power with boys, and the headmasters of several of our large schools to whom he is well known, have given the best evidence of their trust in his method. His method is very simple. He disclaims any rule of thumb and works by personal influence, common sense and an 'infinite capacity for taking pains'. He has devoted his life, and a rare spirit of enthusiasm, to his particular and important work; and he absolutely refuses to consider any of his boys 'bad', or to treat them in the spirit of a martinet.[48]

Devine's devotion was not, however, to be life-long. Glebelands revealed a basic dichotomy in Devine's enthusiasms. He was certainly interested in the problems of disturbed boys and showed great insight in dealing with them, but he was, at the same time, inspired by the vision of Devine as the great headmaster of a reformed public school—not a public school reformatory. With this vision before him he moved in 1896 to Clayesmore, where one of his chief endeavours was to overcome the stigma which he felt to be attached to his former activities. 'It is only by dint of the most strenuous efforts,' he wrote, 'that I have succeeded in overcoming the idea that Clayesmore is a school for the unfit. I have had to make it quite clear that on no account will I receive a boy expelled from school, nor a boy, under any circumstances, without a recommendation from his form master.'[49] Devine's subsequent pursuit of his mission is therefore not relevant to this work, although it is always stimulating.[50]

Devine rationalized his closing of Glebelands by claiming that 'the number of boys who might be called really bad was exceedingly small; the fault of most of them is that they were weak, easy going and easily led'.[51] Boys of this type could not satisfy Devine's ideal of public-school spirit, and he considered that they should be contained (by isolation) in normal schools rather than be given the additional handicap of the stigma of special school education. He had, however, given some idea of what could be done by sympathy and imagination before his light failed.

State education offered little to the disturbed and difficult individual compulsorily instructed in the 3 Rs in large classes by badly trained and underpaid teachers whose meagre salaries, until 1897, depended on the ability of their pupils to perform these basic skills and to regurgitate undigested lessons. The children of the working classes, trained only to retain their depressed status, were without the benefits either of their upper-middle-class brethren in 'reformed' or 'progressive' public schools or of their precursors for whom the ragged schools or the free day schools, less restricted by 'results', had occasionally provided a more humanitarian education.

Private schools, largely for the middle classes, remained and, at the turn of the century, were increasingly influenced by the educational ideas of Froebel or the psychological principles of Sully and Ward but, until after the great watershed of the First World War, had little effect on education in general.

One experiment is, perhaps, worthy of note. In 1888 Mr E. Sargent opened a co-educational elementary school in Hackney, known as School Field, for eighty pupils who paid twopence a week. The regime was one of 'ordered liberty', the top class working on its own to prepare the thirteen- and fourteen-year-olds for adult responsibility. Weekly assignments of work were completed and the punishment for 'unseemly conduct' was 'to follow the headmistress wherever she went for a certain time, short or long in accordance with the nature of the offence'.[52] The staff ratio (1 : 35) was almost twice that of state schools (1 : 60) and the children were allowed to move freely from place to place in class, and the curriculum was imaginative and creative: 'Reading was taught by a really remarkable "Look and Say" method invented by the teacher . . .'[53] and the children were encouraged to produce their own stories, poems and drawings for a school magazine, the production of which formed the basis of club activities and a link between school and home. The school was closed in 1894 for lack of funds.

EDUCATIONAL THEORY

As in the field of mental health, so in education. It was in developing theory, rather than in actual practice, that the greatest hope lay for the deviant child at the end of the nineteenth century.

Educational ideas derived from Rousseau, Pestalozzi, Herbart, Froebel—and later Montessori—put increased emphasis on the needs of the individual child and the importance of experience and volition in education. By the turn of the century, philosophical psychologists such as Dewey were propounding transactionalist theories which were to have profound effects on the methods actually used in schools, and in which the educational needs of the individual child became the focus.

In Britain Dr James Ward, lecturing in psychology at Cambridge between 1878 and 1894, propounded ideas on the process of education which Titchener described as epoch-making and which, through the *Journal of Education,* were disseminated among progressive educationalists. Rejecting still-persistent 'faculty' theories, where memory, intellect, imagination, judgment, etc. were independent mental phenomena capable of being mechanically trained by a process of repetition, Ward posited 'attention' as the one fundamental power (the end to which intellect was the means). In lecturing on psychology as 'the science of individual experience' he put the emphasis in education on 'presentation' rather than on 'training', but went beyond Herbart in stressing the importance of the child's initiating action. Thus the child would be motivated to love work which the adult would direct. The indivisible individual 'ego', or self, integrated experience which was child-chosen and teacher-directed.

The parallel between this and Dewey's transactionalist views and Piaget's later maturational approach is clear.

Ward's pupil, G. F. Stout, author of the widely read *Manual of Psychology* (1898), propounded, although with little empirical support, ideas which could not only be related to later Gestalt psychology but which saw the unconscious as a constantly activated stream progressively organized by sensory and motor experience. Although lacking in scientific method and evidence, the theories of Ward and Stout now appear to be considerably in advance of the primitive behaviourists who succeeded them, although their influence on psychology itself was slight. Their stress, however, on the importance of the whole child as a unique individual (which they shared with Sully) made it possible to find theoretical justification for treating the deviant child as one who had a special educational problem, rather than as one who merely caused special educational problems. It was becoming clear that the problem of the child was more important than the problem in the class.

REFERENCES

CHAPTER 3: Mental Health

1 The Education of the Imbecile and the Improvement of Invalid Youth pamphlet published for 'behoof of the Home and School for Imbecile and Invalid Children, 10 Gayfield Square, Edinburgh'. *p* 10. 1856.
2 Ibid. *p* 12.
3 Ibid. *p* 9.
4 Ibid. *p* 14.
5 *See*, for instance, Strauss, A. A. & Kephart, N. C. *Psychopathology and the Education of Brain-injured Children.* Grune & Stratton, New York, 1955.
6 The Education of the Imbecile, etc. (Ref. 1). *p* 13.
7 WARNER, F. *Lectures on Mental Faculty, 1890,* and Mental and Physical conditions among Fifty Thousand Children. *J. Roy. Stat. Soc.* LIX. *p* 25 *et seq.* 1896.
8 MAUDSLEY, H. *Mental Pathology, p* 188 *et seq.* 1879.
9 TREDGOLD, A. F. *Mental Deficiency, p* 401, for details of surgical processes. 1914.
10 FLUGEL, J. C. *A Hundred Years of Psychology, p* 132. Duckworth, London, 1951.
11 BURT, C. *Year Book of Education, p* 83. University of London Institute of Education. 1955.
12 MINISTRY OF EDUCATION. Report of the Committee on Maladjusted Children (The Underwood Report). H.M.S.O., London, 1955.
13 THOMSON, R. *The Pelican History of Psychology, p* 174. Penguin, London, 1968.
14 KEIR, G. A History of Child Guidance, in Symposium on Psychologists and Psychiatrists in the Child Guidance Service, *Brit. J. Ed. Psych.* XXII, (1.) *p* 14. 1952. (A very useful survey.)
15 SULLY, J., in Keir ibid.
16 FULTON, J. F. Factors influencing the growth and pattern of the child guidance services and school psychological services in Britain from 1900 to the present time. M.A. thesis (unpublished), Queen's University Belfast, 1964. *See also* Keir, op. cit. (To both I am much indebted.)
17 Report of the Conference of Educational Associations, held at University of London, January 1914: (*p* 297).

18 WALL, W. D. (ed.) *Psychological Services of Schools. p* 16. UNESCO Institute for Education, Hamburg, 1956.
19 KEIR, G. op. cit., *p* 15.
20 WALL, W. D. op. cit., *p* 17.

CHAPTER 4: Child Care

21 BALBERNIE, R. *Residential Work with Children, pp* 133–136. Pergamon, Oxford, 1966.
22 HEYWOOD, J. S. *Children in Care, p* 33. Routledge & Kegan Paul, 1965.
23 CARPENTER, M. *Reformatory Schools for the Children of the Perishing and Dangerous Classes and for Juvenile Offenders, p* 340. Gilpin, London, 1851.
24 Ibid. *pp* 339–340.
25 YOUNG, A. F. & ASHTON, E. T. *British Social Work in the 19th Century, p* 241. Routledge & Kegan Paul, London, 1956.
26 Ibid. *p* 243.
27 Ibid. *pp* 245–246. *See also* Carpenter, M. op. cit., Chapter 2.
28 CARPENTER, M. op. cit., *pp* 225–246.
29 Ibid. *p* 245.
30 HEYWOOD, J. S. op. cit., *p* 57.
31 CARPENTER, J. ESTLIN. *The Life & Work of Mary Carpenter*, Macmillan, 1879.
32 FLETCHER, J. Report to the Committee of Council on Education, *p* 279. 1850.
33 CARPENTER, M. op. cit., *p* 159.
34 Ibid. *p* 173.
35 CARPENTER, M. *Juvenile Delinquents, their Conditions and Treatment, pp* 258–282. W. & F. G. Cash, London, 1853.
36 Ibid. *p* 297.
37 Ibid. *pp* 298–9.
38 Ibid. *p* 303.
39 Ibid. *pp* 306–7.
40 Ibid. *p* 5.
41 Ibid. *p* 6.
42 *Ragged School Magazine*, **II**, *p* 61.
43 CARPENTER, M. (Ref. 23). *p* 273.

CHAPTER 5: Education

44 WHITBOURN, F. *Lex: Alexander Devine, Founder of Clayesmore School, p* 79. Longman Green, London, 1937.

45 Ibid.
46 Ibid. *p* 91.
47 Ibid. *p* 117.
48 Ibid. *pp* 125–6.
49 Ibid. *p* 134.
50 *See also* Stewart, W. A. C. *The Educational Innovators* 2, *pp* 18–25. Macmillan, London, 1968.
51 WHITBOURN, F. *op. cit.*, *p* 127.
52 WOODS, A. *Educational Experiments in England*, *p* 82. Methuen, London, 1920.
53 Ibid. *p* 81.

PART THREE

Some Individualists

6

Twentieth Century Originals

WILLIAM HENRY HUNT

In the days before child guidance clinics when the name of Freud had
an unsavoury connotation in the minds of respectable people there
lived a remarkable man called William Henry Hunt, who was in charge
of a large colony of what we should now call maladjusted youths, near
Wallingford.... W. H. Hunt was something of a genius. I remember
him saying very often in his gruff voice as he peered through or over
his oval pebble lenses: 'People are always saying to me, "What do you
do to these boys?" and I say "We don't do anything to them." '[1]

David Wills, who worked with Hunt and who described him thus,
does not find this reaction surprising. He comments that there are
indeed many forms of maladjustment which may respond to a
warm, restful, non-provocative environment.

Hunt, in some ways, appears to form a bridge between the work
of nineteenth-century precursors such as Mary Carpenter, working
with the destitute and delinquent, and later exponents of 'planned
environmental therapy' (see Chapter 15). For the first three decades
of the twentieth century he was superintendent of Wallingford Farm
Training Colony (afterwards Turners Court), which housed about
250 rejects of the Poor Law system. His colony might well be considered to be a forerunner of the 'rehabilitation centre', were it not
for the fact that about three quarters of its inmates were adolescents.
Hunt had no training in social work, being originally a journalist,
and his motivation appears to have been Christian altruism of an
old-fashioned, liberal, nonconformist pattern.

He clearly believed that adolescence is the age of loyalty to the
group. The adolescent boy expressed himself through the group's
common actions. Only by the keen sense of membership of a group
could his deeper impulse be satisfied. More recently, Crutchfield
has detected a strong 'dependency motive' in unstable characters,[2]
although this is not equally true of 'persons with acute psycho-

77

neurotic symptoms'.[3] Hunt's clientele were perhaps more likely to be maladjusted 'displaced persons' rather than suffering from specific psychoneuroses. Be that as it may, Hunt organized the boys in squads of eight or nine, each with an elder 'brother' who shared their life work and was responsible for their well-being. He always insisted that the 'brother' should be the 'stroke oar' of his squad but that his primary duty was to love his charges.

The work was largely farm training and allied crafts considered appropriate to the inmates' lowly social status, and the intention was that they would subsequently emigrate to the Dominions, which most of them did until the war intervened. The 'brothers' were intended to be high-minded and altruistic young men who, after a period of about three years' training at Wallingford, were to go in for other forms of social work. Some of them were satisfactory but many were, in fact, men who had tried other things and failed, and were thus frequently less reliable than their charges. There was much in the colony that was undesirable. It was here that Wills learnt that harsh physical 'discipline' was derived from fear and that aggression only produced aggression; that the strong-arm methods of many of the staff led from violence to violence which 'is seldom more than a transitory deterrent, if that—not a cure of the desire to inflict it', and that the victim identifies with the punisher's strength rather than with any more valuable qualities.[4] Dr Marjorie Franklin raises the pertinent question of how culpable of negligence Hunt was when, despite his humanitarian principles, he gave so little guidance to his staff and condoned, by default, such treatment of his charges.

When Wills speaks of a 'warm, restful, non-provocative environment' it sounds a little like the prospectus of a luxury hotel. The ethos of the Wallingford colony may have been 'warm, restful and non-provocative' but the physical conditions were crude, hard and squalid. Hunt may have seen some virtue in this as a situation in which mastering the environment had some therapeutic value as well as keeping the deprived adolescent in touch with reality. Wills, himself, at the Hawkspur Camp, did not discount this value, although various exponents of 'planned environmental therapy' have always found the exact degree of creative rigour required difficult to determine.

Despite the crises which one would expect to be inherent in the system, particularly with the very large numbers involved, Hunt persisted and both preceded and survived his better-known contemporary, Homer Lane (see Chapter 7). His work was, perhaps, less spectacular, if more arduous, than Lane's, his personality less flamboyant, and his achievement, therefore, less widely known. Although one can trace his progenitors in child care to the founders of the French agricultural colonies or the National Children's Home at Edgeworth (see Chapter 4), he seems to have been little influenced by them. Nor was his influence great, for his model was essentially a nineteenth-century one, appropriate largely for a nineteenth-century poor-law problem in nineteenth-century agricultural terms, although he did cause individuals, other than Wills, connected with the care of delinquents to consider or reconsider the rationale of their work. Among these Frank Foster was in charge of the Borstal after-care service until it was absorbed by the probation service, and was largely responsible for the after-care hostel which Miller described in *Growth to Freedom*,[5] and Wilfred Chinn organized the first Israeli probation service and became adviser in social services to the Colonial Office. This is not to discount Hunt's value to his adolescents, but to place him as an 'original' rather than as a pioneer.

LEILA RENDEL

Although she died only in 1969 the same is, to some extent, true of Leila Rendel, whose origins were in nineteenth-century liberal philanthropy and whose great personal influence made difficult any conceptualization of her methods. She was the granddaughter of Sir Alexander Rendel, an eminent Victorian radical, and niece of Edith Rendel, a suffragette and pioneer girls'-club leader. Her mother was a Paul (the publishers) and the household was a centre for discussion and activity for nineteenth-century liberals involved in twentieth-century political and social reform. Leila Rendel grew up in an atmosphere and in an era of individual 'good works' largely dependent on the interests of wealthy and under-employed upper-class women with strong social consciences — a source of energy in this field which increased after the First World War when, although there was less money, there were more women whose life-fulfilment could no longer come through marriage which had either ended, or been prevented, by the decimation of their generation of men in the war. The original committee of the Caldecott school in 1911 consisted of nine women, eight of whom were unmarried.

Leila Rendel was, at this time, twenty-eight, and had been trained in 'Swedish gymnastics', a subject which she subsequently taught in a teachers' training college and for which she became an inspector. In her early twenties she was greatly interested in Margaret Macmillan's pioneer nursery-school work. She always had a passion for teaching and Baroness Stocks, her cousin, remembers that, while still a young child, Leila Rendel had insisted on teaching her the catechism. Her attachment to the established Church was not fixed. Her religion was of a practical kind and she eventually joined the Society of Friends partly, her co-worker Ethel Davies suggests, as a reaction against her erstwhile colleague Phyllis Potter's involvement with the Anglo-Catholics, and in response to the latter's criticism that she lacked any structural basis for her beliefs.

Leila Rendel's original concern in what was to evolve into the Caldecott Community was in taking gymnastics in a hall attached to her Aunt Edith's girls' club. From this developed first a crèche, then a nursery school, and eventually the Caldecott Community (named after the illustrations from the Rendel's Caldecott reading books which were used to decorate the walls). The first official home of the Caldecott Community, 26 Cartwright Gardens, housed not only Edith Rendel's working girl's club and a day nursery previously run by Phyllis Potter at Whitefields Tabernacle, Tottenham Court Road, but also, by 1914, a mothers' club, an evening play-hour activity and a holiday school. It was also a base for country holidays, medical inspections and a school-meals service. This emphasis on 'the whole child' and the essential interaction of social service and education within the Community was the basis from which all else stemmed.

In 1911 Leila Rendel became secretary and treasurer to the Caldecott Nursery School, where it was hoped 'the children might enjoy that instruction which is usually absorbed by the children of the wealthy in their own nurseries and by virtue of their happier surroundings'.[6] In its present stately home, Mersham le Hatch, this tradition remains unbroken although the world and society (and its attitudes) have changed. No longer would it be possible to record benefactions as they were recorded in 1914 thus: 'The thanks of the Community are due to many people for their help in the past year. . . . To Mrs Britton, Mrs Donaldson, Miss Kelsall, Miss E. Rendel, Mrs Philipson, *Mrs Philipson's Chauffeur's Wife*, Mrs Mooring, and Miss Harrison Rawson for hospitality and care given to various children during the holidays'! (my italics),[7] but many of the compensatory virtues of that supremely self-confident society survived two world disasters. It is still within an essentially secure, ordered and loving framework, and in a gracious environment, that the Caldecott Community endeavours to fulfil its educational and social aim enunciated in 1911: 'To awaken in the children that independence of spirit and joyousness of life which will alone give them the power of realizing to the fullest extent the possibilities of development within their reach'.[8]

In fulfilling its constant aim the Caldecott Community has often changed its external appearance.

In 1917, when it was realized how much the environment of wartime St Pancras frustrated its aim of the healthy development of the whole child, the Caldecott Community was moved to Charlton Court, in East Sutton, Kent (now the home of Red Hill School, see Chapter 11), and so became the first coeducational boarding school for working-class children who were neither 'in care' nor convicted by the courts. Alice Woods gives a very illuminating account of the work there and of its emphasis both on individual development and corporate consciousness.[9]

In 1925, when the Community moved to Cuffley, in Hertfordshire, it was decided that its function would no longer relate only to the socially deprived but to children of any creed, nationality or social class who, by reason of parental death, sickness, divorce, separation or other inadequacy, or through illegitimacy, were deprived of the secure and loving family environment which Leila Rendel had always regarded as essential to their true emotional and personal development.

By 1934 many local authorities were asking the community to accept, as its special concern, the disturbed and difficult children of broken homes, and in 1938 the Caldecott Community became one of the first schools to be recognized by the Board of Education under Section 80 of the Education Act, 1921, as an appropriate establishment for those children whose behaviour problems had led to their exclusion from normal schools. As the inevitable outcome of a conjunction between its care for the deprived and a socially and politically troubled world—in which the breathing space between two cataclysmic wars seemed filled by economic disaster—this function of the Community increased. By 1962 the proportion of maladjusted children in the Community had grown to almost two thirds although Leila Rendel's intention was always preventive rather than therapeutic: 'To rescue intelligent children from disintegrated homes early enough to prevent maladjustment, and possibly delinquency'.[10]

Leila Rendel's interest in delinquency was, doubtless, born in St Pancras before the First World War but it was in the Second World War that the problem was put firmly in her capacious lap. For a few years (1941-5), during which it was in exile on Egdon Heath (Hyde Heath), the Caldecott Community accepted its status of a junior approved school, in response to the increasingly recognized need for a therapeutic rather than a punitive attitude to those many juvenile delinquents whose actions were a clear expression of their social and emotional needs. In a paper, *The Child of Misfortune*, given in 1952, Leila Rendel not only recognized that 'a large proportion of these young offenders are of normal personality, and their difficulties arise through distortion caused by emotional stresses of abnormal home environment' but she also pointed out that they were usually 'the unprotected children of the streets recruited from the poorest ranks of the population',[11] children who, she knew from long experience, shared the psychological problems, but not the supportive and influential backgrounds, of middle-class children. Despite its temporary change of status and the difficulties produced by wartime chaos there was no fundamental change in the philosophy of the Community. The approved-school children, all of whom were under twelve when they arrived, fitted in easily with the resident evacuees, refugees and maladjusted children, and frequently proved much less difficult.

After the war, although the Caldecott Community ceased, at its own request, to be an approved school, Leila Rendel continued to be involved with the needs of the delinquent, as she was with those of all distressed children. In the course of the Curtis Committee's enquiry[12] leading to the Children's Act of 1948, Leila Rendel, together with Dr Hilda Lewis, mooted the idea for 'at least one home in each [L.E.A.] for the temporary reception of children with, in particular, the necessary facilities for observation of their physical and mental condition'.[13]

A pilot experimental reception centre was opened in October 1947 at New House, near Mersham le Hatch, under the general supervision of the directors of the Caldecott Community, which it was hoped would be of help in ascertaining and providing for the individual needs of all homeless and disturbed children. From the first the majority (94 per cent) was composed of children in the care of Kent County Council, most of whom had been remanded from a juvenile court. Maladjusted children, or children disturbed in ways other than delinquent, could be supported only by reference through the school medical officer under Section 48 (3) of the Education Act, and the value of the reception centre was lessened by the absence of any referrals by voluntary agencies or for children temporarily in need because of parental illness, death or poverty. Thus, to the discouragement of their protagonists, the image of reception centres was biased even before they were officially established, although they did succeed in pioneering methods of classifying and assessment which have, subsequently, been of great value in work both with the delinquent and the maladjusted.[14, 15]

In 1956 a 'family group' home was established at Smeeth, Kent, for children who were considered to need greater individual care than the main household could provide. These fifteen children, although cared for separately by a housemaster and his wife, remained part of the whole Community.

Recent development of the idea of community homes and the integration of the social services related to children as envisaged in the White Paper *Children in Trouble* and in the Seebohm Report indicate how far the Caldecott Community has remained a forerunner in methods of social education.

Amid all this change one thing remained constant. From 1911–69 the essential security of the perpetually changing community came largely from the presence in it of Leila Rendel. Although her approach was essentially dynamic, flexible and progressive, she was herself reliable, stable and conservative of the 'good' things from her radical but upper-middle-class Edwardian past. Physically very large, she embodied permanence and, even when the Caldecott Community was homeless and divided during the war, she remained, in the words of Lady Stocks, who was close to her at this period, 'unfluffable'. Through crisis and change Leila Rendel continued to embody the love, comfort and stability which provided the essential therapy of the Community. Her genius 'lay in her ability to make contact with children. Children really loved her and she loved them. She would go to endless trouble with the individual child and, although she was very close to them, she kept a composure and had a lack of sentimentality that they respected.'[16] She remained 'fascinated' by children and every child knew of her interest in it individually, and although she indulged in what Lady Stocks regards as 'the family habit of adopting children' she seems to have succeeded in achieving if not emotional detachment at least emotional egalitarianism.

The effect of her personality and her rejection of dogma makes it difficult to analyse the principles and structure of her work. 'No theory is admitted by Miss Rendel, or her partner, Miss Davies, that has not been tried on the touchstone of many years' experience.'[17]

Leila Rendel was not only a born educator and a trained teacher but she remained essentially a progressive, sensitive and flexible educationalist. Her educational theory had evolved both from the Froebelian and the Montessorian schools of her youth. The main object of the original school was seen as providing 'a garden to test and weed out the new educational theories of which the last decade has been so full. The Community would like to test the new theories that are slowly but radically changing our national education; it would like to be not a universal model but a forerunner. It does not wish to preach community life, nor Montessori games, nor country holidays; but to show by trial what are the good, and what are the bad, tendencies in modern theories of collective life and non-collective teaching'.[18] Although non-collective teaching was assumed to be best for children of all ages—as were self-discipline, spontaneous grouping and free choice within an 'integrated' day—a less absolutely permissive ethos soon developed. One incident was of particular significance:

It was some months before we realized that the children themselves felt restless and lost. The situation reached a climax when a small boy put his head round the door of the directors' sitting room and said abruptly and bitterly, "You seem to forget, Miss Leila, that we are young and you are here to look after us!" ... From then onwards we exercised a somewhat more limited and guarded freedom. For the achievement of balance between discipline and freedom there can be no hard and fast rules. It can be maintained only by an openness of mind, an alertness of spirit, and a willingness on the part of the adult to grow with the children themselves.[19]

It is particularly interesting that although Leila Rendel decided that 'Montessori did not work with "wild children" ', the description which Stewart gives of the essentials of a Montessori class describes exactly Leila Rendel's subsequent approach.[20] He perceives that although the order may appear to proceed from the children's group, the directress is, in fact, *dea in machina* whose job it is to isolate the disruptive child from the group until the group magnetism compels him to return and conform. 'Hers is the ultimate but unobtrusive authority.'

The work of the junior children (the seniors now go to nearby schools) was organized in terms both of group activity and individual work quotas with the emphasis on experience and discovery and the full use of the country environment, and a 'respectable' standard of work was insisted on even from the youngest pupils, since a large part of the object was to build up self-respect through genuine individual accomplishment.

It was typical of Leila Rendel that, as problems changed or became more complex, she was prepared to modify her policy in the light of experience and research. As the Community catered increasingly for maladjusted children so she sought assistance in coping with their educational problems. In 1955 an experimental unit was set up to study the effect of individual remedial education on children who were deemed to be retarded through the effects of their disturbance. It was considered that readiness to learn depended not only on maturation and intellectual ability but on the child's total personal and social experience, and the extent and direction of its motivation. The remedial sessions in reading and arithmetic were conducted through the medium not only of specific books and other material but through a wide range of play and creative materials.

The general results of the two-year experiment were a significant and maintained progress in reading ability, a marked, but seldom maintained, increase in arithmetical ability, and a pronounced and overall improvement in personal behaviour and adjustment—which came, it was concluded, not only through the close personal attention given to each child but also through the discipline of learning and the experience of success.

The following case is typical both of the children involved and the progress achieved:

George came to the Caldecott at the age of 9 years, because of the effects of an unhappy strained home. Both parents were artists, the father being an alcoholic asthmatic and the mother a cold, rejecting woman. George also suffered from asthma and had come to a complete standstill educationally. At the age of 7 years, after two different schools had tried, he was given a private tutor for 2 years, but continued to be an extremely anxious boy, severely blocked with regard to all social or school learning.

At the start of treatment George was markedly lacking in self-confidence, slow in all his reactions, and full of fears.

Response to remedial treatment was slow but steady. As emotional tension gradually decreased, he became able to respond to teaching. However, each holiday provided a setback, as his mother insisted on coaching him which again increased his anxiety. Yet from being a complete non-reader and terrified of the subject, he became able to face his difficulties and persevere despite them.[21]

It was again typical of Leila Rendel that the unit, having been shown to be of value, was continued as an integral part of the Community. Its function was enlarged to include very disturbed children who might profit in other ways from individual attention and the opportunity to play or be creative in an encouraging atmosphere. 'Individual needs could be catered for; the immature could play at a younger level without fear of ridicule; the apathetic or isolated child, unable to respond in a larger group, could find stimulation in the more sheltered environment of a small group; the aggressive could be provided with acceptable outlets without causing harm to people or property.'[22]

In remedial education, as in many other educational innovations, Leila Rendel fulfilled her intention to be a 'forerunner'.

As a therapeutic community the Caldecott has also fulfilled the expectations of its founders who, in 1914 when there was no thought of working with 'maladjusted' children, saw individual adjustment to emotional and social frustrations as their chief experimental aim. 'As far as the experiment has gone . . . it is precisely in this direction that the Community hopes for its most interesting results' (Third Annual Report). Principles were enunciated then which still form the basic assumptions of the Community's therapeutic work.

The environment was to be as harmonious and as free of frustration as possible, for self-control was not to be learnt by overcoming difficulties and confusions, not from the habit of being in trouble, but from character achieved by each child being given a real sense of responsibility for his own actions, the compulsion of inner self-discipline derived from a demanding but loving and secure 'community'. 'There comes a time . . . when the child begins to take up the responsibility for his own life. If at that moment he is helped and encouraged he will find his own individuality and undergo a sort of mental conversion. . . . After that he can face his own troubles as he meets them and it is from there that his discipline will come.'[23]

The actual physical environment was considered to be of great importance and country living and cultured and graceful surroundings were important. It is interesting, in this connection, that an ex-pupil of the Caldecott, an accomplished criminal, once complained to a member of staff that the sort of elegance, comfort and culture which he had experienced as a deprived child in the Community was an inducement to crime—since only through criminal activity could it be subsequently purchased by the 'working classes'. (This view—that special schools, by protecting children from bad environments, unfit them to return to their own social milieu—has considerable, if not such extreme, support.)

Within this secure and congenial environment the interaction of the group was thought to have its own therapeutic value. Leila Rendel said: 'Children come here said to be difficult in behaviour, but before long most of them settle down and find their way. It is the children who help one another.' Children were expected to conform to a fundamentally middle-class ethos in which reasonable standards of quietness, orderliness, good manners and cleanliness were implicit. Noise in the dining room would be muted if Leila Rendel rang the bell and the Community's newsletters are full of gently mocking comments on nonconformists. Children who were too disturbed to cope with normal school work, or a normal mealtime situation, were allowed to 'opt out' and were known as 'special'. It was assumed that community pressure ('How awful it must be to be "special" ') and a desire to be accepted would produce a reasonable degree of conformity which was a strain neither to the individual nor to the community.

Although it was thought necessary for the development of self-discipline that there should be a progressive assumption of responsibility, under guidance, and although Alice Woods describes an early experiment in self-government at the Caldecott in 1920,[24] responsibility was never 'shared' in the later sense of that term (see Chapter 15). School meetings were held at first weekly, then monthly, but did little more than affirm faith in the executive. In direction as in sympathy the Caldecott Community was essentially individualistic.

On one occasion an earnest and puzzled German research worker asked, after a considerable stay, 'But where is the administration?' and was told 'Well, usually, in the girls' bathroom' (where Leila Rendel would often sit and discuss both individual and community problems).

Another apparent paradox was that although great emphasis was placed, in principle, on the importance of the warmth and support of a good family—of which many of these children were deprived— the Caldecott Community, though all-age and co-educational, was not run on any genuinely family basis. The children were divided into age groups both for lessons and for most communal activities, and the boys and girls were not only in separate groups but, at Mersham le Hatch, in separate wings of the building. There was no intention to replace the original families or parents, however bad, if they existed and close contact was maintained through informal visits and school 'occasions'.

Leila Rendel herself did not consider the Caldecott Community the ideal environment for the very deeply disturbed child, although many such children doubtless responded to her care. She recognized her limitations (a rare quality in pioneers) and when children could not profit by staying in the Community they were sent to such institutions as Finchden Manor (see Chapter 10) or the Mulberry Bush (see Chapter 15), which offered a different regime or treatment approach. Others, brought up from infancy in the Caldecott Community, have been sent later to Gordonstoun (of which Leila Rendel was a founder-governor) in order to develop in a new and more challenging environment.

Leila Rendel's appreciation of Kurt Hahn and Gordonstoun was reflected in her policy at the Caldecott. One does not expect in a school largely for socially and emotionally deprived children to find a regime of cold showers, early morning runs, school meetings devoted mainly to ritual re-readings of the 'charter' and reaffirmations of faith. The use of school uniform as a mark of privilege (the uniformed were the trusted and responsible) savours strongly of Gordonstoun's caste system of 'white stripers' and 'colour-bearers'.

On the whole, however, the Caldecott Community avoided extremism while remaining receptive to new ideas. Its strength lies largely, perhaps, in its continuity, which has been maintained by a nucleus of loyal, if underpaid, staff. When Leila Rendel died in March 1969, her co-director since 1931, Miss Ethel Davies, remained in charge. Miss Davies originally came to the Community as an assistant housekeeper in 1928 for a salary of £50 a year and in answer to an advertisement for someone with 'a passion for cleanliness'. The Caldecott continues as an independent primary school and a home for secondary-school children, and has over a hundred pupils. It fulfils many needs and will doubtless continue to act as a 'forerunner' in social-educational care in accord with the spirit of its founder, whom no change of scene, financial crisis, world disaster or advancing age could frighten into a static security.

RUSSELL HOARE

Russell Hoare, the superintendent of Sysonby House, Riverside Village, Melton Mowbray, was another early-twentieth-century 'original' who worked largely through his own personality. Indeed, it would be true to say that this was the sole basis of the work at Sysonby House—one of the three 'juvenile colonies' in existence during the First World War. (The others were the Little Commonwealth and a Berkshire training colony for the reformation of young prostitutes.) The colony, established under the auspices of the Fellowship of Reconciliation, was for adolescent delinquents of above school age mainly from London. They were 'those who for some reason or other nobody else will touch ... the residuum left when the crafts, educational, reformatory, ecclesiastical, social and charitable have sifted their clientele and can attract or will admit no more'.[25]

F. R. Hoare admitted to no 'craft', although before the war he had engaged in considerable relief and club work in East London. He was, by temperament, an anarchist rejecting all forms of organization. His aim was never to turn out good law-abiding citizens but rather rebels who would be capable of retaining their personal integrity in a community dominated by aggression, coercion, economic competition, hunger and fear. Thus he rejected the methods not only of the reformatory school but also of those of his contemporary, Homer Lane, whom he saw as too concerned with conformity and too essentially wedded to a capitalist ethic. He looked for something more 'radical, empirical, personal and spiritual'.

Thus there was at Sysonby no elaborate superstructure of self-government through which the adult could impose indirect authority

or the adolescent community could distort the individual's development by a display of adult forms and adult stability. Radical self-
government by boys and girls he saw as essentially fluctuating
'between the three extremes that make up the triangle of adolescent
polity, tyranny, anarchy, and the golden rule (constitutionalism is
not real to adolescence); it will be both too realistic and too
idealistic to be capable of that continuous process we call development, evolution, progress'. He regarded as a sham any attempt to
foist laws and punishments on the community as its own productions.

Thus he rejected all forms of government and all forms of punishment. He believed that punishment was the most damaging factor
in the establishment of those human relationships through which
he wished to work, and sought to establish that he would not punish,
or hand children over to punishment, under any circumstances.
In his 'police-driven' adolescents he saw an attitude of punishment,
the fear of punishment and the experience of punishment as the
cause rather than the cure of delinquency.

Hoare thus stripped himself of all authority other than that of his
own personality. He believed in the value of adult participation in
the community but only if the adult was capable of remaining an
individual with experience and with more mature spiritual values
without assuming any rights of authority. Above all such a person
had to be true to himself if he was to have any effect on others:

It seems to me that boys and girls need real live grown-ups living
among them, need their help and guidance, need them to be real and
live, and above all *to be themselves*, if they are in any way the right
people to live among them. And so I would say, by all means find a
person who is a real person, a personality, and let him be himself, as big
as his personality, as strong as his personality, but do not let him try to
be artificially bigger or stronger, to rely for discipline or control on
adventitious or external aids, on the prerogatives of seniority, or its
physical or emotional strength, or its worldly wisdom, or an assumed
character, or on institutions or machinery or penal systems. Let him
meet the boys and girls frankly on their own ground, where they can
cope with him, understand him, trust and love him.[26]

Although Sysonby lasted only a few years and Hoare's direct
influence on subsequent developments is not great he was the chief
among idealists and individualists and as such his extreme attitude
is worth examining in some detail as the epitome of an approach
which was fundamental to many subsequent pioneers. His views on

those personal qualities necessary to do effective work with the disturbed are particularly relevant, not less so today.

Self-awareness was crucial. This was to be awareness not only of one's intrinsic personality but also of one's weakness in being an adult. Hoare considered adults to be wedded to mediocrity, limited by conventions and by rules and regulations which became protectively absolute. Sentimentality in adults he thought was derived from the need to protect themselves against reality and the desire to project their needs on to the young. He instanced the failure in adults to recognize the sexuality implicit in their relations with adolescents. 'To hear some of us talk you would think that the adolescent monopolized emotional instability!' A combination of adult emotional need and lack of awareness he saw resulting in incessant appeals to the emotions as disciplinary measures — 'sudden gratification or sudden humiliation; coaxing turned to sudden anger; righteous indignation born in pride; and all the reactions upon ourselves of emotional mastery, as subtle and as horrible as the reactions upon those who punish. And through them all runs the attempt of emotion to evoke responses, not of conduct but of answering emotion, analogous to that which turns little children into toys for ourselves; the profound and hidden egoism of affection trying to evoke affection. Do you know that terrible answer in Meredith's *Egoist*? "Sir Willoughby is really fond of the boy," said she. "He is fond of exciting fondness in the boy." '[27]

Nevertheless, given self-awareness, Hoare attaches primary importance to 'love'. By this he does not mean emotional projection nor 'a sort of general goodwill all round'.[28] He defines love largely in terms of what it is not. It is not a magical panacea which once given is immediately effective. It never bargains, threatens or bribes. It is unaffected by behaviour, whether good or bad. It does not 'alter when it alteration finds'. The strength of love lies not in smoothing things over, in getting passionately involved, but in 'standing by'. Love is 'watchful, understanding, caring, ready, patient. To smooth over is often far easier, but it is not always love; real love, with all its tenderness is one of the sterner virtues'.[29]

As well as the capacity to love, without which one is incapable of helping, Hoare seeks certain other desirable personal characteristics. The capacity to be happy and to generate happiness is essential not only to therapy but to withstanding the stress of living with the disturbed. The ability to enter into the spirit of play, even if it is play of which one disapproves, will rob the play of violence and malice and release tension.

It is, nevertheless, seen as a grievous mistake to appear morally neutral. Hoare attaches great importance to spiritual sensitivity, responsiveness and pliability. By this he does not mean moral dogmatism but a spiritual power expressed in human terms of life and liveliness. He was essentially a humanist.

Hoare's insistence on the child's need of 'space, every sort of space, acreage, time, freedom from repressions, spiritual space', makes any description of static organizational framework at Sysonby impossible. All that one can say is that Hoare lived with a small community of adolescent delinquents at Riverside Village. The colony was concerned with agricultural and domestic work and not with formal education and it existed without compulsion or structure. Hoare considered that every child should be faced constantly with the need to choose and to control his own life. In this way self-knowledge and self-treatment were to be attained. Burt, who stayed for some time at Sysonby, was much impressed by this philosophy, particularly for what he called the 'unrepressed type'. The aggressive child Burt saw as one reacting against restraint who if the restraint were removed would respond initially by violent behaviour. Given freedom the burden of the irresponsible child would be lightened and success in personal adjustment could be anticipated. The adolescent would be guided 'not by authority or rules, but by his own discovery of what is possible and what is not'. The skill lay in avoiding conflict, in asking for nothing which could not be given, in avoiding emotional encounters, in isolating the child from others and in offering him tenderness and support.[30]

Self-discipline through self-awareness Burt thought to be best suited to the needs of the intelligent delinquent, but the best example he gives of its operation at Sysonby is in fact with a dull, apathetic, fifteen-year-old who had perpetually truanted, had been unable to hold down a job, and who had been sent to Sysonby after 'a sexual misdemeanour of a peculiarly senseless kind'.

Jim was at first happy at Sysonby but since there were only two girls there at the time he began to pay attention to two village dairy-maids. Although this was violently resented in the community, Hoare encouraged Jim to invite his rustic girlfriends to tea. In this situation they were so outshone by the resident girls with their metropolitan sophistication and experience that Jim saw the error of his ways and abandoned them. Harmony was restored to the community. Jim, however, had not worked through his difficulties. 'Three days later . . . he resolved to end his grief and heartache by swallowing ink and paraffin. True to the traditions of all disconsolate lovers, the would-be suicide left a letter behind him to explain his fate. He was suffered to consume as much oil and ink as he desired, and the superintendent and myself sat up all night watching his irresolute attempts to drown himself in the stream that ran hard by. We knew, of course, that the first touch of cold water would awake yet another instinct—fear and self-preservation; and so it proved.' This proved to be a turning point in Jim's career. He subsequently turned to gardening and left to become a competent railway porter.[31]

Another aspect of the work at Sysonby which Burt thought effective was the use made of the stable and placid rural background to settle the unsettled. 'The most stable surroundings, both physical and social, are the best for the unstable child.' He admits, however, that the repressed, nervous or sensitive child might be insufficiently stimulated.

Play, too, was important. Sixteen-year-olds arrived at Sysonby unable to play and rapidly regressed to 'babyish buffoonery more appropriate to a child of six, hiding and seeking in the attics and the cellars, parading about with paper helmets and wooden swords, digging smugglers' caves in the garden, or, when all invention failed, merely rushing in frenzy up and down the farmyard shouting vociferously, like infants that have just discovered they can run and scream'.[32]

Sometimes the uncontrolled play went beyond paper helmets and wooden swords in working out aggression. One of the girls wrote to Burt from Sysonby complaining.

I am sorry to say that the boys have been behaving most disgracefully what with smashing doors, windows, crockery etc. we don't know what to do about it there isn't a sound window in the house and they don't seem to realize what they are doing. It seems to me that if there was someone more stricter down here they would not go on like they do — they have every pleasure they want and could wish for nothing better they seem to take advantage because people are easy and I must say they are far *too* easy with us altogether. We would give anything for them to settle down and make this place their future home. . . .[33]

The moderating influence of the girls, which this suggests, was seldom as effective as that at the Little Commonwealth, although another correspondent claims that 'girls have a lot of influence over boys though they are stronger than us'. Indeed, Hoare attributes the failure of the experiment partly to his inability, in a society which was more dynamic and with a more changing population than the Little Commonwealth, to obtain properly balanced groups of boys and girls. Effective coeducation he saw as a prerequisite of a therapeutic community and of the development of the individual. 'After all, sex is perhaps the chief preoccupation of the human mind, certainly of the adolescent mind, and it is only by meeting the other sex on all the fields of life, work, recreation and above all the formation of opinion and rule, that the preoccupation can be diffused and dispelled.'[34]

The chaos and destruction which Burt's correspondents describe —difficulty in coping with an unequal balance of sexes, the changing population, the wide range of difficult cases, including many children who were not intelligent enough to respond to the demands of self-cure—all added to Hoare's difficulties and the doubts of his supporters. Even largely Quaker committees, dominated as they tend to be by middle-class, intellectual 'progressives' from secure backgrounds and private schools, could not tolerate such a complete rejection of society as that expressed by Sysonby's shattered windows or Hoare's desire to produce rebels. Hoare is very critical of 'outward results' expected by committees and of miraculous results anticipated by 'pacifists with the committee mind who do their work by proxy'. Support was withdrawn and funds ran out and Sysonby did not survive the war.

It is impossible to assess Hoare's contribution to therapeutic care. There have been many others who have tried to work in his manner; most, like Hoare himself, have failed. Society has not been able to tolerate the threat to its essential order long enough to allow experiments to continue to the conclusion which their originators anticipated. Sysonby was the first in a succession of apparent failures which have included the Hawkspur Camp, Chaigeley in its original form, Arlesford Place and many similar experiments in the exercise of freedom which have disappeared without trace. Sysonby was perhaps the purest form. The work, based on personal sensitivity and individual skill, cannot be generalized from.

Hoare himself thought that no one who had not had the experience could assess its effect. Only by knowing the individuals concerned, their violence and despair, their backgrounds and their experiences could one evaluate the changes wrought. Many of Hoare's charges returned to crime and were considered failures by society. Hoare looked to 'inward changes', increased self-awareness and rejecting attitudes to unjust society for his justification.

Society in the outside world may never be fit to receive those who have been made aware of its reality. With a certain logic Hoare eventually joined a closed Roman Catholic order.

7

Homer Lane as Archetype

The aim of the Little Commonwealth was to make useful and happy boys and girls. The aim of life to Mr Lane was enjoyed service.[35]

The chief difficulty in writing about 'the ever memorable work of Mr Lane at the Little Commonwealth' is that Lane wrote little about himself and, in his recorded conversations, frequently found it irrelevant to tell the literal rather than the literary truth. He 'was the greatest man thrown up by the [progressive education] movement on the side of personal relationships, though unfortunately he is the least articulate'.[36] Comparatively little has been written about him and what has been written is frequently highly coloured by the author's personal contact with, and fascination by, Lane.

David Wills, his most detached biographer, although one who admits a great debt to his inspiration and example, said of Lane 'He always said to his English friends that he had the greatest difficulty in expressing himself in writing', and in conversation 'he was capable of adding verisimilitude to an argument by referring to the possible as if it were the actual'.[37] Wills cites Lane's autobiographical inventions which have been repeated as real by other biographers (close enough to Lane to be dazzled). These included, among other things, a most eventful childhood during which Lane lived with North American Indians, worked in a lumber camp and grew up on a West Indian sugar plantation. One such fascinated admirer, C. H. C. Osborne, wrote: 'He thought more of the impression he was making on his hearer's mind than of a carefully guarded and balanced statement of ideas. His language was racy; he exaggerated the half-truth he wanted to impress on you and spoke in paradoxes; what he was saying was often more true symbolically for the person to whom he was speaking than a logical truth which was meant for all.'[38]

Similarly it is difficult for us to form any balanced idea of Lane's personality, since no one in direct contact with him seemed able to do so. His chief eulogist, Lord Lytton, wrote of him as 'a man who was so simple that only children could understand him, so good his worth was more apparent to the foolish than to the wise, so generous that no one could injure him, so modest that no one could praise him, so happy that nothing could depress him, so great that no one could for long feel small in his presence'.[39] The classical cadences and the panegyric style continue in Lytton's 1934 tribute *New Treasure,* a much edited compilation of some of Lane's semi-mystical writings, and are an echo of many similar tributes such as that of Miss Bazeley, Lane's biographer and co-worker at the Little Commonwealth: 'Homer Lane was one who expanded humanity for all who knew him. He pushed back the limits of personality.'[40] She describes him as a man of humanity and warmth, of great spirit and integrity, unpredictably reckless and humorous, unself-consciously friendly, powerfully persistent and with an inexhaustible capacity for making people happy. 'As I turn to reflect on Homer Lane's later work, the picture comes before me of a child of twelve, racing along the pavement of Gordon Square after a talk with Mr Lane, crying "Oh, I'm so happy!"'

What this 'simple, perplexing, humble, vain, wise, foolish, tarnished, innocent, happy and tragic man'[41] was actually like is of little importance, even if the apparently essential paradoxes could ever be resolved, compared with the feelings he inspired in other people. It may well be true, as Wills says, that 'Lane was deeply—perhaps passionately—interested in the unhappy and unstable because he, himself, experienced deep emotional conflicts, and was himself an unstable person. He could help them because he could see himself in them',[42] but to those in close contact with him this weakness was transformed into strength. 'Mr Lane gave them happiness and power. He made them trust in themselves and in their own impulses, and thus released for each one huge stores of energy; by sheer force of his own good will and sunny disposition he redirected those energies, once set free, to constructive and altruistic ends.[43]

How far Lane's personality was essential to the success of his experiment, or his system, is of crucial importance for, as Lord Lytton pointed out, to say that the Little Commonwealth was a unique institution run by a unique person is, in one important sense, a condemnation of the institution and the system. Homer Lane believed that to praise him was 'condemnation of the principles in which he believed, the stamp of failure on the work of his life'. It

D

was largely their trust in him as an inimitable genius that led the committee to close the Little Commonwealth in 1918. Lane was not the founder of the Little Commonwealth, nor the first director appointed.

Mr Lane's association with it was quite fortuitous, it could have been established without him, its principles could be applied today with equal success to every reformatory in the world. . . . The results which excited the wonder of puzzled admirers were to Lane but the natural and inevitable consequence of the application of sound principles. He never had the slightest doubt what the consequences would be, provided that he acted according to those principles which the experience of his life had taught him to be infallible, and it was the tragedy of his life that to the end men never said of him 'What admirable principles, let us adopt them' but always 'What a marvellous man, he is inimitable'.[44]

Although Lane was not captured by Indians or brought up in a lumber camp, his life was not without incident. The best short account, replete with legends, is in the introduction which Albert David, Bishop of Liverpool (a former 'client' of Lane's in his analytical period, and a former member of the committee of the Little Commonwealth) wrote to *Talks to Parents and Teachers*, a collection of Lane's lectures and notes published posthumously.[45] The following summary is, however, taken largely from David Wills's more comprehensive and less 'rose-tinted' biography.

Lane came from vigorous New England Puritan stock. His father was a railway worker and Homer had an elder and a younger brother, and a sister for whose death at the age of two he felt partly responsible. At school he was known as a rebel, but his home life, although puritanical, seems to have been good and adequate. He became a grocer's roundsman, married early, and reached an important turning point when Dr Claude Jones (later to be his successor at the Ford Republic) encouraged him to take a course of 'Sloyd' in Boston with a view to teaching. During this period he attended lectures by John Dewey, then teaching at Harvard.

He started a part-time Sloyd school in Southborough after a short period as a vacation teacher of woodwork at the Pennsylvania State Reformatory in Huntingdon. This is where he 'first learnt that the reform school made a bad boy worse'. The Sloyd school, although successful, was short lived, and Lane moved to Detroit where he became a master at the Duffield school, in which he tried to intro- duce his principles of self-government. He was then made superintendent of playgrounds, where he profited by observing the toughest children 'acting out'. At this time he claimed to be influenced by Montessori.

Being blackmailed into resigning this post he took charge of the Solvey Guild—'a kind of settlement house'—moving from here to become a woodwork teacher at the Hannah Schloss Settlement and founding within it several self-governing clubs for the most deprived boys in the neighbourhood. This led to an interest in the Boys' Home and d'Arcampbell Association, which was later to move out into the country as the Ford Republic (named after its chief benefactor), which still exists as the Boys' Republic.

As we have seen in previous chapters, the idea of a community for delinquent, deprived and disturbed children with a degree of independence, a family structure and, sometimes, some form of self-government was not entirely new.

Early reformatory schools in England and Germany, the *colonies penitentiares* in France and the House of Refuge and farm schools in the United States had, almost inevitably in the prevailing ethos, assumed that firm but kindly adult guidance was necessary for moral regeneration. Many, however, like the Rauhe Haus, Dr Stephenson's early children's homes and Mrs Nassau Senior's cottage-homes were organized on a family basis (not unlike that of the Little Commonwealth), in which 'every child as it advances in age, and becomes fitted for the work, takes a part in the management of the household, and in the care and training of younger children'[46] and in which the aim was to 'live together as a family of brethren, cheerful, happy, confiding and, I trust, to a greater or less degree pious'.[47]

This latter description was of the South Boston Reform School (1826) which was followed by many other experiments such as that of the Children's Village, Dobb's Ferry (1855) from which the Ford Republic and later the Little Commonwealth could be thought to have evolved. The most obvious progenitor was 'Daddy' George's Junior Republic at Freeville (1890), with its elaborate structure of 'self-government' and the full paraphernalia of constitution, courts, police, prisons and punishments, many of which were in fact found in the early structure of the Ford Republic—although Lane claimed not to have heard of George until after the Ford Republic was founded.[48] Lane, indeed, appears to have had little knowledge of previous experiments and little contact with existing ones. It is probable that the Ford Republic evolved largely out of Lane's own experience and in terms of his own personality. Like 'Daddy' George's Republic, however, it had a Constitution based closely on that of the United States and although it was more genuinely self-governing its structure was not a spontaneous creation and was, in fact, controlled by a certain amount of authoritarianism and corporal punishment. Nor, at this stage, did Lane see any conflict between his love of a boy and his willingness to 'swipe' him—the term is Lane's—to retain control. Apart from the experience of sharing responsibility, the therapy was largely that of hard manual labour in which Lane was always ready to share. The effectiveness of the Ford Republic was limited by the fact that the dilapidated farm at Clarenceville was used primarily as a remand home and had, therefore, a constantly changing population. Nor did Lane wish to retain the boys in the way he sought to retain the children at the Little Commonwealth.[49] 'I do not want any of the boys to feel at home here. Their home is with their parents. . . . We want the boys always to feel in a hurry to try their new found moral strength in their own family.'[50]

Nevertheless, despite limitations, 'self-government at the Ford Republic was real and dynamic and not merely an ornamental facade erected by the adults.' It was extended into all branches of activity, and here, too, Lane worked out his system of 'economic discipline'.

Life was frequently chaotic and finances confused but Lane continued to inspire confidence and enthusiasm until he admitted to an adulterous relationship with a teacher/secretary and went to work in Buffalo as a navvy. While there he seems to have done a good deal of thinking and possibly reading.

In 1913, at the age of thirty-seven, Lane came to England at the invitation of George Montagu—later Lord Sandwich—to advise on the foundation of a Republic similar to his own or 'Daddy' George's at Freeville. He was not intended to be the first superintendent but became so when the original superintendent, Harold Large, became ill and resigned his appointment.

Lane began his work on a 200-acre farm site with extensive buildings in Dorset (provided rent-free by Lord Sandwich), with some powerful support from a committee which included Lord Grey, the Duchess of Marlborough, Cecil Chapman (a London magistrate), Beresford Melville, chairman of the Montessori Society, and T. Mott-Osborne, chairman of the Prison Reform Commission of New York State. This committee never lost faith in Lane.

The Little Commonwealth was a home for post-school-age adolescents referred either by the courts or by their own parents. There were also some small children placed, as an experiment, by the Montessori Society. The Little Commonwealth was run by Lane on lines similar to, but more liberal than, the Ford Republic and, although co-educational, it was eventually recognized by the Home Office. The withdrawal of Home Office support in 1917, after allegations of sexual impropriety made against Lane by two of the girls, meant that the Little Commonwealth could no longer support itself and it was closed in 1918.

During this latter period Lane came much under the influence of Freud and experimented in a rather amateurish and modified way with the psychoanalysis of some of the girls. One of them wrote to Miss Bazeley: 'Did you know that Mr Lane was a sikeonalies he is taking me ethel carrie and clara for lessions and he does it beautiful ... it is grand being sikeonaniquize.' This led naturally, as Lane acknowledged at length in the paper which he read to the Little Commonwealth Committee after the Rawlinson Enquiry (June 22, 1918), to a transference not to the Little Commonwealth but to himself. 'I sought to secure transference from their own parents direct to their community without any intermediary in myself. ... The events of the last six months have convinced me of the futility of trying to cut psychological corners in educational schemes. I now gladly abandon my beautiful scheme after five years of faithful adherence to it. Mr Rawlinson has completely dissolved my complex.'

Mr Rawlinson was the agent for dissolving not only Lane's complex but also his job. With the collapse of the Little Commonwealth, Lane was established in practice as a psychotherapist of neo-Freudian persuasion (he later discovered Jung), and had many influential clients. He was again destroyed by his handling of the transference situation and the personal contact he maintained with his women patients. He was tried on a technical charge of failing to register as an alien and agreed to go into voluntary exile, in which he died on 5 September 1925. The epitaph by which he is best remembered is that supplied by W. H. Auden, one of his admirers:

Lawrence was brought down by the smuthounds
Blake went dotty as he sang,
Homer Lane was killed in action
By the Twickenham Baptist gang.[51]

It is ironic, and typical of him in many ways, that in the year of his death Homer Lane said, 'The only difference between Jesus Christ and me is that I know how to avoid being crucified.'

After his death, however, his principles, his system, his inspiration and his enigma lived on.

EDUCATIONAL PRINCIPLES

Exactly what Lane's principles as an educationalist were it is difficult to say, for although he was constantly talking about them they were as constantly changing. He was a pragmatist working largely through intuition, but in the course of his varied career he came into contact with many theoretical approaches and, in a pragmatic manner, put them to his own use.

Through 'Sloyd' he absorbed the theories of Uno Cygnaeus with their emphasis on the educational benefits of craftsmanship and manual labour in encouraging independence and self-reliance, appreciation and taste, attention and perseverance. Miss Bazeley said that 'The inventive and masterly doing of things in the workshop and in the open air, exact things with exact and rich results, seemed to me to be the noblest accompaniment, and in the major key, to the profound music of his work with human souls.'[52] Baroness Stocks, who visited the Little Commonwealth and was largely unimpressed by either Lane's personality or his emphasis on self-government, considered that a lot of the undoubted value of the work which he did lay in his ability to communicate his own impeccable sense of craftsmanship.[53]

At the same time that he was studying 'Sloyd' he also heard Dewey speak and, although he did not acknowledge it, it seems possible that his emphasis on democratic processes owed something to Dewey. Certainly his teaching theory had a Deweyite ring: 'The teacher who governs her room through fear of punishment is one of the most potent contributory influences which make for boy antagonism towards modern society. She may teach method and accuracy through arithmetic, expression of thought and self through spelling and reading, but she cannot teach social consciousness through history and geography—the advantage of a republican over a monarchial [sic] system unless her schoolroom is a republic and not a monarchy.'[54] Self-respect through self-government was one of Lane's two invariant principles.

His reputation as a follower of Montessori gains support from the use of her methods with the junior children at the Commonwealth, but as Wills suggests, it is probable that Lane owes his greatest unacknowledged debt to Pestalozzi, who said: 'The Artist who is a genius does not work to rules. He creates something of great beauty, and lesser men derive their rules from a study of the master.' Pestalozzi worked in similar circumstances and put a similar emphasis on skill, and through him Lane was brought to realize the supreme importance of his second invariant principle—the central importance of love and care. 'I know of no order, no method, which did not rest upon the children's conviction of my love for them. I did not care to know any other,' (Pestalozzi) is very like 'Love is the highest form of compulsion known to man, and hope is the only true discipline' (Lane).

The origin of Homer Lane's philosophy appears to be basically Rousseauan in its emphasis on innate good, individual freedom, the reality of social evil, etc., although it was not entirely so. Lane was fundamentally an individualist inspired by a comprehensive hatred of society as it was constituted. To him, not only were the citizens of the Little Commonwealth essentially good but so were their delinquent acts when they were directed at the corrupt society without. The Commonwealth, based on love and co-operation, was Utopian in the sense of being an example to all society; an example which Lane hoped would be followed.

Similarly with education. Despite several attempts, some demand from the inhabitants, and a certain amount of lip-service from Lane, there was never any systematic education in the sense of the learning of academic skills. This, although Lane did not present the argument, was logical and consistent. Formal education was largely the product of the society which Lane hated and rejected, and it was designed to fulfil its ends. Fundamentally Lane expected the citizens also to reject that society, and he wished to prepare citizens for a life which did not exist outside the Commonwealth. Such education as there was within the Commonwealth was directed to this end. During the day the citizens learnt, in a practical way, the skills of husbandry, gardening, cooking, laundering, mechanics or shopkeeping in the process of preserving the Commonwealth's existence. When they were not thus involved they seem largely to have listened to Lane philosophizing, 'psychologizing' or, perhaps, reminiscing. Although he did not rationalize about the process it is possible to see it as a perfectly valid preparation for a society that had, to a great extent, ceased to exist outside the Commonwealth. That it had ceased to exist was largely irrelevant since Lane increasingly saw the Commonwealth as a community of adults and children growing up together in a predominantly alien world. The basic principle appears not unlike that of Dewey. In the rural Arcadia adults and children grew up together, profiting from experience, learning techniques only for use—arithmetic for housekeeping or measuring planks for floors, craft for building, mechanics for repairing machines, botany or chemistry for gardening or agriculture. To Dewey this was essential experience to prepare children as citizens of a world which lacked this natural educational process. To Lane it was valuable, not in itself, but to the community which it served and in whose service Lane thought many of its citizens would remain.

PSYCHOLOGICAL PRINCIPLES

The psychological basis of the Little Commonwealth was even less well defined. Lane thought of himself originally as a Freudian and attempted analysis on some of the citizens, but no one was less temperamentally suited to be an analyst in the classical Freudian sense. As Neill says, Lane was a man of brilliant insights, but he wished always to take an active, indeed the major, role in the process. For Lane transference and counter-transference were not symbolic relationships but actual ones. If the Little Commonwealth was a therapeutic establishment it was not its pseudo-Freudian base which made it so, but rather its sociological structure.

Nevertheless, this was the light by which Lane worked, and although all the parts are borrowed the mechanics, however faulty, were Lane's and deserve consideration.

'During the five years in which he has been in charge of it [The Little Commonwealth] he has made a reputation throughout the educational world as a profound student of the psychology of children and as a leading exponent of the newest ideas and methods in education.'[55] But 'newest ideas' were frequently, as Wills puts it, 'no more than an elaboration and "Freudification" of his long-held idea—expressed before he had ever heard of Freud—that "A bad boy is an example of good qualities wrongly directed"'. Most of his *Talks to Parents and Teachers*[56] were similar 'Freudifications'.

'In the infant I found my clue to the mystery of crime and failure. Even the infant was denied freedom to his self. His very first sense consciousness was perverted through interference.' (A sentiment almost exactly repeated later by Lane's 'pupil', A. S. Neill.) The enjoyment of unhappiness 'will be prevented for any child who is allowed, as the instinctive desires unfold from the "unconscious", to grow up and not to be brought up. Morality is spontaneous.'[57] He emphasized innate goodness, creative freedom, the harm done by the inculcation of conscience.

'The problem of the reformatory school is to resolve these problems which come from the unconscious mind; for crime is fixed energy left over from an earlier period of childhood ... the cause of every purposeful wrong act can be traced to its source by careful analysis and I have found that almost all delinquent children will resolve their own difficulties in an atmosphere of freedom and encouragement. Occasionally special help is required and special knowledge.'[58] This was the principle that took the D'Arcampbell Association to the Ford Republic and which is one of the bases on which most subsequent schools for the maladjusted have been built.

It is of particular interest that in Lane's, in some ways unfortunate, 'apologia' to the Little Commonwealth committee in 1918, he asserts that the organization, education and therapy of the Little Commonwealth were all subordinate to, or dependent upon, its psychoanalytical base. 'Does your boy hate arithmetic? He can be made to love it by analytical pedagogy. Is he rude and ungracious? It is conflict easily removable. Is he purposely annoying? He is suffering from an inferiority complex. His libido can be detached from its unwholesome goal. Does he bite his nails? Fidget in his chair? ...'[59] and so on. Such naive faith in psychoanalysis as an educational panacea is less important than his explanation of his much-vaunted system of self-government—thought by many to be the essential core of his work—as a device for dealing with the problems of 'transference'.

I have always ... felt a strong distaste for the responsibilities involved in making known to my pupil's conscious minds the fact of the transference of their libido to me as the 'nearest parent'. I knew that this transference was inevitable but I shrank from the responsibilities entailed by their consciousness of it. I devised a method of avoiding that responsibility that ... I sincerely believed in. The method was this: by allowing my pupils to create a community of their own, frame their own laws, administer their own courts, they being independent of their own parents' assistance through the wages scheme of the Commonwealth, I sought to secure transference from their own parents direct to the community without any intermediary in myself.... I felt that by making myself a member of the community on equal terms with themselves, that whatever transfer was made to me personally, would be in their conscious minds an added love for the community.... I hoped that the absence of adult and dogmatic moral authority would result in a minimizing of unconscious conflicts in the individual, and that the libido of each citizen would become firmly attached to the vocational, social and spiritual interests of the Commonwealth.[60]

This ingenuous rationalization of the principles underlying the Little Commonwealth was, probably properly, ignored by Lord Lytton when he summarized what he considered to be Lane's universally applicable legacy of principle. He saw this as fourfold:

'First and foremost was the law of love. Lane genuinely believed that you can cure whatever you can love.

'The second great principle—that of freedom.... The freedom which existed in the Commonwealth was not the absolute freedom which is found only in the minds of poets and of anarchists, but the limited freedom both of the individual and of the community to make mistakes, to test for themselves the value of every law and the necessity for every restraint imposed upon them.

'The third important principle which characterized the Little Commonwealth was the principle of self-government . . . at the Little Commonwealth there was no authority to defy except the authority of the whole community.'

The fourth principle (still strongly resisted by authority) was that of coeducation. 'Lane himself would certainly have maintained that the presence of each sex was necessary to the re-education or normal development of the other.'[61]

STRUCTURE OF THE LITTLE COMMONWEALTH

The structure through which these principles were expressed at the Little Commonwealth is most simply stated in a lecture given by Lane in 1918.

The Little Commonwealth is a co-educational community inhabited by children ranging in age from a few months to nineteen years, those

of more than thirteen years of age having been committed for a term
of years for crime – as to a reformatory. . . . The younger children are
those who would in any case be subject to institutional care in asylums
and orphanages. . . . The population of the Commonwealth is five
adults, four of whom are women, forty-two boys and girls of fourteen to nineteen years of age, and nine younger children. This
population is distributed among three 'families' grouped by congeni-
ality. . . . Boys and girls live in the same families, sharing equally in the
responsibility for the welfare of the younger children. The chief point
of difference between the Commonwealth and other reformatories and
schools is that in the Commonwealth there are no rules and regulations
except those made by the boys and girls themselves. All those who are
fourteen years or over are citizens having joint responsibility for the
regulation of their lives by the laws and judicial machinery organized
and developed by themselves. The adult element studiously avoid
any assumption of authority in the community except in connection
with their respective departmental duties as teachers or as supervisors
of labour within the economic scheme.[62]

'The economic scheme' was considered to be the basis of public
morality since the basic punishment was to be unemployed and thus
to become a burden on one's family. A Special Correspondent to the
Times Educational Supplement in 1914 described the working of
the scheme – which had also been basic to the Ford Republic – thus :

We are free to work or loaf as we choose. Our work is paid for in a
currency of our own, equal in value to the coin of the realm, at the
rate of threepence an hour. The diligent citizen earns something over
10s. a week; this pays for his board, food, lodging and clothing, and
leaves him a little sum over which he either spends on luxuries or banks
against his return to the outer world. . . . If the free citizen slacks or
refuses to work at all he gets no wages, and so he cannot pay his way.
But, as he is still supplied with the necessaries of life, somebody has
to pay, and somebody in this case is everybody. He is supported, like
the unemployed without, by the rates and taxes. But not for long. The
rest of the community, who are mulcted of their spare earnings to pay
his weekly bill, soon let him know that he is not behaving as a citizen
should, and in the short history of the Commonwealth the pressure of
public opinion has never yet failed to produce the desired effect.[63]

If the economic scheme was the basis of public morality the
Citizen's Court was its mouthpiece.

'It is in the Citizen's Court that one may get into closer touch
with the spirit of the Commonwealth than in any other community

function and it is here that I look for the true spiritual expressions of our boys and girls.'[64] The court had an elected judge and other officials and included all those over fourteen years of age. Lane considered that below this age they had not yet reached that 'age of loyalty' which gave them discretion and discernment. The court's ostensible function was to hear complaints about work or conduct, discuss some aspects of policy, and award punishment. Lane, however, was not alone in considering it one of the main agencies of therapy in the community through which self-analysis through group criticism of one another would become automatic.

A less dramatic and publicized agency at work in the Little Commonwealth was the family unit. In the three cottages—Bramble, Veronica and Heather (for the little ones)—the members of the Little Commonwealth enjoyed what for most of them was their only experience of stable family life. This was the basis of social training in living together without undue conflict and having a very real responsibility for one another. It was to this family life that Miss Bazeley attributed the vitality of public opinion which was the life-blood of the citizen's court and the origin of that social competence which invariably impressed visitors. It was within these groups, mixed in age, ability and, of course, sex, that the members experienced the giving and receiving of affection. It was here that they came in closest contact with Lane's warm, loving and ebullient personality which was the key to the whole enterprise. Girls who grew up in the Commonwealth stayed on as housemothers and helped others to share their own love of, and confidence in, life. Despite spasmodic attempts to organize formal lessons and church services most of the education and religious instruction which the members received was acquired casually in the evening family meetings—the girls usually with Lane, the boys with Mrs Lane or Miss Bazeley. The latter draws several charming vignettes of these evening meetings, with Lane reading, writing or talking about his largely apochryphal past, or of religion, or of psychology, and the girls learning shorthand, playing the gramophone, reading, sewing or quarrelling. 'We were just a circle of friends gathered round the same lamp and the same fire.'[65]

It is probable that for most of these deprived children this was all the therapy which was needed and even those who were most seriously disturbed appear to have been 're-made' more by identification with their families than by any other agency.

'They had to be taken to pieces by the searching group analysis of the family and community life, to be reassembled into a new and happier being by the healing power of the discovery of personal resource and ability and of personal responsibility to the community.'[66]

Most of the citizens of the Commonwealth were deprived and delinquent. 'Some of them have known the insides of prisons and reformatories; all of them have made the acquaintance of Mr Bumble and the police, and, to speak generally, they have the kind of fingers that would have ensured them ready admission to the school of Fagin the Jew.'[67] Many were clearly very disturbed and some, in fact, came from materially comfortable homes. One such, whom Miss Bazeley calls Leonard, was sent to the Little Commonwealth by his over-anxious and over-protective, but perhaps not over-loving, stepmother. He stole first from his father's pockets, later from missionary boxes. Lane, curiously, attributed this to a desire for power and considered that Leonard's rapid adjustment at the Commonwealth was because he acquired independence. It is, I think, reasonable to speculate that he found in his 'family' more real love than in the company of his stepmother and stepsisters, and no longer felt the need for symbolic gestures of stealing.

Another disturbed citizen was Edmund, a liar and a thief, with a Cockney stepfather from whom he stole. He was so irresponsible and shiftless that he could seldom be employed on the Commonwealth farm, was clothed in rags and was a constant embarrassment to his 'family'. He improved, but after making himself more acceptable to the Bramble household he began absconding. With much encouragement from his 'family' he eventually managed to keep a regular job and with the first 19s 6d which he saved he bought a new suit to wear for his mother's impending visit.

Then a family crisis occurred in Bramble. Several of the newer citizens had been doing badly, and had not earned enough to pay their share of the weekly bills. Bramble's credit in the shop had been stopped and all the food in the house had been finished at breakfast. The older members of the family, who were earning good wages, put their resources to helping the weaker ones to pay their share of the family bills. Edmund had no savings to give, as he had only recently bought his suit. In spite of everybody's struggles, there was still a deficit of 13s. 6d., Chicken's unpaid share of the bill. Chicken was an unmannerly boy at that time, who had made himself disagreeable to most people, and perhaps more especially so to Edmund. Chicken, knowing that he had no money to pay his bills and that no one would be likely to wish to help him, had run away early that morning onto the Downs. The situation became desperate. If Bramble family was unable to pay its way, it would cease to be a Commonwealth family and would become a reformatory house, supported by the Committee, and with rigid institution rules made by the Superintendent.

Without saying a word to anybody, Edmund fetched his new suit, went to the shop with it, said he wanted to give it back, got 13s. 6d. for it, returned across the courtyard to his house-mother and presented her with the sum for Chicken's dues. The family was saved. Long after supper was over, Chicken crept in and up the stairs to the boys' landing to go to bed. To his amazement he found that the score against him had been completely wiped off, that he no longer had to face old troubles, that it was, in a sense, a new family which had re-admitted him, without comment, and in a friendly fashion, to its circle.[68]

This is, one feels, how the Little Commonwealth really worked.

INFLUENCE

Although, as has been shown earlier, both Lord Lytton and Homer Lane himself considered that the principles of the Little Commonwealth could be successfully applied to all schools and reformatories, the former claims that the Commonwealth 'failed only in establishing the general applicability of the principles on which it was conducted ... it was, throughout its existence, and it still remains in the minds of many who knew it, a freak institution associated with the influence of a unique personality'.[69]

It is true that few, if any, institutions have had Lane's principles applied *in toto* but the fact that they have not been applied does not mean that they are not applicable. There have been many successful attempts at partial application both in situations comparable with Lane's own, particularly in residential schools for maladjusted adolescents, and also in normal 'progressive' schools which have traditionally provided a tolerant and congenial environment for 'problem children'. Indeed Boyd and Rawson attribute the idea of what eventually developed into 'the New Education Fellowship' to Mrs Ensor's 'reading of Edmond Holmes's book *What is and What Might Be* and of Homer Lane's *Little Commonwealth*' in 1915.[70] Although Lane wrote no such book it is certainly true that

he was associated with the Fraternity in Education from its inception and lectured at its conferences. Another protagonist of the New
Education—J. H. Badley, headmaster of Bedales—wrote: 'Another
whose work should be mentioned as breaking new ground in this
country is Homer Lane. . . . He showed in the Little Commonwealth
in Dorsetshire . . . what could be done with delinquent children by
sympathy, trust and a system of complete self-government. . . . This
experience of what could be accomplished with delinquents has
shown the far-reaching effect and the value for the young of self-
government in the school under the guidance of one who brought
to the work an understanding of child nature and an inspiring
personality.'[71]

This combination of 'self-government . . . and an inspiring personality' has, perhaps, been the most obvious pattern of subsequent
'pioneer' schools for the maladjusted. Indeed it is largely by virtue
of their application of their own unique personalities that many of
the other leaders can be considered pioneers at all. All took, consciously or unconsciously, with or without acknowledgement, from
Homer Lane, who was not so much a pioneer as the archetypal
figure.

'Group therapy' and 'shared responsibility' are two phrases which
are now cautiously and with a sense of novelty and daring, finding
a place in the vocabulary of those who work in this field (maladjustment), and they are being experimented with as if they were an
invention of our own day. Under other names and without the
encouragement of like-minded colleagues, Lane used these methods
fifty years ago. It has become commonplace to say that offenders
are often people who have been starved in childhood of affection,
and that no healing technique can be successful that does not include
the provision of the affection hitherto denied. This is precisely what
Lane said—and did—at the Little Commonwealth. 'They must
realize,' he said, 'that I am on their side.'[72]

Any Commonwealth meeting was, as Miss Bazeley said, 'an
occasion for searching group analysis' and a prominent modern
exponent of group therapy, Howard Jones, acknowledges this in
writing of his own work at Chaigeley (see Chapter 14). He
recognizes that, directed by Lane's intuitive understanding and
psychological insight, the 'families' as well as the meetings were converted into therapeutic groups.[73] He continues by showing how far
David Wills was influenced by Lane in his own technique of 'shared

responsibility' evolved through spontaneous growth. Wills freely admits his debt and he also, in his first experiment—the Hawkspur Camp—implemented Lane's system of what might be called 'economic morality'.

Even where Wills, and others, disagree with Lane's practice and consider it 'disastrous for the Head of an institution, who is already the centre of a vortex of strong emotions, to practise intensive psychotherapy on the children under his care'[74] there is the apparently successful example of Otto Shaw who, for the past thirty-five years, has been pursuing this policy at Red Hill School (see Chapter 11).

Another pioneer who can, and did, claim direct inspiration from Lane was J. H. Simpson, headmaster of Rendcomb. 'My own acquaintance with the idea of a more truly educative form of self-government dates from a day in September 1913 when I heard Mr Homer Lane describe . . . the Little Commonwealth . . . the most inspiring educational establishment in England. . . . The measure of my personal debt to Mr Lane is incalculable.'[75]

Similar personal tributes could be gathered from a Viceroy of India (Lytton), a Bishop of Liverpool (David), the Reverend Dick Sheppard, W. H. Auden[76] and many other eminent people—but particularly from A. S. Neill, who claims that he was unable to do any really original and successful work until his dependence on Lane was ruptured by Lane's death.

A. S. Neill's first contact with Lane was when a lady in Hampstead who had read the early 'Dominie' books sent him a copy of one of Lane's lectures. When he was in the Army in Wiltshire in 1916 he visited the Little Commonwealth.

That weekend was probably the most important milestone of my life. Lane sat up till the early morning telling me of his cases. I had been groping for some philosophy of education but had no knowledge of psychology. Lane introduced me to Freud. I asked Lane if I could come to work in the Commonwealth after the war and he said he had just been going to ask me to come, but when I was free the Little Commonwealth had been closed by the Home Office.

I owe a great debt to Lane. It was from him that I learnt that unless a teacher could see the child's motives he could not help him to be happy or social. He was a genius although his 'education' was limited. He spoke from his unconscious mostly. He found writing, even a letter, difficult. But with delinquent children he was simply wonderful. I consider it appalling that, since he died in 1925, so far as I can see his great experiment has had no visible influence on the State treatment of delinquent children.[77]

As far as Home Office schools are concerned Neill's pessimistic assessment of Lane's effect has much truth, but in other spheres Lane's optimistic belief that he was contributing something permanent to the science of education—relevant to both normal and disturbed children—is more justified. Wills says, with a conviction born of experience:

In most schools nowadays, and especially in boarding schools, there is a much more free and relaxed atmosphere than perhaps there has ever been. . . . Particularly is this true of special schools for delinquent and maladjusted children. . . . In the new schools for maladjusted children established during the last twenty years or so, free of the disciplinarian traditions of the Home Office schools, Lane's influence is clearly seen. In some cases the debt to Lane is recognized and acknowledged, in some it is present, as it were, second-hand. But no one who knows the best of these schools can fail to see Lane's influence in them.[78, 79]

REFERENCES

CHAPTER 6: Twentieth century originals

1 WILLS, W. D. *Throw Away Thy Rod*, p 18. Gollancz, London, 1960.
2 CRUTCHFIELD, R. Conformity and Character *Am. Psych.* X. 1955.
3 HOVLAND, C. I., JANIS, I. L. and KELLEY, H. H. *Communications and Persuasion*. Yale University Press, New Haven, Conn. 1953.
4 FRANKLIN, M. E. The Work of David Wills, p 23. *A.W.M.C. Newsletter No.* **10**. 1968.
5 MILLER, R. D. *Growth to Freedom*, Tavistock, London, 1964.
6 CALDECOTT NURSERY SCHOOL. First Annual Report. p 3. 1911–12.
7 THE CALDECOTT COMMUNITY. Third Annual Report. p 21. 1913–14.
8 ———— First Annual Report. p 3.
9 WOODS, A. *Educational Experiments in England*, pp 82–9 & 121–4. Methuen, London, 1920.
10 THE CALDECOTT COMMUNITY. Jubilee Fund Appeal, 1961.
11 RENDEL, L. *Child of Misfortune*, The Caldecott Community. 1952.
12 HOME OFFICE. Report of the Care of Children Committee (The Curtis Report). H.M.S.O., London, 1946.
13 'THE CHILDREN'S ACT', 11 & 12 VI, 1948.
14 CHILDREN'S RECEPTION CENTRE—MERSHAM. Interim Report (printed by Headley Bros, Ashford), 1948.
15 LEWIS, H. *Deprived Children*, Oxford University Press, London, 1954.
16 RODWAY, S. Leila Rendel, O.B.E. 1893–1969. *Therapeutic Education*. Autumn, 1969.
17 THE TIMES EDUCATIONAL SUPPLEMENT. 9 November, 1961.
18 THE CALDECOTT COMMUNITY. Third Annual Report. p 20. 1913–14.
19 *The Caldecott Community* (printed by the Swann Press) 1966.
20 STEWART, W. A. C. *The Educational Innovators.* **2**, p 95. Macmillan, London, 1968.
21 KELLMER PRINGLE, M. L. and SUTCLIFFE, B. *Remedial Education—An Experiment*, p 29. Published by the Caldecott Community and the Department of Child Study, University of Birmingham Institute of Education, 1960.
22 Ibid. p 16.
23 Ibid. p 12
24 WOODS, A. op. cit., pp 121–4.

25 HOARE, R. F. Principles of Discipline and Self-Government. An experiment at Riverside Village, *pp* 230–244. Talk given to the Friends Guild of Teachers in Report of the Sixth Annual Conference of Educational Associations, 1918.
26 Ibid. *pp* 241–242.
27 Ibid. *p* 240.
28 cf. WILLS, D. W. *The Barns Experiment, pp* 64–5. Allen & Unwin, London, 1945.
29 cf. LYWARD, G. L. in Chapter 10.
30 BURT, C. *The Young Delinquent* (4th Edition). *pp* 520–2. University of London Press, London, 1944.
31 Ibid. *pp* 325–330.
32 Ibid. *p* 91.
33 Ibid. *p* 615.
34 HOARE, R. F. op cit., *p* 233.

CHAPTER 7: Homer Lane as Archetype

35 BAZELEY, E. T. *Homer Lane and the Little Commonwealth* (introduction by the Earl of Lytton) *p* 139. Allen & Unwin, London, 1928.
36 PERRY, L. R. (ed). *Bertrand Russell, A. S. Neill, Homer Lane, W. H. Kilpatrick. Four Progressive Educators.* Collier-Macmillan, London, 1967.
37 WILLS, W. D. *Homer Lane, a biography, p* 76. Allen & Unwin, London, 1964.
38 Quoted in Wills, ibid. *p* 145.
39 LYTTON, Earl of. Introduction to Bazeley. op. cit.
40 BAZELEY, E. T. op. cit, *p* 142.
41 WILLS, W. D. op. cit., *p* 20.
42 Ibid. *p* 71.
43 BAZELEY, E. T. op. cit., *p* 168–9.
44 LYTTON, Earl of. op. cit., *pp* 12–13.
45 LANE, H. *Talks to Parents and Teachers.* (Introduction by Dr A. A. David). Allen & Unwin, London, 1928.
46 HEYWOOD, H. S. *Children in Care, p* 74. Routledge & Kegan Paul, New York, 1959.
47 CARPENTER, M. *Juvenile Delinquents, p* 212. W. & F. C. Cash, London, 1853.
48 WILLS, W. D. op. cit., *pp* 108–109.
49 *See* Miss Bazeley's account of Lane's conversation with Margaret (Bazeley op. cit, *p* 85).
50 Letter from Lane to Miss Pauline Laddie, July, 1909, quoted in Wills, (op. cit.,) *p* 84.

51 AUDEN, W. H. *Poems* No. XXII. Faber & Faber, London, 1930. (Bazeley op. cit., *p* 85).
52 BAZELEY, E. T. op. cit., *p* 168.
53 PERSONAL COMMUNICATION.
54 WILLS, W. D. op. cit., *p* 87.
55 Report of the Committee on the Closing of the Little Commonwealth, July 1918.
56 LANE, H. op. cit., *p* 116.
57 Ibid. *p* 124.
58 Ibid. *p* 162.
59 ———. Paper read to the Little Commonwealth Committee after the Rawlinson Enquiry, 22 June 1918. *See* Wills, W. D. op. cit., *p* 262.
60 Ibid. *pp* 265–6.
61 LYTTON, Earl of. op. cit., *pp* 13–19.
62 LANE, H. *Talks to Parents and Teachers*. (Ref. 45) *pp* 188–9.
63 SPECIAL CORRESPONDENT. *The Times Educational Supplement*. *p* 6, 6 January 1914.
64 LANE, H. op. cit., *p* 192.
65 BAZELEY, E. T. op. cit., *pp* 59–76.
66 Ibid. *p* 145.
67 SPECIAL CORRESPONDENT (Ref. 63) op. cit.
68 BAZELEY, E. T. op. cit., *pp* 109–114.
69 LYTTON, Earl of. op. cit., *p* 10.
70 BOYD, W. and RAWSON, W. *The Story of the New Education*, *p* 67. Heinemann, London, 1965.
71 BADLEY, J. H. *A Schoolmaster's Testament*, Blackwell, London, 1937.
72 WILLS, W. D. op. cit., p. 19.
73 JONES, H. *Reluctant Rebels*, *p* 21. Tavistock, London, 1960.
74 Ibid. *p* 22.
75 SIMPSON, J. H. *An Adventure in Education*, Sidgwick & Jackson, London, 1917.
76 AUDEN, W. H. and MACNEICE, L. *Letters from Iceland*, *p* 210. Faber & Faber, London, 1937.
77 NEILL, A. S. My Scholastic Life—2. *Id, Journal of Summerhill Society*, October, 1960.
78 WILLS, W. D. op. cit., p. 139.
79 For a less well-known description of Lane, *see*: Doty, M. Z. *Society's Misfits*. *pp* 227–255. Unwin, London, 1914.

PART FOUR

The New Era

8

The New Education

Activity, versatility, imaginative sympathy, a large and free outlook, self-forgetfulness, charm of manner, joy of heart – are there many schools in England in which the soil and atmosphere are favourable to the vigorous growth of all these qualities? I doubt it. – Edmond Holmes: *What Is and What Might Be*, 1911.[1]

For my own part I honour the teachers as a body, if only because here and there one of them has dared, with splendid courage, to defy the despotism of custom, of tradition, of officialdom, of the thousand deadening influences that are brought to bear upon him, and to follow for himself the path of inwardness and life. Ibid. *p*. 147.

The pioneer is abroad in the land. Ibid. *p* 87.

It is as easy to over-estimate the effect of educational philosophers and psychological theorists on the process of education as it is to underestimate the contribution of the schools themselves both to the cause and to the cure of maladjustment in their pupils.[2]

Edmond Holmes, a prematurely 'retired' H.M.I., made neither of these mistakes. While acknowledging the importance of theories derived from the work of Rousseau, Pestalozzi, Froebel, Montessori and others, which gave intellectual support and impetus to the educational experiments which began to flourish in the dynamic climate of the twentieth century, he did not over-value their con-tribution. He looked rather to practical teachers to cure the malaise in English education derived from an over-emphasis on results, mechanical obedience, systems of punishment and reward, infor-mation imparting and the failure to recognize the growth of the whole child as the basis of the educational process.[3, 4, 5]

He saw mechanical education as singularly inappropriate for a mechanistic age. A child who had not developed his full growth-potential as a human being at school had little hope of achieving it later or elsewhere as he might have done in that more human and varied rural environment—the passing of which Dewey also regretted and sought to substitute for. This failure, Holmes thought,

119

would lead both to social and personal maladjustment. He saw vandalism and other forms of 'naughtiness' as the inevitable result of the release of that tension which was caused by 'inactive' educational method. 'Malignant egoism', a viciousness, sensuality, untruthfulness, insincerity—even timidity—Holmes attributed to unhealthy environments both at home and at school which discouraged natural growth, enforced immaturity and failed to recognize that 'most . . . vices are virtues in the making'.[6]

Holmes's effect on the New Education which promised so much hope, not only to the maladjusted child within the existing system but also for the prevention of maladjustment, was two-fold. He encouraged and publicized the work being done within the State system by pioneers such as Miss Finlay Johnson (his 'Egeria' in *What Is and What Might Be*), and E. F. O'Neill, and he inspired and supported the efforts of those in the 'private sector' such as Mrs Ensor, Homer Lane, J. H. Simpson, Caldwell Cook and A. S. Neill not only through his writings but also through his work for those various bodies which developed into the New Education Fellowship.

Since prevention is clearly preferable to cure, and since much of this early work in 'ordinary' schools is acknowledged as a source of inspiration to those who later worked in special schools for the maladjusted, a brief review of some of this pioneer activity may perhaps be considered relevant. Indeed it might be argued that had we learnt the educational lessons of the first decades of this century well enough, and had we applied them in our schools, very few special schools would have been necessary. There seem to be few approaches current in modern 'maladjusted' schools which could not be found in early 'progressive' schools whether State or private. Shared responsibility, psychoanalysis, art-therapy, environmental therapy, activity methods, child-centred programmes, permissivism, small-group activities, close staff-pupil relationships, 'compensatory' education—all had their advocates and practitioners before the first special school for maladjusted children came into being.

EXPERIMENTS IN ORDINARY SCHOOLS

Holmes described Miss Johnson's work as headmistress of Sompting village school in Utopian terms and stressed that Utopia had

been realized.[7] Before the First World War, when the majority
of elementary schools still suffered from the aftermath of 'payment
by results', she sought to liberate the full potential of her 120
children by activity methods, guided discovery, encouragement of
arts and crafts, a Socratic method and an atmosphere of love and
sympathy. Education became the 'foster nurse' rather than the
'destroying angel' of the child's expanding life. Maladjustment
(although the term was not used) was seen largely as a social
artefact—the chief agent of society being the normal school. 'Goodness' and harmony (i.e. adjustment) are considered to be the almost
inevitable end of a process in which 'the one end and aim of the
teacher must be to stimulate and direct this process of spontaneous
growth'. Miss Johnson's pupils are found to be active, versatile,
imaginative, sympathetic, broadminded, self-forgetful, charming
and joyful. Their 'goodness' and 'harmony' are apparent.

While still an inspector of schools, Holmes had noticed and
approved of the work of E. F. O'Neill, then a student teacher too
imaginative to be successful. When O'Neill later became the headmaster first of Oswaldtwistle Knuzden Saint Oswald's and then of
Prestolee in industrial Lancashire (1918) he continued to pursue his
private vision of education as involving the whole school and the
whole community. He cast the entire school routine overboard, dis-
pensed with all timetables, mixed all ages and as far as possible
allowed children and teachers to choose each other on a basis
of mutual sympathy. He freed the children from rote learning,
based all work on creativity, activity and discovery and pioneered
many experiments in the 'integrated day', 'activity methods', 'team
teaching' and parent-teacher co-operation in the half century before
Plowden. The school, both during the day and throughout the evening, became the centre for arts and crafts: the library, the social
club, the reading room, the playing field, the evening institute—and
even the public gardens for both children and adults. This was
achieved despite continuous, and at times savage, opposition from
local reactionaries.

As well as the inspiration which he gave to contemporary workers
with disturbed children, it is clear that one of O'Neill's educational
aims was the active prevention of maladjustment and delinquency.
He was given to axioms (which he displayed in the school) such as:

'Children are only "little devils" when they cannot find something
legitimate to do.'

The life force is there
Do something they must
Or else they will bust.

or:

Man was made to master himself first
then. . . .

or:

Take care of the children and later on the adults will take care
of themselves.

His colleague and biographer, Gerard Holmes (nephew of
Edmond), noted that when, at the beginning of the Second World
War, the community activities of Prestolee were temporarily sus-
pended 'this multitude of children and young people, used to very
active lives in handicrafts rooms, cookery rooms, gyms, in dancing
rooms, with access to player pianos, libraries, and apparatus of all
kinds, found themselves with no other outlets than darkened streets,
darkened shop doorways and rubbish dumps' and that 'very soon
"juvenile delinquency" began to make its appearance in the
neighbourhood'.[8, 9]

PRIVATE SCHOOLS

The contribution of the private sector to that educational renaissance
which promised so much is well known. L. B. Pekin, the author
of *Progressive Schools* (1934) had no doubt that it was the continuation of repressive and psychologically unsound methods in ordinary
schools which produced many of the 'problem children' with which
the 'new' schools were asked to deal. 'So far from it being the case
that progressive schools get rid of their "difficult" children on to
ordinary schools' he reveals rather bitterly 'they are constantly being
asked to help or heal children with whom the latter have shown
themselves incompetent to deal'.[10]

Annabel William Ellis, another protagonist of progressive education, wrote in the introduction to the *Modern Schools Handbook* of
1934 that she was assured by a well-informed foreigner—'Twenty-
one progressive schools! But there are only two in the whole of
England.' In the 1920s there were, in fact, many more than the
twenty-one which Miss Ellis had mentioned, ranging from private
ventures such as the Russells' school at Beacon Hill, Norah Lay-

cock's 'farmhouse school', Winifred Nicholl's 'garden school', to the
original New Education schools of Abbotsholme and Bedales; the
Theosophists' St Christopher's, Letchworth, Frensham Heights, King
Arthur's School, Edinburgh; and, of course, the Quaker schools.
All served the needs of upper and middle-class normal and maladjusted children and many were run by individuals who—had they
not been quite so individualist—might have pioneered valuable new
methods. Priory Gate School, in Suffolk, was designed to test the
psychological theories of its founder, Major Theodore Faithfull,
but like the Malting House School founded by Geoffrey Pyke and
used by Susan Isaacs as a basis for her early experiments in educational psychology, it did not last long enough, in its original form,
to prove anything. Many, however, survived, and some, like the
Theosophist and Steiner schools, were to make a direct contribution
to the education of the emotionally handicapped.

Mrs Ensor, another dissatisfied H.M.I., was influenced both by
Edmond Holmes and by Homer Lane into forming a group of
teachers within the Theosophical Society. This group became, in
1915, the 'Theosophical Fraternity in Education' which was later to
merge into the New Education Fellowship. Its educational beliefs
were, like those of Edmond Holmes, based largely on the conviction
that human life was growth towards goodness which education was
to stimulate rather than suppress. The latent spiritual powers of
the child were to be released by an educational process which
followed the practice of Miss Johnson, the theory of Montessori, and
the philosophy of Theosophy. Schools such as Arundale (later St
Christopher's, Letchworth) and Frensham Heights (of which Mrs
Ensor was joint headmistress) were co-educational, democratic,
practical, non-punitive, largely open-air and vegetarian. The value of
this sort of regime to handicapped, disturbed and deprived children
was realised by Mrs Douglas-Hamilton, who founded Brackenhill
Theosophical Home School at Bromley for handicapped and normal
children from broken and undesirable homes. Its aim, not unlike
that of the Caldecott Community, was to provide a secure and
healthy environment within which the child, given the maximum of
individual attention, could grow towards physical, emotional and
spiritual self-control. The experiment, although taken over by the
Theosophical Society, was short-lived and Brackenhill was closed
in the early 1920s. The closure was, to some extent, logical since it
was felt that the majority of such children could be helped almost

equally effectively in such normal progressive schools as Frensham Heights which Mrs Douglas-Hamilton was largely instrumental in founding in 1925.

Steiner schools also, although numerically never of great importance in England, were based on a philosophy which in many ways appears to have much to offer to the unbalanced child. The principles of Anthroposophic education as originally enunciated by Steiner in 1911 (shortly before his final break with the Theosophical Society) [11, 12, 13] are the basis of a practical programme in which child nature is methodically nurtured through stages of physical, moral, rational and spiritual growth. Since growth could be hampered or distorted at any stage through inappropriate treatment it was inevitable that Steiner schools, as well as catering for normal children, should develop a curative function. Steiner himself became increasingly interested in certain medical applications of anthroposophical theory, and in 1921, in collaboration with Dr Ita Wegman, founded the Clinical Therapeutic Institute in Arlesheim, near Dornach in Switzerland, where they developed systems of Curative Eurythmy and Curative Education. These were thought to be particularly effective 'in the treatment of disturbances of the metabolic system and difficulties of movement and posture, especially in children'.[14] Curative Homes (of which there are now over twenty in England) were established for handicapped children thought to be 'in need of special soul care', and the Lauenstein and Sonnenhof institutes were founded to propagate the principles embodied in Steiner's and Wegman's book *Fundamentals of Therapy*, published in the year of the former's death, 1925.

Since these Curative Homes were primarily for mentally-handicapped children and since the first Steiner schools specifically for maladjusted children were not founded until after the Second World War, further consideration of Steiner's contribution to the education of maladjusted children will be left until a later chapter concerned with attempts at 'conceptualization'.

Margaret MacMillan, who presided over a course of lectures which Steiner gave at Ilkley in 1923, seems to have been much impressed by him but she was, of course, primarily significant in another sphere which has some importance to this study. Her pioneer nursery-school work at Deptford in itself had important implications, only now being realized, for the prevention of maladjustment. Her belief in the therapeutic value of 'open-air' education had, perhaps, a more immediate effect as we have seen—for instance, in the impetus it gave to Leila Rendel and others concerned with the education of the deprived.

THE OPEN-AIR MOVEMENT

The open-air and 'back to nature' educational movements so prevalent in the first decades of this century had many origins. The MacMillans were primarily concerned with the healthy body without which the healthy mind could not grow in circumstances of urban squalor. To the theosophists, the experience of nature and the open air were a necessary part of spiritual growth and the communication with supra-human forces. To Dr Reddie, at Abbotsholme, the natural environment meant a challenge greater than that posed by the playing fields of Eton, a belief which was exported to Germany in the form of county boarding schools (Landerzie-Hungsheime), free school communities (Freie Schulgemeinde) and Wandervogel camps, and reimported later by Kurt Hahn to Gordonstoun. Other organizations such as those of the Boy Scouts and the Woodcraft Chivalry stressed the importance of *mens sana in corpore sano*.

It appears that, from the first, schools created from these principles have played an important part in the education of deprived, delinquent and (even more) mildly maladjusted children suffering from neurotic disturbances, psychosomatic conditions such as asthma, and what may still be known as 'nervous debility'. Indeed until, in the 1930s, such people as Dr Fitch found ways of manipulating the 1921 Education Act to make the State support children at special schools for the maladjusted (see Chapter 9) open-air schools were almost the only 'special schools' available for such children—who could be sent on the recommendation of the school medical officer. 'Nervous debility' must have been a very flexible term.

Delamere Forest School, which celebrated its fiftieth anniversary in 1970, is typical of such schools. Miss Langdon, its founder and still the chairman of its governors, is also characteristic of the period. She was born in 1891 into a wealthy Jewish family which had been engaged for many generations in a variety of philanthropic activities. Her mother and her aunt were particularly active, the latter having founded in 1892 a holiday home for babies and working girls at Chinley, in Derbyshire. They were also very active in the

Ladies' Public Health Association, which concerned itself with home visiting, social work and housing conditions. This gave Miss Langdon early experience of severely deprived families when she visited the most depressed areas of Manchester with her mother. Her social concern was further stimulated when she was sent abroad at sixteen and, while completing her education, visited schools, hospitals and 'tramp wards' in Germany, France, Italy and Switzerland. She spoke with many of the leaders of the open-air movement and was also greatly influenced by a brother with whom she did much cycling and mountain climbing.

When she returned she became secretary to the Chinley venture, where her efforts were mainly expended on extending the customary length of stay from five days to three weeks, which she thought was the minimum effective period. She also managed to obtain support for six children to stay for six months with such satisfactory results that she became determined in 1912 to found a permanent open-air school. She formed a committee of enthusiasts none of whom was over twenty-one (her own age) and in response to a challenge from her chief supporter, Alderman Frankenberg, she raised £1,000 for the project. At this point the war intervened.

During the war she worked largely as an untrained health visitor, trying to improve standards of baby care and practising the effect of massage on the limbs of children with rickets. This experience convinced her further of the importance of fresh air and sunlight and when in 1916 a Manchester schools holiday camp was closed she undertook, with several equally inexperienced friends, to take sixty-nine boys camping in Derbyshire. She was much impressed not only by the effect of the experience on the boys but also by the boys' ignorance of nature. One highly intelligent boy was reluctant to climb a mountain with a group because he imagined that there would be no room for them all on the point! The camp became an annual event and eventually a permanent site was established at Prestatyn, in North Wales, to which groups of schoolchildren could go with their teachers.

At the end of the war Miss Langdon immediately revived her plans for an open-air school and eventually an appropriate site was found on the edge of Delamere Forest. 'The Jewish Fresh Air Home and School for Delicate Manchester and Salford Children' was founded in 1920 with Miss Landor, an idealistic and convinced teacher from the Jewish Free School in London, in charge. Miss Landor stayed for thirty-nine years.

Initially, 'delicate' children meant, in particular, children suffering from the effects of malnutrition and poor and overcrowded homes. The majority had rickets, gland-trouble, anaemia or bronchial conditions. Maladjustment, which was not, of course, ever the sole cause of admission, appeared to be largely the result of the over-protection of delicate children, the limitation of their experience in social relationships and sometimes a neurasthenic listlessness and withdrawal. There was the added factor that many of the children had been without their fathers during the war and many fathers had been killed.

Faced with these problems the staff placed its confidence in the therapeutic effect of open-air life and of a liberal, sympathetic and 'non-school' regime. Work was done out of doors whenever possible and special equipment such as collapsible desks and a portable piano were used. Sun-ray treatment was also given.

With the development of school health services and some improvement of living conditions the type of child referred to the school changed. There were fewer cases of acute malnutrition, rickets and pre-tubercular conditions and there was more 'nervous debility'—a term which, as has been mentioned, was often used euphemistically to secure placement for a disturbed child under the conditions of the 1921 Act. An increasing number of children came from middle-class families. This change in the pattern of need was attributed to such general causes as the depression and the change in the pace of life, but was probably largely the effect of the law of supply and demand. As fewer children required treatment for physical disorders so the needs of those suffering from nervous disorders could be met. The majority of open-air schools, like Delamere, had a clear therapeutic policy and a liberal regime based on the principles of 'progressive' education. This, combined with their healthy physical surroundings, appears to have made them particularly suitable for children suffering from a variety of neurotic conditions, particularly those which, like school phobia, are often associated with some form of psychosomatic illness. Staffing ratios were also high compared with those in ordinary schools, and this meant the maximum of individual care. Continuous social work, family case-work and aftercare provide at Delamere a supportive structure and minimize problems of reintegration.

Within recent years Delamere has evolved into a school dealing with all forms of handicap—physical, emotional and educational. Its apparent effectiveness supports a widely held view that the conditions needed for most handicapped children—individual attention, small groups, a liberal regime, psychological supervision, remedial instruction—are so similar that our present fragmentary provision of 'special' schools for 'special' handicaps is illogical.

A belief in the value of the open air and the challenge of nature in re-educating the urban delinquent child has been part of a long-established tradition going back to the Philanthropic Society's school at Redhill in 1849. This tradition continued through the Little Commonwealth, and many other less remarkable rurally situated approved schools, to experiments such as the Hawkspur Camp (see Chapter 12) and the present-day Cotswold Community (see Chapter 21). The assumptions behind this treatment have never been fully tested or conceptualized although the Planned Environmental Therapy Trust has to some extent clarified the aims and systematized the practice (see Chapter 15).

One such experiment which attracted much attention after the First World War was Thorp Arch School for Delinquent Girls, near Leeds. This industrial school on a rural $13\frac{1}{2}$-acre site was conducted on the best 'open-air' principles. Classes and meals were taken out of doors whenever possible and washing facilities were also 'open-air'. The girls 'wore brown tunics and knickers and were allowed bare legs and sandals, giving many of those "square inches of flesh exposed to the air" which some doctors hold to be so essential to health'.[15] Hair was worn long and free to diminish any feeling of institutionalization.

Apart from normal school work the girls were engaged both in gardening and animal husbandry and there was considerable freedom in the use of the estate. The girls were largely unsupervised during the country rambles, on visits to the seaside, and while walking to church. One effect of this regime of trust was that, apart from specific sums of money, it was not found necessary in the school to keep anything locked up.

SHARED RESPONSIBILITY

Since 'shared responsibility' and other forms of self-government have also been part of the pioneer tradition of institutions for the maladjusted at least since the Little Commonwealth, it is interesting to see also the movement towards such regimes in experimental schools of all types at this period. For many Homer Lane was the supreme originator.

As early as 1915 he had inspired the superintendent of Montefiore House—a Jewish institution for sixty-six delinquent and deprived girls—into instituting a system of self-government. This was introduced 'after the superintendent had carefully studied the subject and spent a week at the Little Commonwealth. The self-government is of a simple character, and is at present [i.e. 1920] confined to the questions of faults and their punishment.'[16] The superintendent had clearly not spent long enough at the Little Commonwealth to understand the principle. She might otherwise, perhaps, have become a notable pioneer in the neglected field of the education of maladjusted girls.

Other modified forms of 'shared responsibility' developed in both private and State schools, but in general during this period the real authority lay in the hands of the head teacher in a way of which Homer Lane, to whom many paid lip-service, would not have approved.

Of particular interest is the career of J. H. Simpson and the foundation of Rendcomb College. Simpson, as a young teacher at Rugby, had been encouraged by Homer Lane, Norman McMunn, and by his headmaster, Dr David, who was a member of the committee of the Little Commonwealth, to experiment with forms of self-government.[17] Rendcomb, of which he became headmaster in 1919, was originally founded as 'a boarding school for promising boys from the Public Elementary schools of the County of Gloucester' and might be considered the prototype of the 'county boarding school' which today plays an important part in the education of children who are mildly maladjusted, usually as the result of incompatible home circumstances. Simpson's inspiration and Rendcomb's example were also important to such later workers as N. B. C. Lucas, who, as headmaster of Midhurst Grammar School, instituted a system very similar to that of Rendcomb as part of his policy of helping the highly intelligent maladjusted boys who were sent to him (see Chapter 14).

The form of self-government which Simpson introduced into Rendcomb was a much modified version of the Little Commonwealth

E

model, since it excluded all members of staff other than Simpson and it was not equated with an extension of the family circle since it not only applied to a much larger group but was based on a formal constitution and the rule of law. Like Lane, Simpson also excluded the junior boys from the process. There were weekly General Meetings of all over thirteen years of age under an elected chairman. Most of the normal functions of a school were run by elected committees, including a finance committee the job of which was to organize the Laneian (Homeric?) 'economic moral structure' of the school. There was an elected judicial committee of seven members to enforce the decisions of the General Meeting.

Simpson retained the essential power over all major matters of school policy and himself says 'The organization of Rendcomb was emphatically a diarchy'.[18] While he claimed that this saved the school from his own potential despotism he also recognized that self-government was a medium through which the liberal headmaster could express his personality. 'Anyone visiting a democratic school will be struck by how far more closely its atmosphere manifests the personality of the Head than in authoritarian establishments.'

Simpson did not, however, see self-government merely as a way of projecting his own image. He also recognized it as a way of helping the precociously clever boy, the neurotic and maladjusted. 'The nervous boy . . . who, probably owing to some form of repression in childhood, is shy of expressing his opinion and is incapable of assisting himself.' Self-government was seen as, above all else, a way of using the energies of the rebel by, to some extent, removing his *raison d'être* ('the most anarchic boy will adopt a new attitude to the law when he himself is the legislator'), and by valuing those qualities which frequently put him in opposition to society. 'He more than anyone will profit by the membership of a self-governing community. All that is enterprising and constructive in his ideas will be expressed and appreciated.'[19]

EDUCATIONAL THEORY

The principles of the educational movements of these dynamic years which were to be significant when the subsequent 'slow down' of educational change made special schools increasingly necessary were largely pragmatically derived. Although Alice Woods considered that 'Our awakening to the need of interest in education was largely due to Froebel and Herbart. Our methods of developing interest received a wonderful impetus from Dewey, and our growing sense of the need of freedom, which is perhaps our most national asset, came to a climax through the influence of Dottoressa Montessori',[20] most of the pioneers of this era could probably say with A. S. Neill that they were not consciously affected by any of them. The type of educational theory which these early pioneers evolved has been well described by O'Connor as 'more like the empirical insight of the herbalist in the early stages of medicine. Practice comes first; but its theoretical justification has to wait for the scientific development that can explain its success. Thus educational theories which preceded the rise of scientific psychology were more or less acute guesses at explaining successful practice.'[21]

The pioneers learnt largely from one another and their practice was adventurous and experimental. Indeed, schools which were founded too rigidly on theory tended not to survive, while those which drew their life from a dynamic human being frequently did so. Perhaps theories tend to change and decay rather more quickly than men.

9

The New Psychology

> In the greater freedom of expression which it gives to the child, and in the establishment of more friendly relations based on sympathy and understanding rather than on authority and compulsion, the new education seeks to give effect to the findings of modern psychology.
> Badley J. H.: *A Schoolmaster's Testament*.[22]

The psychology to which Badley refers above was not that 'scientific psychology' to which O'Connor looks for precise answers to educational problems or precise expositions of educational theory (to which teachers paid, and still pay, little attention), but rather the child psychology derived from Sully, the pragmatic social psychology of Dewey and the psychoanalytic theory of Freud. Moreover, since the millenium of universal progressive State education did not materialize, despite the ardour of its protagonists, it was necessary for a dual system of ordinary and 'special schools' to emerge to cope with, among others, the casualties of continued 'unenlightened' upbringing in homes and schools into which Freudian—or any new—psychological ideas were slow to percolate or were, later, to be generally misunderstood or misapplied.

'The findings of modern psychology' were mainly to be applied in the 1920s and the 1930s to the maladjusted children of the middle class in private 'progressive' schools which would tolerate them. Here they found the sort of environment which even Freudians like Susan Isaacs (obsessed as they were by the traumatic experiences of the first five years) thought offered hope of recovery to children to whom analytical treatment was not available and even to those whose neurotic difficulties were not in any way attributable to an unfavourable environment. Susan Isaacs recognized that 'environmental influences and real events are nevertheless of great importance chiefly in determining whether or not a child will grow out of his early difficulties'.[23] Thus children from favourable economic environments could, and still do, 'grow out of' their difficulties by finding tolerable and tolerating conditions in a large number of private, fee-

132

paying normal schools such as Summerhill. (This may be the only occasion on which Summerhill has ever been referred to as 'normal'. I am using the word in the sense of 'not exclusively for maladjusted children', i.e. 'special'. Indeed A. S. Neill 'gave up specializing in problem kids years ago').

A. S. NEILL

There are many essential differences between Summerhill and other progressive schools as was apparent when, in the early 1920s, Neill and Mrs Ensor were for a time co-editors of *New Era,* the journal of the New Education Fellowship. Neill rejected the high ideals of what he considered to be 'crank' schools, considering that, whatever the ideal, it imposed a restriction on child development as potentially harmful as those restrictions imposed by any religious or moral code. He rejected the psychological mysticism of Jung, which the Theosophists and other new educators found attractive as a rationale for their 'Higher Life' attitudes, and based his approach primarily on Freud. Sexual prohibitions, from which Neill had often suffered in his childhood, were seen as the ultimate cause of unsatisfactory personal development and, while other progressives thought in terms of the social sublimation of sex through coeducation and healthy living, Neill believed in complete freedom of sexual experience. For practical reasons he was never able in his school to be entirely consistent with his aim. Sexual freedom was little more than the freedom to masturbate.

Nor did Neill have any particular educational objectives. He did not experiment with new methods or new subjects, he did nothing and does nothing to encourage interest in conventional areas of knowledge. Drawing on his own unhappy and unproductive academic educational experience he adopts a 'take it or leave it' attitude and has been accused of being obstructive rather than encouraging to his teachers.[24] Most progressive schools, on the other hand, while rejecting much which was traditional in the content and method of academic education, have seen the teacher's role as that of encourager, stimulator and guide. For the latter, education offered an expansion of experience in thought, in art and in craft which presupposed the presence of an adult who had more to offer than could be derived only from the child's inner processes.

While other progressive educators sought to learn from the work of Dewey, Froebel, Montessori and other teacher-theorists, Neill's rejection of authority included this in its scope. He claims never to have read any educational theory and says that 'If I found myself studying Rousseau and Pestalozzi and Montessori I should give up my job as a failure. To be a good mason one does not require to learn the history of masonry.'[25] Nor did he take note of the educational methods of his progressive contemporaries. Of an article on new educational methods and theories which appeared in *New Era* he wrote in 1936: 'It makes me sad to see people struggle with compromise things like Dalton Plans and pseudo-self-government schemes. . . . The articles . . . are over twenty years late in appearing. They should belong to the time when Edmond Holmes and Caldwell Cook and Norman MacMunn were writing of their new experiments. None of them is as arresting as the new educational methods of E. F. O'Neill nearly twenty years ago. . . . I am a better man than any of them but I claim no original experimentation in education because education is a thing which does not interest me. . . .'[26]

It is ironic, therefore, that for many people A. S. Neill and Summerhill were, and still are, the New Education.[27] Robin Pedley, for instance, writes:

Neill, more than anyone else, has swung teachers' opinion in this country from its old reliance on authority and the cane to hesitant recognition that a child's first need is love, and with love the free growth of his personality; free that is from the arbitrary compulsion of his elders, and disciplined instead by social experience. . . . Today's friendliness between pupil and teacher is probably the greatest difference between the classrooms of 1963 and those of 1923. This change owes much to Neill.[28]

That Neill rejected both compromise and authority, and threw away the baby of education with the bath-water of repression, seems to be largely the result of his early experience as the unsuccessful son of a Scottish dominie. After being completely unable to learn at school and after being employed in a number of menial clerical jobs, it was decided that he was fit for nothing but to become a teacher. His early teaching experience in Kingsmuir (1902), Kingskettle (1903–6), Newport, Fife (1906–8), and Gretna Green (1915–7) further convinced him of the futility of both the content and methods of traditional elementary education. He established himself as an educational iconoclast not only through his teaching but also through his books. *A Dominie's Log* (1915) and *A Dominie Dismissed* (1916), were the first of a long and continuous series of autobiographical diatribes attacking formal and traditional education.

In 1919 he moved to the New Education day school, King Alfred's at Hampstead, London, and fell increasingly and naturally under the influence of Homer Lane, who he had first met at the Little Commonwealth in 1916. Lane further intensified his convictions. 'As we listened to him [Homer Lane], our critical faculties were in suspense. He made the most extravagant assertions and we accepted them.' King Alfred's, although progressive of its type, was too authoritarian in structure for Neill. Mrs Lane wrote: 'Our poor Mr Neill is having an awful time here in King Alfred's school, where he has just started self-government.' The informant was possibly Lane's son, Allen, who was in Neill's class at the time.

From London Neill went to Germany to assist in founding the International School, Hellerau, Dresden (1921–3), moving to Sonntagberg, Austria (1923–4). Although the educational experience was not altogether satisfactory, since Neill rejected the formalism of German methods and the academic emphasis on traditional culture, the psychological thinking of postwar Austria was much more congenial. He was greatly influenced by Wilhelm Stekel, with whom he went through a lengthy process of psychoanalysis. To a protegé of Homer Lane, Stekel's active Adlerian approach to psychoanalysis, with its emphasis on the analyst's insight attacking the patient's neurosis, must have seemed familiar. What Neill learnt from Lane, Stekel and Freud was incorporated into both the theory and practice of Summerhill, the school which he founded on his return to England at Lyme Regis (1924–7), and, later, moved to Leiston in Suffolk, where it still remains with the octogenarian Neill at its head.

Of Summerhill's foundation he said: 'Freud showed that every neurosis is founded on sex repression. I said "I'll have a school in which there will be no sex repression". Freud said that the unconscious was infinitely more important and powerful than the conscious. I said "In my school we won't censure, punish, moralize. We will allow every child to live life according to his deep impulses." '[29] With such principles and such a background it was inevitable that Neill and Summerhill should attract maladjusted children, and Neill has an important place as a pioneer headmaster, theorist and propagandist. Summerhill offered new hope to children full of hate for parents, teachers and authority, for books, study and learning. 'Their enrolment at Summerhill represents a traumatic and sudden "decompression" in the scholastic environment ... this interval Neill calls "recovery time".'[30]

Between 1924 and 1938 Summerhill's survival frequently depended on Neill's willingness to take 'problem children' for whom he represented a last hope. Consequently many were too deeply neurotic and too late in their development for simple freedom to succeed as therapy. Neill went beyond freedom to the extent, for instance, of rewarding children for stealing in order to assure them of his friendship and approval of themselves. He sought not only to remove moral restrictions but also to attack them. He endeavoured to release the child's pent-up emotions through psychoanalytical sessions known as 'private lessons'. Delinquency he thought to be the product of a natural hatred of a society which prevented the self from developing naturally. In an atmosphere of freedom, love and trust the disturbed and delinquent would become happy and honest. Morality he thought produced conscience, conscience operated through guilt, guilt distorted personality. The child had only to regulate himself in accordance with his needs (if his needs had not been distorted by regulations) to be both happy and good. In his rejection of all external agencies in the development of the ego, Neill went beyond Freud and eventually found in Reich a more satisfactory theoretical exponent of his own intuitive practice.

During this early period his reputation for understanding problem children was increased by his writing *The Problem Child* (1926), *The Problem Parent* (1932) and about the work he was doing in *That Dreadful School* (1937). He was not, however, entirely happy with the reputation which he created. Increasingly he wished not to cure children of problems but to prevent the problems from occurring by creating an environment for normal children in which 'self regulation' was possible.

There appear to be many reasons for this change of emphasis. The most remarkable, for Neill, was admitted failure. He writes in *The Free Child* (1953): 'Like others I have always considered the problem child a bright child with a creative energy that had to come out in an anti-social way because there was no positive way for it to come out. Make him free from inhibitions and discipline, I thought, and he will most likely turn out to be clever, creative, even brilliant sometimes. I was wrong, sadly wrong. Years of living and dealing with all sorts of crooks and swindlers and liars showed me that they were one and all inferiors. I can think of only one who made good in later life.'[31] This disillusionment, expressed in Neill's customary dogmatic manner, was not the only sign of, or reason for, change.

He had discovered also in practice that he could not play the roles both of psychiatrist and principal—'most pupils cannot do much work with the man who is their father confessor.... The psychic doctor should not really live in the school at all; the children should have no social interest in him.'[32] He gave up his psychoanalytical sessions and concentrated on prophylaxis rather than cure.

The most marked change came with his introduction to Reich in 1937. Neill had never been entirely happy with Freud or with Freudians. The latter declined to send children to Summerhill on the grounds that Neill neither understood nor applied Freudian principles.[33] To Freud the patriarchal family was the instrument of a necessary process of socialization operating originally through direct suppression of instinctual drives and then through the conscience. Sublimation meant civilization. Only when primitive energy was diverted was culture possible. Neill opposed suppression and had little use for culture. This attitude was the product of his own life experience, but in Reich it was given theoretical formulation. To Reich suppression, particularly of sexual energy, was the source of all neurosis, productive only of social and sexual impotence.[34] The family was the origin not of social competence but of social and personal emasculation. Psychoanalysis and other therapeutic techniques could do little unless parents could be prevented from inflicting the initial damage. Teaching parents became more important to Neill than curing children; the children he could only hope to save before the malignant conscience became embedded.

Whether it was, as Skidelsky suggests, this new insight which 'freed Neill from his need to work with "problem" children'[35] is doubtful, although Reich's importance cannot be questioned. This is, perhaps, to underestimate the significance to Neill of the six weeks of therapy which he received from Reich and which he describes as of more importance than years of 'talky' analysis.[36] The object of Reichian therapy was to free the personality by unblocking sexual energy so that complete surrender and fulfilment was possible.[37]

Neill was, on his own admission, severely sexually repressed when young. He married late and had no children by his first wife, who died in 1944. After her death he remarried and at the age of sixty had his first child, who was to be the prototype of the 'self-regulated child' and who was the subject of *The Free Child* (1953).

It seems possible that Neill had found a solution to his own problem and with it lost the need to work out his own difficulties by projecting them on to problem children. This has important implications when one considers the personalities of those who work with maladjusted children. Perhaps a degree of frustration and sublimation is necessary if one is to expend one's energies on the arduous task of adjusting those whose failure to adjust has made them neurotic. It may, on the other hand, have been no more than that as Neill got older he became less capable of withstanding the daily strain of living with disturbed children.

However much Neill's theories may have changed, the structure of Summerhill remained constant. Neill writes: 'My association with Reich, however, had no effect on my school work. ... I had run Summerhill for twenty-six years before I met him, and the meeting did not alter my school in any way. Indirectly it may have done, for Reich's therapy helped me enormously.'[38] The clearest exposition of this abiding structure is given by van Cleve Morris, who interestingly, and with much justification, claims that Neill's philosophy was Existential and his school 'the Paradigm school' for Existentialists. He describes Summerhill — now forty-seven years old and having about as many children, mainly American, in terms of the following 'hazardous hypothesis':

Suppose you had a school in which there were no rules, no requirements, no homework, no regulations, no roll-taking, no grades, no academic expectations, no tests, no institutional code of decorum, no social conventions. Suppose all you had were a small 'campus', some living quarters, some classrooms, half a dozen teachers and forty to fifty youngsters ranging in age from five to seventeen. It would be a small but thoroughly free and open society, with no institutional ethos to adjust to and no organizational hierarchy to please. It would be, rather, merely a collection of separate individuals dealing with one another, old and young alike, as free and autonomous persons. Could anything like 'education' possibly occur there? Neill has found that the answer is 'Yes'.[39]

Van Cleve Morris is not alone in pointing out subsequently that rules do, in fact, exist in this 'existential' school, but they are made by the self-governing General School Meeting of all Summerhill citizens. As Pekin says: 'Neill for instance writes that every disciplinarian is a humbug when he isn't a sadist, but he attends a disciplinarian jury of his school-children every Saturday evening, and he believes in the existence of this discipline in his school [for], after all, Neill is not a fool: he happens to be an educator of genius. In one of his books he modestly disclaims this title, but nothing else will describe the gentleness and good humour, combined with the uncanny flair for child psychology which go to make up this most remarkable of Headmasters.'[40]

However much Neill may categorize maladjusted children as 'destructive, thieving, hateful brats' and claim that his school is engaged in preventive education for normal children rather than treatment for abnormal ones, Summerhill is a therapeutic establishment. It is engaged not only in preserving children from society's contaminating touch but also in curing them of the ills which society has implanted. In Freudian terms the emphasis is on preserving a healthy 'id' rather than on developing a strong 'ego'. In these terms, if Neill were to succeed in what appear to be his therapeutic aims one would expect to find the 'id' largely uncontaminated by the 'super-ego'. The child would have been shielded from the essential conflict which may not only overwhelm the ego but also strengthen it. If Neill, in fact, abrogated an external super-ego role then one would expect his pupils to remain immature, impulsive id-creatures whose personality development is incomplete (lacking in one essential element). David Holbrook commented in 1965 in the Summerhill Association journal *Id* (a significant title): 'I've known some [former pupils] in whom this lack of self-discipline is disastrous; and others in whom the same lack of strong identity, of resources, and of energy has been their weakness in personal relationships. They lack organization in the reparative impulses, and their inward struggle between love and hate isn't lively enough.'

Although this accusation is made with some reason Neill clearly does not, and cannot, entirely abrogate the super-ego role. For all the freedom and the self-government, the absence of fear and guilt, the acceptance of the selfish needs of the child and of his essential goodness, the rejection both of religion and psychoanalysis, Neill remains to be identified with, to love and to hate, and to develop the ego. It is a god-like responsibility.

NORMAN MACMUNN

If Neill was atypically typical of pioneer workers with maladjusted children in 'normal' schools Norman MacMunn, partly because of his idiosyncratic methods and his consciousness of himself as an individual, may be considered the first in, and typical of, a line of pioneer workers with disturbed children in private 'special' schools.

MacMunn had no doubt of his pioneer status and it appears curious that Boyd and Rawson should say of him: 'He himself was perhaps not aware of the tremendous influence of his own character and of that love of his children which supported their steps towards freedom, and was inclined to think that they only needed to be given the opportunity to be creative and spontaneous for all to work out as it should. The result in the case of severely repressed children is often astonishing, and no doubt had he lived (he died in 1925) he might have come to realize his own influence more clearly'[41] — although it may be true that he elevated the effect of his methods above that of his character, a failing which he shared with many pioneers.

MacMunn was, from the first, a propagandist for his own methods. Reviewing educational experiments which followed from the First World War, he said: 'However rare relatively, they are absolutely quite numerous, though, with the exception of Mr O'Neill's school at Manchester, that of Mr Arrowsmith in Lincolnshire, the ever memorable work of Mr Homer Lane at the Little Commonwealth and our own venture at Tiptree Hall, most of these efforts to adapt education to the ascertained needs of the times are sporadic rather than formative.'[42]

As an assistant master at West Downs preparatory school during the war and later at King Edward VI School, Stratford on Avon, MacMunn, whose own school experience had been extremely unhappy, became a very vocal protagonist of the New Education in general and his own teaching techniques in particular. By his book *A Path to Freedom in the School,* first published in 1914 and later extensively revised, he attracted a great deal of attention to his activity methods of teaching foreign languages and mathematics, in particular through the medium of co-operation rather than competition in the class and the use of ingenious visual aids.[43]

After the war he set up a community of war orphans at Tiptree

Hall, in Essex. At this time MacMunn, a typical educational optimist of the period, wrote: 'The past ten years [i.e. 1910–1920] have been so fruitful in educational discovery and in striking experiment with defective, delinquent and normal children that it can hardly be doubted that we have reached in educational science much the same state as that reached by medical science and art after the discovery of the circulation of the blood.'[44]

MacMunn's war orphans could not have been classified as mal-adjusted, since no such classification existed, but most had suffered violent traumatic experiences and extreme environmental depriva-tion which had resulted in a variety of neurotic disorders which MacMunn describes, e.g. Little Jack: 'A phthisical boy with a nervous system as sensitive and raw as bleeding flesh. . . . Jack was not only a bundle of nerves but he was strangely unresponsive to his freedom. . . . He was grasping and had been very cruel. . . . But even he was inspired on that first night when everyone suddenly seized the meaning of freedom.'[45]

MacMunn could seldom afford to educate more than ten boys. All were from the working classes. He claimed that 'it ought to be generally known, and it is the opposite of the general opinion, that children of the poorer classes are infinitely more nervous than children from comfortable homes'. Partly from necessity and partly from conviction his approach was basically Pestalozzian and pater-nalistic. All furniture and equipment for the school was made by MacMunn and the boys, and his teaching not only involved one boy instructing another but, after the small school had moved to Italy in 1924, was expanded to include the appointment of boy 'professors' as experts in different subjects in which it was their responsibility to guide the studies of the others.

In treating neurotic and maladjusted boys MacMunn's technique resembled Homer Lane's in that, although largely intuitive and pragmatic, it was later rationalized in pseudo-Freudian terms. 'Psychic sickness is always more complicated than physical, and always dates further back. It is all traceable to early suppressions. X [i.e. MacMunn] first tries the shock of extreme gentleness and generally this is enough.'[46] This refers to his technique for dealing with neurotic aggressiveness which, not unnaturally, he found the chief symptom among his war orphans.

Like Neill, MacMunn believed in the value of a period of 'decompression'—'recovery time'. 'During the period of transition the misdemeanours due to the inhibition of the children's work play activities will be looked at as sympathetically as possible, and the "difficult" boy may well be turned over for increased scope in the experimental class and in the workshop. The graver offences will be treated as symptoms of nervous disease and as requiring analytical or suggestional treatment or both.'[47]

Although it does not appear that MacMunn attempted to analyse the boys himself (although they were doubtless subjected to considerable 'suggestional treatment') he believed strongly in the value of psychoanalysis. 'The believers in a great extension of freedom for the child owe much gratitude to the new study of psycho-analysis. Not only have the evils of repression been traced and relieved by the removal in a clinic of nearly all the suppressions which nearly all of the old-time and many of the present-time schoolmasters have considered it their duty to encompass, but we are probably on the eve of discoveries which will help to provide a rational analytical technique which can be passed on for use by teachers.'[48]

It would probably have depressed the optimistic MacMunn to realize how few teachers were interested in extending analytical techniques or of carrying on the sort of work for deprived and maladjusted children which he had pioneered. Of those people who attacked the problem of maladjustment frontally, as it were, in special schools during the 1920s and 1930s very few were of the teaching profession.

If Neill and MacMunn were teachers who used psychology as a tool, Dr Dodd and Dr Fitch were psychiatrists who used education as theirs. Their pioneer work was derived from the inadequacy of the emergent child-guidance system to achieve work of lasting effect in a society which was lamentably lacking in the provision of education suited to the needs of the disturbed—or even nonconformist—child.

MEDICAL APPROACHES

For doctors to concern themselves with the work of education was by no means new. Apart from the work of Dr Howe and others referred to in Chapter 3 whose work pioneered new ways of educating the mentally defective both in America and in England, there was the more immediate example of such European practitioners as Dr Decroly and Dr Claparède. In 1901, after considerable research into the psychological problems of mental abnormality in children, Decroly took some mentally defective children into his own home for training and observation. From this small beginning there not only developed the Institute for Abnormal Children in Uccle but also a whole system of education based on 'centres of interest' and a 'play' approach to learning. The Hermitage school was opened in 1907 to apply Decroly's methods to the education of normal children. The classroom was looked upon as a workshop in which the task, from planning to execution, was chosen and engaged-in freely by the children while being organized not only round the individual needs of the child but also round the four main 'centres of interest' — the need of food, the need of shelter, the need of defence, the need of work. This approach not only inevitably became a source of inspiration to the New Educators but, partly because of its origin, it influenced others whose work lay with problems of abnormal children.

One such person was Edouard Claparède, who in 1912 was largely instrumental in the foundation of the Rousseau Institute in Geneva. Claparède, who as a young doctor had worked in the psychological laboratory of the University of Geneva, had, like Decroly, originally been interested in the problem of educating the defective and abnormal child in special schools. He realized increasingly, however, that the psychological principles which applied to their education were part of the problem of general education (a lesson which we have not yet sufficiently learnt). It is interesting that the Faculties of Arts, Science and Medicine combined to prevent his *Seminaire de psychologie Pedagogique* — a course of lectures for teachers on educational psychology, physiology, health, and the pathology of childhood. After 1912, with the foundation of the 'Ecole des Sciences de l'Education', Claparède was able to pursue his vision of a science of education based on child study and to build up a team of teachers, psychologists and social workers which resulted ultimately in the foundation of a school psychological service in Berne (1920) and Basle (1928).[49]

DR F. H. DODD

In England the influence of Freud's work and the advent of the First World War changed the focus of attention from the needs of the subnormal and retarded children to the phenomenon of the neurotic and emotionally unbalanced adult. Attempts were made to treat the hysterical condition of 'shell shock' by various psychological and psycho-analytical means and MacMunn was not alone in realizing the application of some of these techniques to severely disturbed children.

In 1920 the Institute of Medical Psychology (the Tavistock Clinic) was founded under Dr Crichton Miller to study and treat the functional nervous disorders of adults but its work inevitably focused attention (as Freud's had done), on the significance of childhood experience and on the nervous disorders of children themselves.

Frederick Henry Dodd was one of the doctors at the Tavistock Clinic who became increasingly concerned with this problem and increasingly frustrated by the absence of provision for treating the neuroses of childhood. It is interesting that while other doctors were finding a new rationale for treating disturbed children within their discipline Dodd's solution was educational.

Dr Dodd, born in 1892, was trained as a surgeon and physician and, before joining the Tavistock Clinic, had been physician-in-charge of the psychological department of the Eastern Dispensary in London. He became interested in the relationship between physical ill-health and psychological disturbances and concluded that more help could be given to children in a natural home atmosphere. Encouraged by Dr Hector Cameron,[50] whose understanding work with children he admired, he set up a small residential school for disturbed boys at Blackheath in 1920. He married and, in 1924, moved to a larger house and continued his work with about twenty boys and girls between the age of five and fifteen. In 1940 he moved to Dorset and did much work with children disturbed by the process of evacuation. He died in 1950. His school which, wherever it was situated, appears always to have been known simply as 'Dr Dodd's', can be claimed as the first to cater specifically for emotionally disturbed children—without any other necessary corollary. Its aim was, from the first, both therapeutic and educational and although

his widow, Mrs Kathleen Dodd, who worked with him, considers
that he was 'an empiricist not a theorist' he did, in fact, write one
book, *Commonsense Psychology and the Home,* which explains his
theoretical attitude.[51] Mrs Dodd considers that 'the work of Adler
had considerable bearing on his approach'. This is true of many contemporary Continental workers with maladjusted and delinquent
children. To Dr Dodd the parental attitude, as represented by himself and his wife, was of supreme importance. This was to be firm
enough to be supportive yet not so strong that it mutilated the personality of the child by over dominance.[52] Dr Dodd was not an
exponent of permissivism. 'This tendency to give the child freedom
for complete so-called self-expression and development is only the
swing of the pendulum from the opposite extreme of over-domin-
ance by fear of the father, or over anxiety on the part of the
mother.'[53]

Possibly because he was himself fatherless from the age of twelve
and was brought up by a loving but over-protective mother, he lays
great stress on the psychological state of what he calls 'the mother's
darling' and considers that 'though it is our duty to understand our
children, it is also our duty to encourage them to appreciate the value
of the principles involved in a Spartan attitude to life, to encourage in
them the romance of bravery, healthy endurance and achievement.
From the beginning of its life a child must be accustomed to reasonable discipline and training, endurance and acceptance of facts.'[54]

Fear is regarded in the early stages of growth as a substratum
'which will be sufficient to reinforce the love motive and so compel
the child to act rightly'. In this way the child grows to a knowledge
of what is socially acceptable and the love factor permeates the whole
relationship of the individual world. Punishment reinforces the
developing 'conscience' but it is essential that the child shall understand and be in essential agreement with the limitations imposed.
The repression of creative urges is wrong and if their expression
is socially unacceptable an alternative outlet must be found. The
boy who attracted attention by openly urinating in the garden would
be encouraged to work with the hose 'which was much more fun as
the fountain produced was far larger'.

Education must, nevertheless, be essentially 'a drawing out and
developing of the child's own personality, rather than an impression
of the adult on the child'. I think it is with some feeling that Dr Dodd
continues: 'Although probably almost everyone would accept this

fact in theory, it is not so easy to carry it out in practice. Only too often we try to impress our own adult views on the child and so distort its normal development.'

The practice at 'Dr Dodd's' agreed with the theory in that it was loving, secure, practical and Spartan. There was little direct psychotherapy but a great deal of what might now be called 'work therapy'. Mrs Dodd, who was clearly of vital importance as the doctor's co-worker, writes: 'In our work we always tried to solve problems indirectly through education and all sorts of out-of-school activities, community life, and getting the children to help and understand one another.... Always our desire was to create a normal, full, interesting life, and not to label the children as maladjusted.... Freedom was something which gradually increased, we did not believe in unrestricted freedom, which can make a child more anxious and less able to cope with its environment.'[35] In a later letter Mrs Dodd emphasizes 'the commonsense, practical attitude which my husband took in unravelling psychological "problems" which he sometimes felt were tackled too "intellectually".'

Dr Dodd continued his work at the Tavistock Clinic, which in 1929 established a most important precedent by advising that an eight-year-old girl, described as nervous, emotional and restless, should be sent away to a private home which took children suffering from rickets, debility and nervous disorders. The local education authority concerned asked the Board of Education to sanction the payment of the fee of fifteen shillings a week charged by the home. The board agreed to sanction the proposal as an experiment, regarding it as an arrangement under Section 80 of the Education Act, 1921, 'for attending to the health and physical education' of the child. The girl did not, in fact, go to the home, but went instead to a foster-mother who took a few difficult children, and the sanction already given was allowed to apply to the new arrangements. In this way the power of local authorities to board out maladjusted children was established.[56] Thus Dr Dodd helped to create an administrative instrument which Dr Fitch was, soon afterwards, to use most effectively.

With the rapid growth of interest in psychoanalytical techniques and the slower spread of psychologically based educational services, increasing attention was being paid both by doctors and educators to those children who were still regarded in the terms of the Mental

Deficiency Act (1913) as 'morally deficient'. The 1913 Act referred to 'Moral imbeciles, that is to say, persons who from an early age display some permanent mental defect coupled with strong vicious or criminal propensities on which punishment has little or no deterrent effect'. The 1927 Mental Deficiency Act modified 'moral imbecile' to 'moral defective' i.e., persons in whose case there exists mental defectiveness with strongly vicious or criminal propensities and who require care, supervision and other control for the protection of others'.

Burt claims that 'the traditional notion of an innate "moral faculty" or "sense" though still upheld in the 1920s by most psychiatrists had long ago been discarded by nearly all psychologists' in favour of explanations derived largely from social psychology, views which were confirmed by the work of Burt and others in his psychological laboratory in Liverpool before the First World War.[57, 58] Some enlightened magistrates in the juvenile courts (set up under the Children's Act of 1908), were already seeking the help of psychologists and psychiatrists before making decisions about the children brought before them, but were hampered not only by the uncertain status of such authority at the beginning of the century but also by the absence of any facilities for the treatment or placement of children who were considered psychologically disturbed rather than criminally inclined or 'morally defective'. Such child guidance centres as existed within the general aegis of university 'psychological laboratories' were largely informal bodies concerned primarily with research and teaching. The London County Council's example in appointing an educational psychologist had not been followed (and was, indeed, temporarily abandoned by the L.C.C. itself after Burt's resignation in 1931).

It was during the indecisive years which followed the First World War that a critical change in the directions of educational psychology in England occurred. The work of Galton's followers in America was reimported in an alien form at first to buttress and then largely to destroy the native product derived from both Galton and Sully. The psychological clinic begun by Galton's follower Cattell in Pennsylvania in 1896, with Witmer in charge, was originally based largely on the English model, but Witmer's work was not encouraged. The approved emphasis was rather on clinical treatment within a hospital setting derived largely from the work of Meyer and having as its aim the treatment of mental disease. 'Since they operated on the assumption, prevalent at the time, that mental disease was caused almost entirely by organic factors, these clinics had little to offer to maladjusted children. It was only when the social and emotional origins of mental illness began to be taken into account that the clinics began to accept maladjusted children as patients.[59] The tendency to think in terms of mental illness was strongly reinforced not only by the immense impact of Freud on American thought but by the foundation of the National Association for Mental Hygiene in 1909.

The year 1909 was also the year in which Cattell's pupil William Healy opened a clinic in Chicago which became the Juvenile Psychopathic Institute. Healy's clinic, although not the first, rapidly became the best known for its work with juvenile delinquents and greatly influenced those who, in 1922, set up the first demonstration clinics 'to develop the psychiatric study of delinquent and difficult children, to develop sound methods of treatment, and to provide courses of training'.[60] These and similar American foundations under the aegis of the National Committee for Mental Hygiene and financed by the Commonwealth Fund had what came to be regarded as the classic clinic structure of a psychiatrist-in-charge, a psychologist whose main function was testing, and a psychiatric social worker.

Thus when Mrs St Loe Strachey, a London magistrate, sought the aid of the Commonwealth Fund to promote similar work in London she unwittingly imported a structure which was based on a fundamentally different concept from that of the school-based psychological service which Burt had laboured to construct. Mrs St Loe Strachey's aim was primarily the prevention of delinquency but both Burt and Sir Percy Nunn urged a wider view. While London County Council representatives urged the extension of provision to 'every type of mentally subnormal child, not merely delinquents', Nunn asked: 'Why must a child be subnormal before he can claim the psychologist's help? Every child at some time or other may need guidance; and, as often as not, we shall be concerned with "guidance" given to the teacher or the parent as well as to the child. Above all it must be realized that the work of such a "clinic" will be educational and social more frequently than medical or clinical in the strict sense.'[61]

With the example of Burt before them, the protagonists of the new child-guidance clinic established at Islington, London, in 1928 saw no discrepancy between what was proposed and what Nunn suggested as desirable. When, however, Burt declined to become the head of the new clinic and Sir George Newman, the Chief Medical Officer of the Ministry of Health and Board of Education, insisted that if children were to attend the new clinics in school hours the head of the clinic should always be medically qualified, it was clear what function was envisaged. Moreover, the new director of the clinic, Dr William Moodie, made it obvious that he saw a clear distinction between the psychiatrist who treated and the psychologist who tested. 'Knowledge of the essential mechanisms involved in all forms of behaviour, normal as well as abnormal' was accorded to the doctor, knowledge of the 'structure and operation of the intelligence' to the psychologist.[62]

In the following twenty years the inter-disciplinary quarrelling was one of the chief reasons for the slow development of a service which could have offered much to maladjusted children. Psychologists lacked interest in playing a subordinate and tedious role as testers and there were, in any case, too few trained psychiatrists to expand facilities thus organized.

The particular significance of the London Clinic, other than this fundamental alteration of approach, was that the L.C.C. was a party to its foundation and regarded it as an integral part of its school health service. This had little immediate effect outside London and clinics were not recognized for grant purposes by the Board of Education until 1935, when child guidance services became an official part of school medical services. Moreover 'since maladjusted children were not officially recognized as a category of handicapped children any boarding out arrangements thought necessary by the clinics were approved under Section 80 of the Education Act 1921, which allowed authorities to attend to the health and physical education of children'.[63] These powers were, however, seldom invoked before the 1930s, and, in any case, local authorities had no power to provide schools for the maladjusted. Had it not been for the altruism of individual pioneers no special provision would have been made until the Second World War demonstrated its necessity.

The Child Guidance Council was founded in 1928 'to encourage the provision of skilled treatment of children showing behaviour disturbances and early symptoms of disorder', but its appeal was responded to rather by concerned individuals than by local authorities. Two such 'concerned individuals' were Drs Steven and Muriel Barton-Hall who, in 1924, set up a 'voluntary' clinic in St James's

Road, Liverpool. Dr Steven was responsible for psychiatric work and Dr Muriel, who was, in fact, a bacteriologist by training, pursued her growing interest in psychology. There was no social worker and the work was inevitably medically orientated although the Barton-Halls shared Mrs St Loe Strachey's interest in Burt's work in psychometrics and on the problems of juvenile delinquency. Initially much of the work was with adults, but in 1929 the first properly constituted child-guidance clinic outside London was set up in Nile Street, Liverpool, with a council under the chairmanship of Charles Booth, a Liverpool philanthropist, who shared his grandfather William Booth's concern for the deprived. The chief instigator of the work of the clinic and the council in Liverpool was, however, Dr Alfred Fitch, a dynamic physician, a biochemist, a skin specialist and, at one time, a medical journalist employed by William Randolph Hearst of the *Chicago Tribune*. In the 1920s Fitch turned his attention to psychiatry, in which he appears to have had little formal training, and diverted his considerable energies to promoting the idea of what he called 'habit clinics'.

DR ALFRED FITCH

In his psychiatric work with children, Fitch met the same discouraging experience which had induced Dr Dodd to found his school. So many of the behaviour problems with which he was called on to deal were the result of harmful and intractable home conditions combined with inadequate schooling that he realized that much of his work was being wasted.

It is characteristic of him that his interest was immediately diverted to education, a sphere in which he had had no previous experience other than some schooling in France after he had been expelled from Monmouth School for throwing an ink-bomb at a master. Nevertheless in 1935, at the age of forty-eight, he took over—with great enthusiasm but few funds—Dunnow Hall at Newton in Bowland, a large mansion on the Yorkshire-Lancashire border, to see what 'a controlled environment and regular life' could do for maladjusted children. He is of interest not only because he was one of the first 'special school' principals to make extensive use of the loophole provided by the 1921 Act to secure financial support from the local authority to maintain and educate maladjusted children but also because he was one of the few pioneers who saw sufficiently beyond his own institution to propose a comprehensive general scheme for the establishment and management of residential schools for the maladjusted.

Apart from his *Memorandum on the Establishment of Schools for Maladjusted Children* in 1948, which was never published, he seems to have written little, but both his widow and some of his surviving colleagues have been very helpful in providing me with material related to his life and work. He started his school at Dunnow Hall with three children and a staff of four, and at first had great difficulty in finding sufficient children who were diagnosed as maladjusted, and who could afford the fees, to add to the numbers. His first, unwelcome, expedient was to accept educationally sub-normal children. This made for great difficulties particularly, he found, in out-of-school activities. He then secured the support of St Helen's L.E.A., who were prepared to pay thirty to thirty-five shillings a week for children who required 'special' education. *The Clitheroe Advertiser and Times* (20 November 1936) announced that 'Dunnow Hall is ... to be recognized by the Board of Education as a school for all that large field of pupils whose existence has been very briefly and inadequately hinted at, i.e. those who are neither delinquent nor defective but in need of special forms of education. The School Medical Services are to make themselves responsible for the cost as an extension of their normal medical activities and thus one more attempt is being made to stop the waste of human activity, and increase the sum of happiness by training childhood in stabilized and intelligent adult life.' The number of children increased and the intelligence level rose.

At the beginning of the war the problems caused by evacuation resulted in a large increase in the number of children and a considerable decrease in the number of members of staff, most of whom were 'conscientious objectors' with little academic training. The school, however, survived, partly through the help of the Quakers in Yorkshire, and when it was re-organized under an Educational Trust in 1945, in accordance with the provisions of the Educational Act, the Society of Friends was represented on the committee together with L.E.A. representatives. Dr Fitch became the director.

In June 1948 the school was moved to Ledston Hall, near Castleford, an Elizabethan mansion which required a great deal of conversion to house the sixty children and ten teaching staff. When Dr

Fitch retired in 1952 the school was moved to Breckenbrough, near Thirsk, and a schoolmaster was appointed as head. The school still survives as a secondary special school for maladjusted boys.

> Lo! who dares say 'Do this,' who dares call down
> My will from its high purpose? Who say 'stand'
> Or 'go'? This mighty moment I would frown
> On abject Caesars – not the stoutest band
> Of mailed heroes should tear off my crown.
> Chip of organic members!
> Old Scholar of the Spheres!
> Thy spirit never slumbers
> But rolls about our ears.
> For ever and for ever!
> O what a mad endeavour
> Worketh he.

This Keatsian tribute to Dr Fitch appeared in the *Dunnow Hall Magazine* in July 1935. Already Dr Fitch had established himself as a somewhat authoritarian figure who, although he claimed to be a 'great believer in personal liberty', said in the same speech (7 August 1936): 'With the extraordinary swing in the opposite direction from Victorianism, with its repressive and inhibitive methods, the swing has been far too great, and there is an idea abroad that you have only to put knowledge in front of a child, and by some mysterious means it gets into that child. If that is the case then all I can say is that education is, and has been, entirely useless. . . . It [the child] has to be told many things and must learn what we all have to learn from statements of fact on the one hand to ordinary discipline on the other.'

There was a fixed timetable at Dunnow, although compulsion to attend classes was not absolute. Of discipline Mrs Fitch writes: 'In all things we sought a middle way between repressive discipline and entire and unguided freedom—aiming at tolerance and patience with the obstructive minority so far as it was compatible with the protection of the peaceable majority.' A school council of all senior pupils sat weekly at which school problems were discussed and weekly staff meetings were held 'when details of the children's social life, physical conditions, hereditary tendencies, and reactions were typed out and discussed in detail', and a plan of action evolved. It appears that in both meetings Dr Fitch frequently found himself 'giving detailed instructions' although in theory he objected to doing so.

Some of the instructions given to individual teachers about individual children read rather strangely to the modern ear, but at least reveal Dr Fitch as a man with his feet on the ground, not too concerned with the niceties of psychological jargon:

A. 'Backward and babyish. Shirker and piffler. Needs a firm hand and if need be a hard hand. Should never be allowed to get away with anything.'

B. 'A very firm hand. Incredibly untidy and slapdash. A nice child but needs keeping at a distance.'

L. 'Much more capable than he appears. Lazy, inert and slack (partly owing to early disease). Needs pushing hard. No notice should be taken of tears.'

R. '*Very* average mentally. In all ways a complete fathead. Will try to be the dear little girl if allowed.'

His largely untrained staff were further lectured on many aspects of modern psychological and psychopathological theory and practice which, together with their instructions, were doubtless modified in the light of that intuitive sympathy which is so essential to, and fortunately so often found in, workers with maladjusted children.

As one can see, one of Dr Fitch's most insistent contentions was that he was not dealing with abnormal children but with normal children who, when they could profit by the improved environment offered at Dunnow or Ledston, could be treated in a more or less normal way. Although a psychiatrist he did not attempt any intensive psychotherapy with his children. As Mrs Fitch says: 'Psychiatry with him was not a thing taken in sessions in a self-conscious way, but something that pervaded his whole life'; treatment was an apparently casual affair given 'as they needed it without their knowing they were having it'. When asked what he did with the children in his charge the answer was usually the same as W. H. Hunt's: 'Nothing at all!' 'The stimulation of personal interests and the removal of sources of chronic irritation were in themselves sufficient to cause maladjustment to disappear, or to disappear to a large extent.'[64]

As an administrator and organizer Dr Fitch must have had considerable ability and many of the organizational ideas which he put forward in the 1930s and 1940s were still being discussed and newly put into practice in the 1960s: co-education welcomed by the Underwood Report but still rarely implemented; the four-term year to prevent the regression that almost inevitably occurs when maladjusted children return to unsatisfactory homes for over-long summer holidays, and his interesting and original plan for the establishment of groups of schools for maladjusted children forming one unit with facilities for student teaching and psychiatric and psychological support.

A memorandum which he produced on this fundamental subject was in its scope and originality far beyond the possibilities of his own time, but not of ours, and was a distillation of many years of thoughtful practice. He envisaged units of three co-educational schools, junior, middle and senior, within easy reach of one another in the country but with the senior school, at least, within reach of a sizeable town. There would be accommodation in the senior school for probation, social science, medical and teaching students and there would be full-time psychiatric and psychological staff to oversee therapeutic, diagnostic and remedial work. A seaside hostel would be available to those children unable to go home during the holidays.

The staff should have a strong personal concern in the work but also well-developed lives of their own. A high proportion should be married. 'A deep belief in the human race, a wide tolerance, a profound love of children and a willingness to learn' are considered of more importance than academic or psychological qualifications. Discipline should, as far as possible, be based on the inculcation of normal social behaviour and it should be seen to exist as a necessary structure within which the individual child may feel secure. It should be 'a condition rather than an event and should be present throughout a carefully thought out and controlled milieu'. Punishment, where necessary, should take the form of voluntary expiation, unresented correction and logical restriction. It should be the 'logical consequence' of the act. Religion, acceptable to the children, should provide the 'external standard of reference'.

Dr Fitch considered that children of above average intelligence would profit most from the experience offered but stressed that intellectual attainment would be affected by the basic emotional disturbance, the origins of which he saw as stemming essentially from previous abnormal and 'illogical' environments. He hoped that, with the extension of child-guidance clinics, the majority of children would be referred early through local education authorities. Each school, containing no more than forty to fifty children, would be sub-divided for small-group work in academic and practical subjects and social activities. There would be considerable emphasis on remedial teaching in the basic subjects and arts and crafts would be encouraged as curricula and extra-curricula activities. Social activities would be carefully planned on the basis of family-groups guilds, which would also form the basis for discussion of school matters to be raised at the general meeting.

Looking beyond his time and its limitations he saw the immediate needs of work with maladjusted children as more such schools, more teachers, more psychologists trained in remedial teaching, more training facilities, and a clear administrative and lay distinction between the needs of the sub-normal and of the maladjusted.

Above all, where Drs Decroly and Claparède had stressed the value to normal children of methods evolved in work with abnormal children, Dr Fitch emphasized the importance of treating and educating maladjusted children as normal children with some special needs derived from their experience of abnormal circumstances.

REFERENCES

CHAPTER 8: The New Education

1 HOLMES, E. *What Is and What Might Be*, p 195. Constable, London, 1911.

2 For a more modern assessment of school as a factor in producing maladjustment *see* Scottish Education Department. *Pupils who are maladjusted because of Social Handicap*, Section 31, H.M.S.O., Edinburgh, 1952.

3 HOLMES, E. *Give Me the Young*, p 137. Constable, London, 1921.

4 ———. *In Defence of What Might Be*, Constable, London, 1914.

5 ———. *The Tragedy of Education*, Constable, London, 1913.

6 ———. *What Is and What Might Be*, (Ref. 1) p 247, 1911.

7 Ibid. *pp* 153–308.

8 HOLMES, C. *The Idiot Teacher*, Faber & Faber, London, 1952.

9 *See also* Woods, A. *Educational Experiments in England, pp* 143–155. Methuen, London, 1920.

10 PEKIN, L. B. *Progressive Schools*, The Hogarth Press, London, 1934.

11 STEINER, R. *The Education of Children from the Standpoint of Theosophy*. Theosophical Publishing Co., London, 1911.

12 EDMUNDS, L. F. *Rudolph Steiner Education*. Rudolph Steiner Publications, London, 1962.

13 STEWART, W. A. C. *The Educational Innovators*, 2, Chapter 8. Macmillan, London, 1968. (Excellent summary of Anthroposophical theory and practice).

14 CARLGREN, F. *Rudolph Steiner*, (2nd Edition) p 37. The Goetheanum School, Dornach. 1964.

15 WOODS, A. *Educational Experiments in England*, p 185. Methuen, London, 1920.

16 Ibid. *p* 106–107.

17 SIMPSON, J. H. *An Adventure in Education*, Sidgwick & Jackson, London, 1917.

18 ———. *A Schoolmaster's Harvest*, p 171. Faber & Faber, London, 1954.

19 ———. *An Adventure in Education*, (Ref. 17) p 188.

20 WOODS, A. op. cit., *p* 76.

21 O'CONNOR, D. J. *An Introduction to the Philosophy of Education*. *pp* 108–109. Routledge & Kegan Paul, London, 1958.

CHAPTER 9: The New Psychology

22 BADLEY, J. H. *A Schoolmaster's Testament*, Blackwell, London, 1937.
23 ISAACS, S. Some Notes on the Incidence of Neurotic Difficulties in Young Children. *Br. J. Ed. Psych.* **2.** (part 1) *pp* 71–91. 1932.
24 FRANCIS, L. in *Neill and Summerhill,* Walmsley J. (ed). Penguin, London, 1969.
25 NEILL, A. S. *Is Scotland Educated?* *p* 21. Herbert Jenkins, London, 1936.
26 Ibid. *pp* 25–26.
27 BOYD, W. & RAWSON, W. *The Story of the New Education, p* 26. Heinemann, London, 1965.
28 PEDLEY, R. *Comprehensive Education—A New Appraisal,* Gollancz, London, 1956.
29 NEILL, A. S. *Summerhill, p* 294. Gollancz, London, 1967.
30 MORRIS, VAN, C. *Existensialism in Education, p* 148. Harper & Row, New York. 1966.
31 NEILL, A. S. *The Free Child, p* 31. Herbert Jenkins, London, 1953.
32 ――――― *Summerhill,* (Ref. 29) *p* 296.
33 ――――― *The Free Child,* (Ref. 31). *pp* 133–4.
34 OLLENDORFF, I. *Wilhelm Reich.* Elek, London, 1969.
35 SKIDELSKY, R. *English Progressive Schools, p* 177. Penguin (Pelican), London, 1969.
36 NEILL, A. S. On Reich, in William Reich and the Sexual Revolution. *Anarchy* 105, *pp* 332–3. 1969.
37 REICH, W. *The Function of Orgasm.* Penguin, London, 1965.
38 NEILL, A. S. On Reich, (Ref. 36).
39 MORRIS, VAN. C. op. cit.
40 PEKIN, L. B. *Progressive Schools, pp* 156–7. Hogarth, London 1934.
41 BOYD, W. & RAWSON, W. op. cit., *p* 64.
42 MACMUNN, N. *A Path to Freedom in the School.* Curwen & Sons, London, 1914.
43 YOUNG, E. H. *The New Era in Education.* Phillips, London, 1920.
44 MACMUNN, N. op. cit., *p* 7.
45 Ibid. *pp* 114–7.
46 Ibid. *p* 115.
47 Ibid. *p* 134.
48 Ibid. *p* 7.
49 WALL, W. D. *Psychological Services for Schools, pp* 19-20. UNESCO. Institute for Education, Hamburg, 1956.
50 CAMERON, H. *The Nervous Child,* Oxford University Press, 1918.
51 DODD, F. H. *Commonsense Psychology and the Home.* Allen & Unwin, London, 1933.
52 Ibid. *p* 27.

53   Ibid. *p* 52.
54   Ibid. *p* 131.
55   PERSONAL COMMUNICATION.
56   The Underwood Report. Section 43, 1955.
57   BURT, C., in *The Year Book of Education. pp* 91–2. 1955.
58   ――― *The Young Delinquent.* University of London Press, London, 1925.
59   FULTON, J. F. Factors influencing the growth and pattern of the child guidance services and school psychological services in Britain from 1900 to the present time. *p* 57. M. A. Thesis, unpublished, Queen's University, Belfast, 1964.
60   STEVENSON, G. and SMITH, G. *Child Guidance Clinics*: a quarter century of development. Commonwealth Fund, New York, 1934.
61   NUNN, P., quoted in Keir G. A History of Child Guidance, *p* 23. *Br. J. Ed. Psych.* **xxii.** (1). 1952.
62   KEIR, G. Ibid. *p* 24.
63   PRITCHARD, D. G. *Education and the Handicapped 1760–1960, p* 194. Routledge & Kegan Paul, London, 1963.
64   *The Clitheroe Advertiser and Times*, 7 August, 1936.

PART FIVE

Contrasting Communities

10

Finchden Manor and George Lyward

If men are made the recipients of understanding love, they may learn to accept the interests of others as equal to their own, submit to the rule of law and be admitted in common fellowship. — T. S. Simey, The Concept of Love in Child Care Oxford University Press: 1961.

Although the general rethinking of education and psychology had a considerable and sometimes direct effect on the treatment of mal-adjusted children, the inter-war period was marked mainly by the growth of a number of communities notable for their differences in basic ethos. Although one can perceive certain antecedents, precise chronology is of little significance when considering work of such an individual nature. The pioneer at the centre of the community owed only one debt to time. Experiment was at first tolerated and then appreciated and encouraged by an increasing number of people aware of the problems. Moreover, new approaches based on personal ideologies were still, at this time, free of the necessity of academic empirical justification. Individuals were, therefore, free to demon-strate the effectiveness of communities derived from their beliefs, and were not inhibited, as we may now be over-much, by a com-pulsion to await research evidence in a field in which such evidence has always been negligible.

George Lyward is rare in this field in that he was, for sixteen years, a schoolmaster. Education, in the widest sense, was his means and end, transmitted through a person who was not only deeply educated but inspired by a profound love of others. Although he began his career in the 'new era' of education he did not so much rebel against traditional schooling as realize its inadequacies. He taught with an intuitive recognition of the needs of other persons and conceived education to be a co-operative and creative enterprise aiming at the quality rather than the quantity of the response. This he found led not only to better 'results', in the conventional sense, but also the development of understanding in depth — a process

161

F

which took 'time, growth, and inner consolidation'. Thus, as a house-master at Glenalmond in the 1920s he found that he could use his position as a sixth-form teacher, a rugby coach and a housemaster to create an atmosphere in which real education was possible. He remarks that: 'It is an irony of my life that I came to healing through a discovery of how to use "subjects" to release and emotionally re-educate young people, but now have so frequently to plead or insist that they should be protected from subject-teaching in so far as it can do harm.'[1]

For Lyward the step from education to therapy did not exist. His object was to teach, and to allow, his pupils to think. 'To think is to be released from the tyranny of feelings. Head and heart together is the way to fuller life and richer relationships.' Again: 'We should teach to the feeling for the sake of the thinking, for the sake of the subject, and still more for the sake of the child. It is only what he makes his own that helps him to think clearly; to live not posses-sively. To make his own he must see, synthesize, and seek and find unity. He must not merely analyse or accumulate and so lose gradually the power of keeping alive to the "mysterious, threaten-ing soul-searching realm of being which lies behind and within the sphere in which organization achieves its ends".'[2] The alternative is a schizophrenic disunity of thought and feeling.

It is this belief in the unknowable and inexpressible, in the mysterious and poetic nature of life, and in the almost incidental existence of organizational substructures, which makes Lyward's work so difficult to describe. It has to be viewed in metaphysical rather than sociological or psychological terms. Superficially, as I have suggested, there is a chronology and there are certain discernible characteristics.

Lyward left Glenalmond in 1928 having, according to the chairman of the governors, raised the standard of work by 40 per cent in the fifteen years he was there.[3] In 1930 he began his therapeutic re-educational work with two boys in a Kentish farmhouse—Guild-ables—and, five years later, moved to Finchden Manor. Finchden is a small Elizabethan manor-house near Tenterden with a particu-larly peaceful air of having grown from the soil. As Lyward says, 'not adapted but lovingly adopted'. It now houses a community of fifty-five young men, normally of between sixteen and twenty-four years of age. Before the Second World War his work was mainly with ex-public school boys but after the Education Act of 1944 money became available to widen his clientele. The staff, one or two of whom have themselves been boys at Finchden, also include adults who are glad to share, for a longer or shorter time, the therapeutic environment of Finchden Manor. Others come drawn to the experience of working with Lyward.

Because Lyward holds 'strong wishes about the dead wood in education, about pressure, about early specialization, of the way in which subject teaching of a certain kind can rob a school community of depth of group life; and how the subject teaching suffers also',[4] academic education at Finchden is at first indirect and then tutorial, and dependent on the varying skills and experience of the members of staff and, even more, on the members' ability to learn for themselves. Study, like the discipline of relationship, is based on individual need and especially on spontaneous sharing, as are other aspects of the community's life. Drama and the arts are encouraged and some very interesting work is done in pottery. Individuals take public examinations but any pressure to do so comes from a healthy recognition of the needs of ordinary life. The emphasis remains always on therapy.

Michael Burn, the author of *Mr Lyward's Answer,* who himself spent a considerable time at Finchden, said that Mr Lyward made no claim for his community other than it was one. Burn nevertheless claims that in the first twenty-two years of its existence 290 people —men, women and children—had lived in the community and that, apart from ninety who left before treatment was completed, 'nearly all ... have settled down, some in distinguished careers, many in jobs which would have appeared fantastic when they came'. These are not 'hard' figures but they impress particularly in relation to the severity of the 'cases'—often sent to Finchden as a last hope.

Many of the members have suffered in various ways from the inadequacy of substitute parents and from disturbance largely occasioned by failure to adjust in adolescence to the demands of the so-called adult world. With many the disturbance was very severe, causing trouble with the police or making the youth completely unacceptable either in his own or a substitute home. They are immature because they have never experienced the reality of childhood. They come to Finchden because 'however they may look, and however big and cleverly they may talk, they may in truth be no more than seven-year-olds with an L sign'. It is Lyward's task to reduce the unbearable tensions of adolescence by easing the transition from childhood to adolescence in a relaxed atmosphere which enables them to re-live and to re-grow. Such an adolescent is tied to his childhood because the problems of this period have not been resolved and yet he is conscious of the demands of adolescent status. While inwardly there is confusion, doubt, guilt and humiliation, 'outwardly there is chiefly a vague sense of confusion, frustration and defiance and a determination at all costs to keep hold on the adult world in which he feels he must at all costs maintain a stake'.[5] The adolescent must not only be allowed to experience his past but its hold on him must be relaxed. Within the tolerant atmosphere and emotional security of Finchden both processes are possible and fear and guilt can progressively vanish away.

In the early years at Finchden deep analysis played an important part in treatment, but increasingly the deepened group life was allowed to loosen the bonds. At the beginning the boy was allowed to regress to the fullest extent necessary in an atmosphere of almost complete acceptance. He was then gradually 'weaned' towards the joy of interdependence within the body politic of the community.

This concept of 'weaning' away from childhood and towards a rebirth into adulthood is central.

At puberty the child becomes something of an adult physically. But the word adult should not really be used about anybody who is only physically changed and who has yet, himself, to play his part in the translation of his childhood experiences. If he is to move towards a full life, he must so grow that these experiences shall no longer hold him to a life in which they are merely repeated in a disguised form, but shall be revised (seen anew) and recognized for what they *were* as distinguished from what he felt them to be at the time. Otherwise he will remain in bondage to the past and be, for the most part unconsciously, a good boy or a rebel, both something less than a man.

It takes the whole of the period of adolescence for this bondage to be cleared. Or rather – and this alteration is important – until it *is* cleared the child has not become an adult, whatever be his age in years and however sound his intellectual valuations.[6]

The boy must first be given his childhood back. He must not remain unchildlike merely for fear of sometimes being childish and doing childish things. 'If they don't do them now they'll do much worse things later.' The process of rehabilitation started, boys who for a long period have perhaps wandered aimlessly around attach themselves to a person or an interest. The members of staff become mediators. At this point challenges become inevitable and a boy's adjustment is frequently tested by a sudden or gradual arrival at what may well seem a merely arbitrary restriction. An attitude towards one's self as part of a community is nourished until eventually the boy is involved in what is seen as a surrender. 'It is at such a moment that insight is important, insight rather than any planned technique. The challenge may come in the refusal of . . . money, while he sees his friend receiving ten shillings, or it may come in the sudden gift of twenty pounds to start a hobby. A reasoned argument may be met by a reasoned reply, or by an apparently irrational quip, a deliberate deflection or frustration of thought. Insight sees beneath the request, the argument, the rude remark, to the need from which these spring; and the action meets the need not the gesture'[7] — although it may, at other times, and for the same purposes, meet the gesture.

The boys' ideas of themselves are challenged and a rebirth is required. Unhampered by a fear of criticism they are forced back upon the unknown self. The acceptance of the community is almost complete. One boy wrote to Mr Lyward: 'You began the operation of stripping off my outer skins. Life has removed most of the others. I feel singularly naked but I am beginning to enjoy life.'[8]

This dynamic process involves certain special approaches to 'discipline' and to 'love', which Lyward considers necessary if the adolescent is to be regulated into some creativity. 'Self-government' Lyward rejects as 'an extra, liable to be served out in little parcels, and no solution for the boy's tautness, being only another kind of imprisoning formalism',[9] although he recognizes that self-government may have some value as a sort of institutional compost: 'It is as recurring opportunities of breaking up the institutional soil that "self-government" should chiefly be welcomed and emulated.'[10] On the other hand, formal discipline which brings about a premature crystallization is considered suspect. 'The secret of discipline lies largely in being casual, for that leaves both parties on the same side. . . . True discipline is that which maintains fellowship.'[11]

Great emphasis is put on flexibility, play and humour, and sometimes sheer nonsense, in maintaining the necessary 'flow'. 'Let us see to it that our children's communities are real havens, sensitive to rhythm magic circles within which the children can meet with uncertainties and unfairnesses and as a result become aware of the giver and thus know our membership one of another. Then they will not cling to the gift. Then they will develop a strength which will allow them to re-dedicate themselves to something more challenging than any system or than any state.'[12] Certain arbitrarily chosen 'possibilities' recur as part of the game. 'If you read a paper at mealtime you are liable (not certain) to have it torn up—this is part of the tradition. If you were there and I walked in, you might see the paper quickly sat on, but again the atmosphere is not made tense by rules and sanctions! If you are found smoking in bed, you are liable to have a bucket of water thrown over you, because you are on fire. The play is not lost, even then. Sternness need not be moralizing.'

The essence is to keep a rhythmic flow in people who are 'everything by starts and nothing long' and so to work towards analysis and synthesis. 'Prior to analysis the elements are sustained in a vital rhythmic connection, and it is that vitality which we need to maintain in community life.'[13]

To Lyward the development of a sense of individuality, however important, is but a first step to the development of a sense of 'oneness'. In this development the community acts as a microcosm of humanity and ultimately of universal existence. The process of analysis and synthesis is not scientific but poetic, the aim being the unification of disparate but related parts, both in and out of time and space, to create a 'one-ness' of the logos of the soul which, in Heraclitus' term, has no discoverable frontiers. In this pursuit, Lyward sees not only the hope of the fulfilled, because related, individual but the only hope for the continuance of civilization.

In terms of daily living this alchemy often transmutes through conditions of 'much admired disorder', within a security which is the product of, and promotes awareness of, love as a reality.

'Stern love' is a term which Lyward uses frequently. In stressing the need for stern discipline in therapy Lyward cites as interview with a 'tough guy' seeking admission to Finchden.

'I asked him straight away what he would really choose if I could give it to him and he blurted out immediately: "An 'ome and I'd 'ave one if that bloody lodger hadn't gone off with my mum."

' "Would you like to have stern love here?" (adding to myself, "as distinguished from strict rules")....

' "I've never 'ad that kind: it sounds a better kind as long as it's still love." So he had it in a community where, as in all true communities, the psychological and moral approaches can to some extent be left to weave themselves together, so that the moral is not abrogated but deepened in meaning; given meaning, I would almost say.'[14]

'Love is not love which alters when it alteration finds,' although the demands that it makes will change as the members' needs alter. Some of the demands will appear inconsistent for, as has already been mentioned, Lyward frequently refuses 'reasonable' requests from a boy who, he feels, is, as it were, asking to be tested and challenged in order to establish for himself 'a secure relationship between two people who know how to give and take'. The rationale of this part of Lyward's technique, which is often misunderstood, he explains thus:

The real secret of living in a House with children is to know how to be creative in taking away and in being 'unfair' and haphazard, so that the gift shall never deny the children increasing awareness of the giver. Most people know what we must give to the children. But the kind of giving that can include 'taking away' and yet be known for giving — that is what is needed. Else you have missed the 'deeps'. Such 'unfairness' can be one of the chief ways of producing a deeper sense of security, and where this is being successfully achieved, 'please' and 'thank you' are not so much polite words frequently heard from those under an obligation, as echoes (sometimes shy, sometimes exuberant) of something heartfelt.[15]

The atmosphere becomes one of challenge to break the restrictive barriers of self and ultimately to accept the obligations of an individual in society. 'Love of the strong kind is surely an act of creation.'[16]

Through understanding and love the will is finally 'baptized into reality'. 'Behind frailty and the trouble it causes is love and its power —love locked out or loved locked in, whichever you will. Our love, yours and mine, can, it is true, open the door. Their wills—or shall we say their power of willing spontaneously and intelligently—will become more certainly theirs to surrender to the Highest they know.'[17]

11

Red Hill School and Otto Shaw

Otto Shaw's role as a father-figure is a less Olympian, because a more specific, one in that, as a psychoanalyst, it is a role projected on him in the 'transference' stage of analysis. It is complicated, however, by the fact that he is also the principal of his school and is thus inevitably cast in a more general paternal role by those under his direction. This duality occasions considerable comment from those who, like A. S. Neill, Shaw's earliest educational mentor, have discovered from experience that 'man cannot play both of these roles'. Slavson writes 'among difficulties one encounters in the practice of interview group therapy in institutions is the inevitable contacts that the patients and the therapist have with each other at times other than the regular, set, sessions, and that the patients find it difficult to dissociate the therapist from the restraining and sometimes punishing role of other members of staff. This situation greatly complicates the transference relation, mobilizes its negative aspects, intensifies and prolongs resistance.'[18] How much more true this must be of individual analysis particularly if it is conducted by someone who is himself the ultimate source of authority.

Shaw himself is fully aware that 'we are extremely vulnerable to this danger' and agrees that 'It is unfortunately a practical and well established and documented fact that it is desirable that an analysand has little or no social contact with the analyst outside the treatment situation.' He endeavours to maintain this social distance with a boy at least until the treatment is nearly completed and relies on other members of his staff to fill the gap. 'Hazards necessarily occur in the practical situations arising from analysis, but the devil must be allowed to score a few points sometimes. As a successful analysis proceeds, the pitfalls become more a matter of routine and cease to provide difficulties and, with a complete analysis, the difficulties neither arise in private nor in public. That, of course, is the result we aim at and which good fortune allows us to accomplish so frequently.'[19]

Although, I think, there is now no other analyst headmaster in Britain, a dual role is found in current American practice, and Bruno Bettelheim points out in justification of his own counsellor therapist organization in the University of Chicago Sonia Shankman Orthogenic School that the procedure 'follows the classical first case of the psychoanalytical treatment of children—the case of Little Hans, where the father himself was the therapist'.[20, 21]

RESULTS

Shaw's real justification lies in the apparent success of his method. This is systematically and thoroughly documented in a way which is unfortunately most unusual in special schools. Since 1934 contact with local education authorities, psychiatric social workers, probation officers, parents and former pupils has provided data for the annual report on what has been achieved at Red Hill School. The criteria of adjustment are clearly stated in general terms. 'The term "cured" means that a radical resolution of the child's maladjustment took place and the after-history shows the boy to be balanced, happy and contented. To be "improved" means that the child now earns its living usefully, has not been in trouble with the law and is most unlikely to be in that trouble, but that the resolution of its conflicts is incomplete. Superficially the "improved" cases seem well and orderly.'

The 1968 report on those children with whom effective contact had been maintained (almost all since 1934) reveals:

Cured	242
Cured/improved	29
Improved	44
Improved/failures	6
Failures	40
Withdrawn prematurely	28
Dead	7

Shaw also reports that 'During the same time, ninety-eight boys have married fiancées to whom most had previously introduced us. Of these we find all are successful and happy families in what seem to be a loving and religious sense, except in six cases. Fourteen others have consulted us from time to time about marriage difficulties which fortunately appeared susceptible to our counsel. Of the six bad cases, two have re-married and we feel all will go well.'[22]

The success which this impressive record illustrates has not been confined to those aggressive, extraverted boys who appear particularly suited to analytical techniques, but have included many passive, introverted, anxious boys who have responded to a more gradual, and sometimes less specific, psychotherapy. Only with schizophrenic children does Shaw admit the absolute failure of analytic techniques to effect cure.[23]

When it is realized that the vast majority of the children treated arrive at Red Hill suffering from acute emotional disturbances derived largely from broken, harmful or inadequate families or traumatic experiences in early childhood, the methods used demand study.

PSYCHOTHERAPY

Formal psychoanalysis is undertaken in the school by Shaw himself and by two other lay analysts on the staff, and is supplemented when necessary by a consultant psychiatrist, who is not in any way involved in the structure of the school, and by some work done in hospital clinics. The child himself must express a wish for treatment and all material uncovered in analytical sessions is strictly confidential and is never referred to in the general context of the school. The period of treatment varies but may last for most of the four or five years which the boys normally stay at school since it is continued beyond the point at which the superficial signs of disturbance have disappeared in order to secure a fundamental readjustment. Therapy takes precedence over all academic work—which cannot normally be tackled successfully until the underlying disturbance is dealt with—but creative art work is encouraged not only as valuable in itself but for the light which it may throw on the child's condition.

The aim of all analytical work, of whatever persuasion, is to achieve in the analysand an understanding of himself through the uncovering of his unconscious motivation. This, as far as the analyst is concerned, may be a largely passive process in which his chief role is to act as the focus for his client's projection, through the process of 'transference' (as in classical Freudian analysis), or it may involve more active interpretation direct to the client as a means of encouraging understanding to be interpreted in action (as in the Adlerian and Kleinian approaches).

Shaw's analytical approach derives basically from Melanie Klein, although his own analysis was Jungian. This orientation can clearly be explained in terms of the special position which Klein gives to the mother-child relationship as an explanation of the neuroses of very many seriously disturbed boys. To a Kleinian the origins of profound disorder are likely to lie in the pre-Oedipal relationship of mother and child in the first two years. At this stage the infant, it is suggested, being completely dependent on the mother for all that appears good (satisfying) or bad (painful), projects on to her innate feelings of aggression which can then generate more aggression (derived from fear) or depression (derived from guilt) which are subsequently both internalized, to damage the maladjusted child, or externalized in a delinquent way, to damage society.

It is the analyst's job to explore a wide range of aggressive and sexually-derived fantasies stemming from this infantile experience and often becoming more specific in the Oedipal terms of the desire for sexual experience of the mother and destruction of the father. These fantasies are often either internalized into a desire to have the characteristics of motherhood—breasts, vagina, etc.—or the physical potency of the father, or a pathological urge to destroy those maternal attributes which have failed to supply adequate comfort.

In exploring the fantasies and the behaviour derived from them (sexual-sadism, anal eroticism, transvestitism, homosexuality, murderous aggression, fetishism, pornographic attitudes to sex, stealing for symbolic purposes etc.) the analyst seeks to give the analysand the insight which will enable him both to understand his behaviour and to modify it.

Shaw gives many detailed examples of his work in his two books, *Maladjusted Boys* and *Prisons of the Mind,* and a brief summary of one of his cases may help to clarify his approach.

Donald, originally referred for stealing, unable to make satisfactory relationships with his peers or teachers and unable to apply himself to academic work, was for two years coped with in the understanding and tolerant atmosphere of the school. At this stage, when he had acquired some status in the school, he was caught stealing female underwear and was persuaded to consult Shaw. In analytical sessions the boy revealed extreme transvestite behaviour in which he would induce orgasm by dressing in female garments and strapping his penis to himself in such a way as to conceal it. His delinquent and anti-social behaviour he explained as a form of protest against his own abnormality.

The first explanation offered for his behaviour was intense jealousy of his younger sister, whose feminine attributes he envied. This jealousy produced intensely sadistic sexual fantasies in which these attributes, or alternatively his own masculine attributes, were mutilated or destroyed. In particular, at this stage, he referred to mutilation of the breast and this he was shown as arising from an original agression against his mother. Envy of his mother's maternal powers had transferred to jealousy of his sister, as female, and to a desire to un-sex himself.

At this point Shaw explained that Donald could modify his behaviour only when he realized

that your mother really does love you in a way now suited to your age, just as she loved you by feeding you at her breast when you were a baby. You will stop it too when you realize that your sister has a right to her breast as well, and that right was not won by excluding you. The right was taken up when you no longer had need for your mother's love to be expressed in those terms. So let us try hard to see what is after all only the truth, that your mother does love you and in a metaphorical way is prepared to give you her breast, though obviously at your age you cannot expect to suck a nipple. Of course, you try to do it sometimes by pinching cigarettes. Sometimes you try to do it by nibbling your pencils, and by all the other little phallic tricks like the nightly fantasy of getting people to suck your own 'do it youself nipple' (his penis).

After two years of analysis the boy seemed well adjusted in his behaviour but then developed an acute hostility to Shaw which was interpreted and resolved in terms of an Oedipus complex and the transference of the hated and envied father's role to the analyst.

Outside the context of Kleinian theory these interpretations may sound at best speculative but they were sufficiently accepted by the boy as explanations of his agonizing disorder that he made a startling improvement, both socially and academically, secured a place at university, became an industrial chemist and achieved a satisfactory emotional balance.[24]

Shaw gives many other comparable examples within the context of the same rationale and it is necessary to accept the rationale before it is possible to agree with such assertions as 'When maladjusted children commit such offences as breaking into cigarette machines or any box or container of objects they consider to be of value, it is a reasonable assumption that they are subconsciously breaking into some female part they regard as locked against them',[25] or that the stealing of bicycles is a symbolic theft of the desired breasts in the form of two round wheels.

One can, however, say with some conviction that the techniques used appear to succeed and an enquiry conducted by Shaw between 1943 and 1945 indicated that the children (at this time both boys and girls) saw psychotherapy as the most important reformative influence of all those at work within the context of the school. Some of their comments are interesting:

I have found that with analysis I have been relieved of many a worry which could not be quelled by presents or pleasant words. Also I have found help in troublesome matters which would have remained on my nerves or which I would be continually thinking about. Also matters which I was not competent enough in doing or in which I might have slipped up in. Advice and knowledge has been given to me through analysis too.

I think analysis is a good thing as you get all the worries off your mind in confidence and therefore can be dealt with constructively.

Analysis undoubtedly heads the list, the opportunity to strengthen difficulties is invaluable.[26]

Shaw also speaks of analysis as 'a solution which goes right to the bottom of the difficulty'. He says 'We seek not only to understand the child, but to make the child understand himself, so that his relationships with other people may be improved, and the resulting contentment will allow genius to show itself; he will be able to make a successful marriage which will bear fruit in the happiness of his children.'[27] The process is difficult and the child has to accept that in the pursuit of the child's happiness the analyst 'will discover the deeper strata of even more confusing and even more sinister ills' but the process will be accompanied by love, the burden eased by confession, and the child given mastery of himself.

Shaw is not a purist and admits to the use of many unorthodox procedures. He resorts, if he thinks it necessary, to what he calls 'trick psychology' and he has been much criticized for his technique, in one case, of rewarding a boy for stealing in order to demonstrate the symbolic nature of the act. His justification in this and similar cases is that it works. 'The child's welfare is paramount, and when it is felt that different techniques might promise results even if they disobey the rules of analysis those techniques are promptly brought into use.'[28] Above all he ignores the Kleinian injunction not to seek the co-operation of parents and, in fact, values their contribution to his understanding of the total situation.

He does not, moreover, despise other forms of therapy and is concerned to establish a total therapeutic environment. 'Informal therapy is, ideally, a part of all relationships between adult and child from the time of waking up in the morning to falling asleep at night.'[29] At Red Hill the staff, while not rejecting the real parents, accept a parent/guardian role expressed in terms of love, care, tolerance and concern. The homes of staff members are used readily by the boys and the staff have the advantages over 'real' parents in that they are on the whole more trained in therapy, they are without parental feelings of guilt, they have the advice and support of colleagues, and the school 'court' and other representative organizations remove from them much of the responsibility of everyday discipline which may, in normal families, produce conflict.

ORGANIZATION

The court, in which the boys are encouraged to talk out their problems and grievances, also applies sanctions (normally in the form of acts of restitution) against those boys who have offended against the pupil-generated laws or who have committed delinquent acts which are considered to be within their control. Even when delinquent acts are seen as an inevitable part of a pupil's condition such reasonable sanctions may be applied to 'keep the matter alive in the delinquent's mind, and perhaps emphasize to him the very real nature of his problem and the even greater urgency of an effective solution to it'.[30] The court is one part of the elaborate self-governing structure of the school which performs the multiple function of running the day-to-day affairs of the school, giving intelligent boys meaningful experience of responsible government, acting as a form of low-level group therapy and relieving the headmaster/ analyst of some of the onus and peculiar difficulty of being the centre of authority in the school. The functions of chairman and committee secretaries are regarded as of great importance and there is underlying belief in the principle of 'cabinet responsibility'. The organizational structure is unusually complex and may, perhaps, best be explained diagramatically.

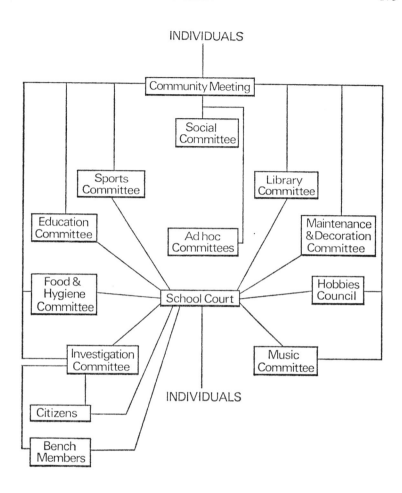

INDIVIDUALS

Community Meeting

Social Committee

Sports Committee

Library Committee

Education Committee

Ad hoc Committees

Maintenance &Decoration Committee

Food & Hygiene Committee

School Court

Hobbies Council

Investigation Committee

Music Committee

INDIVIDUALS

Citizens

Bench Members

Self-governing Structure of Red Hill School

TITLE	COMPOSITION	METHOD OF ELECTION	FUNCTION	MEETINGS	POWERS	Category
Community Meeting	Chairman & two Deputies; Chairmen of Committees; Whole School (pupils & staff)	Nominated by Meeting; Elected by committees; Selected by Otto Shaw	To receive reports, suggestions and complaints on committees; To make recommendations to committees	Fortnightly	To enforce community control over administrative committees	Legislative
Bench Members Meeting	10 senior boys	Co-opted with ratification by staff	Judicial; Introducing new boys to school system; Leadership of committees; Administrative Duties	Fortnightly; Separately and jointly with citizens	Control of citizen membership and court; Some executive function	Executive
Citizens Meeting	12–14 boys	Co-opted; Ratified by bench members	As for bench members	Fortnightly; Separately and jointly with bench	Share general functions of bench	
Food & hygiene	Co-opted member of staff; Elected chairman and secretary; Sufficient other members	Selected by existing chairmen and secretaries; Meeting as ad hoc committees every 6 months	Responsibility with cook for kitchen & dining room	As often as necessary but not less than once a week	Organisation and Administration of particular areas of activity	Administration
Sports			Fixtures, use of facilities etc.			
Social			Indoor pastimes, parties, entertainment			
Library			Administering Library			
Maintenance Decoration			Furniture, fittings, repairs etc.			
Hobbies council			Clubs, Hobbies other group activities			
Music			Music practice & performance			
Education						
Ad hoc Committees	Chairman; Secretary; Sufficient others	Election by Community Meeting	To investigate particular problems, e.g. smoking; Selection of committees at 6-monthly intervals	As required	To suggest a course of action and methods of enforcement	
School Court	2 bench members; 1 citizen; all pupils and staff present	Rotation	To investigate complaints and school offences; To give advice	Twice weekly; Setting as a judicial court	To impose fines or loss of privileges	Judiciary

ACADEMIC WORK

Another unusual aspect of Red Hill School as a school for maladjusted children is the importance attached to academic work.[31]
'The classroom is considered a basis for academic work and procedures should have as much resemblance as possible to those in
other schools'. The classroom atmosphere is free and pleasant and in
the classroom teachers are vested with all the authority found in
normal schools. There is a fixed timetable, lessons are compulsory,
and standards of punctuality, neatness and general attitude are
expected to be high. GCE examinations at A and O levels are
attempted (sometimes in stages to overcome tension), and in the
upper forms work becomes increasingly formal, particularly—
apparently—in history, geography and maths. Creative activity in
art and writing is encouraged by the staging of London exhibitions
and by the production of a monthly school magazine. Music, since it
imposes a more exacting discipline, is a minor and voluntary activity
largely functioning through informal 'pop' groups.

  In only two important ways does the structure appear to differ
from that of the normal, fairly progressive grammar school. Classes,
which are graded largely on a basis of verbal ability, contain
normally not more than from eight to twelve boys, which allows for
an individual approach in teaching; secondly (or rather of primary
importance) academic work is considered subordinate to the therapeutic process and conditions must allow for particular disturbances
of intellectual functioning, e.g. inability to do maths, which it is
anticipated will adjust themselves as the pupil acquires insight into
his own difficulties. The classroom is, in fact, considered as a testing
ground for the level of adjustment achieved. The whole delicate
machinery is kept in balance by the headmaster/analyst who is the
only one who has the full knowledge of all the subtle factors involved.

  As in other aspects of the school's work results are impressive.
In the academic year ending in June 1968, not an exceptional year in
this school for forty boys, GCE results were as follows:

ADVANCED LEVEL

	Pass	Fail	Total
English	3	0	3
History	3	0	3
French	1	0	1

ORDINARY LEVEL

	Pass	Fail	Total
Art	11	3	14
Chemistry	2	1	3
English Language	4	11	15
English Literature	2	8	10
French	5	2	7
Geography	5	3	8
History	4	4	8
Mathematics	5	1	6
Physics	1	1	2

In the subsequent year thirteen pupils were included in one or more A level courses, involving all subjects in the general curriculum except geography. Of these, seven were working on three subjects each.[32] Many pupils then go on to university.

It is obvious, and Shaw freely admits, that such success can be partly attributed to the original selection of pupils of very high potential ability with I.Q.s of 130 plus. Most of the pupils, however, enter the school unable to release their full potential, and academic successes are as much the result of successful therapy as of excellent teaching and innate ability. Pupils are selected not only for their potential ability to profit by an academic education but also for their appropriateness for the type of therapy available. Shaw writes: 'There seems to be nothing unfair and improper in choosing only gifted children for our treatment: we should be adding to general folly if we chose children who could not be cured, and attempted to cure them.'[33]

The freedom which Shaw has in the selection of his pupils is crucial to the whole operation. The boys are selected not only because their high intelligence makes analytical interpretations and verbalizing more possible but also on a basis of the sort of presenting neurosis which Shaw considers particularly suited to his interpretation. Essentially, the boys have to wish to seek the sort of help which Shaw offers and to co-operate in the process. Although this may greatly narrow the range of the work at Red Hill it allows for considerable depth of approach to one very significant area of disturbance.

This may also help to explain the success of the school as a social and educational institution. Since the problems were emotional and personal in origin they may well be less disruptive to the elaborate school organization of responsible government than problems largely of social origin, and less disruptive to educational structure than problems arising directly from learning experiences.

Shaw, born in 1908 into a conventional, conservative and stable family, was not by profession either a schoolteacher or an analyst. Until the early 1930s he was a petroleum technologist and then, as he describes in *Maladjusted Boys,* he 'read, by chance, a book on education in freedom by A. S. Neill. Reeling from the iconoclastic impact [he] read more by the same author' and visited Summerhill 'The freedom, joy and contentment of the school laid the foundation for a change of vocation.' Inspired by Neill and 'reading of Freud, Stekel, Fenechel, Glover, Heyer, Jung, Adler, Reik, Aichhorn, Groddeck and many other lesser but pioneer lights followed, ballasted by studying the records of St Vincent de Paul, St John de Bosco, St Ignatius and St Francis, who all discovered ways of loving unlovable people'.[34] After himself being psychoanalysed and after an intensive study of delinquency and current methods of dealing with it he felt ready to begin Red Hill as a residential school for intelligent maladjusted boys and girls of secondary-school age in 1934. He began 'with the strong belief that to understand is to cure. Later years modified that naiveté.' In truth it would be impossible for anyone of Shaw's temperament to try to practice a technique appropriate to Neill. In the treatment of maladjusted children one golden rule stands out above all others — 'This above all: to thine own self be true' — and this is one reason why pioneer work with maladjusted children has been so difficult to generalize from. Particularly in the 1920s and 30s each school was first an expression of the personality of its director and it is perhaps fortunate, since there were so few schools, that there were so many different personalities being expressed through them.

Originally founded in suburban Chislehurst, the school moved to its present site at East Sutton, near Maidstone, in 1935. It was supported by the local education authority (under the 1921 Act) in 1941 and, like Dunnow, was reorganized as a charitable trust in accordance with the provisions of the 1944 Education Act, and was recognized by the Ministry of Education as 'a Grammar School for the education and psychological treatment of maladjusted boys of very high intelligence'.

Few have attempted to follow Otto Shaw's example directly, few are qualified to do so, but his influence has been considerable—directly, through his writing, and through his work for the Association of Workers for Maladjusted Children, of which he was a founder and the first secretary. His work as a magistrate has also been notable and influential. His school has not been widely imitated but he considers that, given the analysts, it could and should be. In urging the extension of the principle he is appropriately echoing the words of Melanie Klein, who looked towards a Utopian future when 'child analysis will become as much part of every person's upbringing as school education is now'.[35]

12

The Hawkspur Camp and David Wills

David Wills began his career as a 'brother' in W. H. Hunt's Wallingford Farm Training Colony in 1922 at the age of nineteen and, to some extent, retains the mark, brotherhood rather than paternalism remaining his objective although inevitably others have cast him in the role of father. His experience at Wallingford was traumatic and of the greatest significance both to him and to all who have accepted his principles of education. Being frightened of losing the 'respect' which he had been led to believe was essential, and being new, inexperienced 'and in a state of despairing terror', Wills became a tyrant and a bully. Eventually understanding came and he saw that ' "discipline" derives largely from a fear of the persons on whom it is imposed. It arises also, of course, from the satisfaction we derive from having power over our fellow creatures.'[36]

This was no sudden 'road to Damascus' conversion. Wallingford, which had been preceded by Wills's own unhappy elementary-school experience, was followed by much further study. After a Social Study Diploma course at Birmingham University, Wills became the first Englishman to complete training in America as a psychiatric social worker, as a Willard-Straight Fellow of the New York School of Social Work. This was followed by four years in adult education in which Wills continued the evolution of that Christian humanism which characterizes him. The publication of Miss Bazeley's book on Homer Lane[37] and Lane's own *Talks to Parents and Children* coincide with the progress of his thought 'at a time when I thought I was, so to speak, alone'. He was subsequently much encouraged by reading of Aichhorn's work with delinquents in Austria,[38] and sharing his 'aloneness' with a friend, Stuart Payne, with whom he evolved a plan for a therapeutic environment for problem children, and in particular for young offenders, which was later published in *The Friend*.

THE HAWKSPUR EXPERIMENT

This plan attracted the attention of Dr Marjorie Franklin (see

181

Chapter 15), the inspiration behind the Q Camps committee, which was formed in 1934 to put into practice with disturbed social misfits the principles of the Grith Pioneers, an organization promoting camps for normal youths to demonstrate the benefits of 'pioneering' and self-government as an educational experience.[39] The Q (for query or quest) venture was specifically directed to the needs of delinquent youths, and the chairman of the committee was Cuthbert Rutter, an ex-Borstal housemaster who was, at the time, endeavouring to experiment with progressive methods in his own Forest School. The Grith Pioneers were represented by Dr Norman Glaister, a man of original ideas on the organization of communities, which stemmed to some extent from his work in the field of mental health, although owing much to early ideas of open-air education and therapy (see Chapter 8).

David Wills was asked to become 'Camp Chief' and after resigning his job as co-warden (with his wife) of the Risca Educational Settlement in Wales, and gaining further experience as housemaster at Rochester Borstal, he accepted this appointment in 1936. A twenty-six-acre site was found at Hawkspur Green, Great Bardfield, with no buildings or facilities of any kind other than good soil and natural springs of water. During the inclement summer of 1936 the members of the community lived in tents and, while a skeleton staff supplied technical knowledge, all those capable of doing so laboured to provide more adequate accommodation.

The incentive was originally that of survival and the community spirit which it sometimes generates but, increasingly, it became necessary to put some pressure on individuals who were not 'pulling their weight' and a system of economic sanctions was evolved by the council of members (the Community) by which regular work in the mornings was paid for and 'slackers' not only lost their 2s 6d weekly pocket money but became the financial liability of the community. This use of economic and social pressure resembles that of Homer Lane, and Wills said 'Homer Lane was the root and inspiration of all our work at the Hawkspur Camp.'

This was not entirely true, and Wills also pays tribute to the vital importance of the role played by the Selection and Treatment Committee[40] and of the use of medical psychology as an integral part of the Q method. This committee, of which Dr Marjorie Franklin was secretary and convener, consisted of a body of physicians and psychologists including two medical members of the Institute for the

Scientific Treatment of Delinquency—which latter body was much concerned with both the selection and treatment of camp members. Dr Hermann Mannheim, a member of the committee and of the institute also, considered that the way in which 'the difficulties inherent in the psychological treatment of delinquents' was tackled 'may be regarded as one of the most original and valuable features of Q Camps.' He pointed out that the three-tier system of treatment at Hawkspur by the Camp Chief, the treatment committee, and the outside treatment experts, working together with a full understanding of the institution and knowledge of its needs, avoided both the tensions caused by entirely externally based treatment, and the even greater tensions often caused if the treatment is given by a resident specialist.[41] This ideal state of affairs, as Mannheim says, could exist only 'through utter devotion and mutual understanding between those concerned'. An acceptance of role is clearly important and it was helpful that Wills, while trained as a psychiatric social worker and recognizing the value of psychological aid, was without Homer Lane's passion for psychoanalytic meddling. He says: 'I am not a psychologist. I am that most noxious of creatures, a layman dabbling in psychology. Although I may refer to psychological phenomena and attempt to draw conclusions from them ... I speak not as a psychologist nor as a scientist, for I am neither. I speak as a Christian.'[42]

Wills did not psychoanalyse anybody. He considered that 'consciously probing in the murky depths of anyone's unconscious ... would ... be a mistake, even if I were qualified to do it.' This did not mean, however, that what analysts would call 'transference', negative or positive, to Wills, did not occur. Most of the inmates had some degree of 'transfer' to the Chief, who lived in the centre of an 'emotional vortex'. Within this centre he worked like a psychoanalyst with twenty clients in one consulting room, all demanding attention. Therapeutically it was a very rewarding situation if one had the courage to take advantage of it. Wills, as Camp Chief, was inevitably the father figure to whom the youths transferred the thwarted hate or love which they felt for their own inadequate fathers or father substitutes. It was true of Hawkspur, as it was of Finchden and Dunnow, that there 'psychoanalysis was not done but lived'.

Nevertheless camp members were not without specific psychological treatment, if necessary of a psychoanalytical persuasion. This was the function largely of the Selection and Treatment Committee, with the support of the I.S.T.D. The former 'were concerned with all aspects of behaviour and with every member, and not merely in giving advice about abnormal situations', while the latter were more concerned with sharing the work of psychiatric interviews, specific medical treatment, and varius forms of therapy, including 'glandular therapy'.[43]

The committee was also responsible for admissions, which were normally based on social reports, physical examinations, psychometric tests and psychiatric interviews. The intention was not only to choose members most likely to profit by the Q process but also to suggest treatment. In selecting members the committee had in mind 'young men . . . who seem likely to respond to an unconventional but carefully thought-out open-air life . . . but who nevertheless are not sufficiently advanced in citizenship to fit as ordinary members into an unmodified environment'. Some categories of delinquents were considered unsuitable—those who had been for a long time under prison discipline; severely psychotic or neurotic persons requiring extensive analytical treatment; women, whose presence, although desirable, would have added immensely to the difficulties of running the camp; and young children, for whom the practical running of the camp would have had to be modified.

Despite these criteria the range of personality and symptom was wide and the committee was under constant pressure to accept very deeply disturbed youths with whom others had failed. Of the sixteen acknowledged failures among all the fifty-six members who were subsequently followed up[44] ten were clearly psychotic and five showed deep-seated symptoms which, had the committee rigidly maintained its policy, would have excluded them. Of the remaining forty almost all had made good progress and had become stable and self-supporting, although a number continued psychological treatment and showed some recurrent signs of neurotic behaviour or delinquent proclivities.

It is difficult to evaluate the results as, with the coming of war, the majority of the leavers were absorbed into the Forces, where conditions of life were abnormal and where effective follow-up was difficult, but a number of things must be borne in mind. Almost all had come to Hawkspur after all else had failed, many were accepted although considered unsuitable for treatment, and many had left before treatment was completed. It was considered a prerequisite of

Q Camp therapy that members should be free to leave if they chose, and nineteen stayed for less than three months, eighteen for less than a year and only nineteen for more than a year. On the other hand 60 per cent had I.Q.s of over 100 and 40 per cent had received secondary education which represents a very atypical delinquent population, although the relevance of this factor to the success of the treatment is not clear.[45]

LOVE AS THERAPY

The treatment, including the specific psychotherapy already mentioned, was basically that of the concept of 'planned environmental therapy' (to be discussed more fully in Chapter 15). It is necessary, however, to take into account certain aspects when considering Wills's particular and varied contribution to therapeutic education in a number of different milieus. For him faith, love, work and 'shared responsibility' were the essential criteria of any therapy in which he was involved.

As a Quaker, Wills's faith was a profoundly Christian belief in a god of love, which was a constant guide to his own 'light within'. This gave him confidence in his own rightness throughout the innumerable moments of stress which were an inevitable part of his work. 'Faith not . . . in myself and my own abilities. That has always been in short supply, not without reason, but absolutely invincible faith in the healing and redeeming power of love.'[46]

Although in recent years the importance of love as a primary condition for the successful treatment of the maladjusted has been critically re-assessed (e.g., Bettelheim, *Love is Not Enough*), few pioneers did not see it as central. Wills considers it the unconditional prerequisite of any therapeutic work. He says: 'You may talk as much as you like about aggression and projection and transference and counter-transference and unconscious motives and all the rest of it. And I do, and we must, and it is all very valuable and useful. But they're only recently elaborated techniques which will tomorrow be replaced. They're just the best that we can do in that line up to now. But *Love* is the dynamic that makes them work, and the psychoanalyst, in his curious roundabout way, says this very thing himself.'[47]

Indeed Ferenczi in paying tribute to Freud on his seventieth birthday said: 'Psycho-analysis works ultimately through the deepening and enlargement of knowledge; but . . . knowledge can be enlarged and deepened only by love.'[48]

In using the word 'unconditional' Wills echoes Homer Lane, who believed not only in loving the child and its good actions while disapproving of its bad actions, but of loving the bad actions themselves as symptomatic of the good qualities that were innately in the child. Delinquent actions to Lane were 'positive virtues wrongly expressed'.

Wills does not, in fact, go so far as this and in saying that all of the fifty or so misfits who came to Hawkspur found 'approval', he qualifies it by saying: 'Approval, not necessarily and always of their acts, but always of themselves.' He acts on the assumption that 'He's a good boy, yer honour, bar what he does.'[49] The therapist 'must back his intuitive judgement all along the line. Give the lad unstinted approval in spite of everything he may say or do, approving him always, even if what he does cannot be approved. . . . Our chief aim is to make the boy feel that whatever others may think of him, whatever he may have done—or be doing—we approve of him. We are on his side. It is not easy.'[50] Acceptance, love, kindness is not enough unless there is enough of it and, in this sense, it must be unconditional and limitless. 'Kindness isn't a patent medicine of which one takes a couple of doses just to confirm one's suspicion that it is useless. It must be "instant in season and out of season". It "suffereth long". It must be continued for months and if need be for years. You cannot eradicate the effect of ten or fifteen—or more— years of brutality by a couple of weeks of kindness. It must be applied in something of the spirit of that faith which can remove mountains.'

Another important prerequisite of therapy at Hawkspur was work. Work, which was shared fully by the staff, was not only necessary for survival but under these pioneering conditions was seen as having value as 'inspiration, encouragement, adventure, education and discipline'. Work under such circumstances was an act of creation whether it was making a garden from virgin soil or building shelters. 'It would have saved us some real hardship, and have sometimes been cheaper, to buy doors, windows and other joinery ready-made or ready-milled. We did not do so, even though this meant our working in the midst of winter covered only by a roof in a shelter with neither walls nor solid floor, which it was impossible to warm, because we wanted to build the camp as nearly unaided as we could. We also avoided using metal bolts and other sundries for the making of which we had not yet the equipment. This meant the invention of gadgets which would serve the same purpose, or a reversion to the methods of craftsmen of the days before machinery.'[51] Work was thought to develop not only the powers and abilities which would have vocational utility but also self-respect. It expressed faith in the judgement of members, a feeling of community, an appreciation of the individual's contribution of effort and skill, and a sense of responsibility. It was achieved with the minimum of compulsion, and what compulsion there was came from the community of workers themselves in the exercise of 'shared responsibility'.

SHARED RESPONSIBILITY

As practised at the Hawkspur Camp and in subsequent institutions with which David Wills was associated, 'shared responsibility', differs from the popular concept of self-government in that the elected councils have a limited—but absolute—sphere of action and, beyond this sphere, the responsibility is recognized of whoever is appropriate, e.g. in the appointment of staff the headmaster, arrangements for bedtime the matron, provision of meals the cook. In the legislative body adults not only have equal rights with children as members of the community but, by virtue of their greater experience, are likely to be able to exercise considerable control over the meeting. Wills says, and one can well believe him : 'Indeed if I really press a point hard the decision never goes against me.'[52] The occasions when such pressure is used are deliberately rare but the adult is aware of what is going on and whether the machine is running efficiently or not, and is able to manipulate or stimulate its action as seems necessary. He must accept the responsibility of his role while at the same time 'he must be able at the drop of the hat to divest himself of all authority and become just another citizen with a single vote and subject to the authority of the community'.

Wills emphasizes that 'self-government' may be imposed but that it is essential that 'shared responsibility' shall grow naturally. Self-government may become static with an immutable constitution but shared responsibility is dynamic, changing constantly with the changing needs of the community which it serves. 'I say to newcomers: "This is how we do things at present. If you don't like it try to change it—you have only to get the majority to agree with you." '

Wills enumerates eight main advantages of a system of shared responsibility:

1 It is a natural vehicle for group therapy.
2 It is a means by which the children may learn that socially acceptable behaviour is demanded of them not only as a result of adult prejudice but by their peers.
3 Under shared responsibility the adults are less pre-occupied with disciplinary matters than under a more orthodox regime, and can therefore more easily maintain the friendly, affectionate relationship which is so necessary.
4 It enhances the authority of the adult, i.e. the fact that the adult so seldom says 'Thou shalt not' or 'Thou shalt' tends to make his authority more effective when he does.
5 Shared responsibility is a device for encouraging and making constructive use of the herd instinct which in maladjusted children is apt to be either anti-socially directed or pathologically inhibited.
6 Shared responsibility helps to protect the weak and the small from the big and aggressive without the stigma of tale-bearing.
7 Shared responsibility satisfies the need that all children have to feel that their side of the question is being heard.
8 Shared responsibility is a means by which the child can be helped by practical experience to learn that laws exist for our mutual protection, and that the price of freedom is eternal vigilance— or in other words that if he wants the place to be a good place, he will have to make his contribution.

A further point emphasized by Howard Jones in *Reluctant Rebels*[53] with relation to the Hawkspur experiment is that in a society of neurotics and delinquents such as existed at the camp 'shared responsibility enables the group members to impose that degree of discipline on themselves which they feel able to support'; moreover unless that discipline involves a great deal of personal choice and freedom any accurate diagnosis of a neurotic condition would be impossible. 'It is possible for a person under discipline never to display a single symptom, and go out into the world again quite untouched. But in the freedom of Hawkspur we see them as they really are.'[54] This degree of freedom and responsibility was for many of the occupants of the camp the hardest part of the treatment to bear. 'Having to discipline one's self, instead of being disciplined by others, is a burden. . . . So now we can see self-government in a new light. It is not merely a privilege that is bestowed on them because we superior mortals think the experience might be useful for them. It is an absolute necessity to enable them to set a term to the horrors of personal self-discipline which we have thrust upon them by refusing to be authoritarian.'[55] Moreover it is perfectly fair to point out that 'in the main people do not care to accept responsibility unless they are well rewarded'; it is easier to sit back and watch others make a mess of things and feel no guilt about it.

Unless shared responsibility served a therapeutic function there would clearly be no use for it. No one who has practised it would claim that it was either an easy or an efficient method of government. 'Do not look for efficiency. If you want that you must provide it in the good old way.'[56] Wills's only justification is that in the circumstances it is necessary.

At the Hawkspur Camp the council grew spontaneously and its authority was limited to the domestic affairs of the camp and was 'concerned primarily with people's relations to one another, and the day-to-day conduct of family life'. It combined both the legislative and judicial function but its chief importance was as a vehicle for the expression of public opinion which was, in essence, its most effective sanction.

The Hawkspur experiment lasted for only four years, closing in 1940 for a number of different reasons. As funds ran out attempts to get the Home Office to accept some responsibility for the camp failed. Wills says that he 'was told, very politely, that we should have to have much more discipline before we could ever be recognized by them'. Staff tensions increased as wartime conditions made continuation more difficult. An attempt to continue the work with difficult evacuees was frustrated by official interference which the staff could not tolerate. The Q Camps committee eventually withdrew from the project—although remaining in existence—and Wills accepted an offer from Peebles to become the warden of the Barns Hostel.

THE BARNS EXPERIMENT

The Barns Evacuation Hostel for disturbed and unbilletable

evacuees began in July 1940 under the general authority of the Peeblesshire County Council. The actual direction was in the hands of a committee of management consisting mainly of Quakers with a belief in David Wills and his methods. Since all the boys, however, came from Edinburgh and the Edinburgh Education Authority paid the teaching staff they, too, had a considerable influence—although less faith. A teacher was appointed from Edinburgh who was the only person at Barns who accepted the advice offered to Wills by a member of the education committee—'A strap behind the door, Mr Wills—you should keep a strap behind the door.'[57]

Thus a curious situation was established in which the schoolroom was the only place in the hostel in which there was any punishment since Wills—who was the warden but not the headmaster—felt that only by removing all fear of punishment could a valid sense of morality emerge in boys who, at the beginning, were, at best, amoral. He gives four reasons for avoiding punishment:

1 It establishes a base motive for conduct.
2 It has been tried and has failed.
3 It militates against the establishment of the relationship which we consider necessary between staff and children—a relationship in which the child must feel himself to be loved.
4 Many delinquent children (and adults) are seeking punishment as a means of assuaging their guilt feelings.[58]

During the first four months of the experiment of 'no punishment', while the boys were testing out its reality there was, as Wills readily admits, chaos, surging unrest, destruction. 'The chief game seemed to consist of charging wildly through the house howling madly and slamming all the doors on the way. Any kind of organized activity was almost impossible. Crockery would be dashed on to stone floors, games destroyed, furniture broken, stones hurled through windows. Mealtimes were an indescribable babel, and there were mass truantings from school.'[59]

In this process the boys were clearly seeking the only sort of security most of them knew—that of imposed discipline. Wills refused to give it to them and, as he anticipated, self-discipline emerged. Convinced of the sincerity of the adults, and of their unconditional love and acceptance, the boys began to work with the next major problem, since he found that the emerging system of adults rather than against them. This, in fact, became for Wills the 'shared responsibility' gave the adults too great a share of control. He therefore, as Homer Lane had done, precipitated a situation by establishing a dictatorship which was ended by the establishment of the Citizens' Association—a voluntary organization of 'all those willing to work for Barns'. The 'association' accepted the full responsibility of organizing and controlling the Barns' routine, including that at bedtimes, mealtimes and, eventually, in the school-room.

This (and succeeding systems of 'shared responsibility)[60] is all the more remarkable when one considers the boys involved. 'They were all difficult boys, hating school, prejudiced against adults in general, punished often but not wisely, fearful, suspicious, aggressive, untruthful, uncared-for and in the main unloved.' Only two out of fifty had normal and satisfactory parents and these two were brothers. All the boys had been sent to Barns because it had been found, or was considered to be, impossible to billet them with normal families. Their chronological ages varied from nine to fourteen and their 'mental ages' from about six to sixteen—but the majority were of 'low-average' or 'high sub-normal' intelligence. Most had missed considerable periods of schooling. They had little idea of conventional morality, particularly with regard to private property.

These were the boys who eventually governed themselves in most of the ordinary affairs of the day, but for whom Wills asked for, and to whom he gave, not only tolerance but love. One can well believe that 'shared responsibility' was at times 'no picnic for the adults' and, even more easily, that to love the aggressive, ill-mannered enuretic, encopretic, maladjusted boy required more than being 'awfully fond of children'.

It is not just a matter of being 'awfully fond of children'. Anyone can be that. It is a matter of being 'awfully fond' of Johnny Jones whose table-manners are nauseating (he sits opposite you and crams as much food into his mouth as he possibly can; this he chews with his big mouth wide open; presently he lets out a loud guffaw, ejecting his breath powerfully through his overfull and open mouth. . . .); it is a matter of being 'awfully fond' of Willie Smith whose nose is usually in a condition such as to make one retch almost every time one sees it; it is a matter of being 'awfully fond' of Jimmy Brown, who stinks because of his encopresis; or even of Tommy Green who has all of these failings and a foul and nasty disposition thrown in. It consists of loving this Tommy Green in spite of all that, of making him feel that this affection is always

there, is something on which he can absolutely rely, which will never
fail, whatever he may do. It consists in establishing a relationship such
that, however much a child may wound his own self-esteem he cannot
damage the esteem in which we hold him . . . when that relationship is
established therapy has begun.[61]

BODENHAM MANOR

One way in which Wills differs from most other 'pioneers' is in the
range of his activities. As well as his varied early experience,
ventures over which he had charge embraced the Hawkspur Camp
(delinquents aged sixteen to nineteen); the Barns Hostel (difficult
evacuee boys, average age ten to twelve); Bodenham Manor (maladjusted boys and girls aged eight to sixteen), and Reynolds House
(hostel for ex-pupils of special and approved schools in need of
aftercare, aged fifteen to nineteen). The principles of management
were essentially the same although different situations required some
difference in practice.

At Bodenham Manor, to which Wills went at the end of the war
at the insistence of Frank Mathews, who died before the project was
started, he was, from the first, faced with certain problems. Although
envisaged as a coeducational establishment this was made meaningless by the Ministry of Education's absurd insistence on the boys
leaving when they reached secondary-school age. This made the
practice of 'shared responsibility' difficult since, as many people have
observed, girls seem less prepared to accept political and administrative responsibility than do boys. Moreover since the average age
was about ten-and-a-half and Wills considers that children below the
age of ten—particulary if maladjusted—are unable to understand
or to profit fully by self-government, the system was necessarily much
modified. Nevertheless the adult share of 'shared responsibility'
remained as small as the children would allow it to be.

Wills was at Bodenham Manor for eleven years (see *Throw Away
Thy Rod*)during which many of the patterns of the Barns Experiment
were repeated. It was, however, during this immediately postwar
period that bold experiment was most hampered and misunderstood
by officialdom, which considered schools such as Bodenham and
Chaigeley too out of touch with the requirements of society at large
to be given unqualified official approval. The restrictions imposed by

the Ministry, e.g. on effective co-education, and by the controlling body—the Birmingham Society for the Care of Invalid and Nervous Children, e.g. over staffing, led to frustration, disagreement and disappointment, and Wills left. Bodenham Manor continues as a school for maladjusted children.

While at the Barns Hostel School, Wills had been concerned, as are all workers with maladjusted children, about the need for a system of after-care to ensure that the work done in special schools is not wasted when the child leaves and is either returned to the home which produced the original problem or, leaving the home the school has provided, is left homeless. For the latter in particular, i.e. those left to fend for themselves in a largely indifferent world, the 'Barns Flat' was established. This, the first specific attempt at 'after-care' associated with a special school, was, however, inadequately pro- vided for, insufficiently integrated with the parent body, and, although clearly fulfilling a need, 'was the source of endless trouble and worry to all concerned with it'.

At Bodenham, however, the function of the hostel founded in 1961, the year in which Wills left, was more specific, acting—as is now frequently the case in special and approved schools and mental hospitals—as an intermediate station between the institution and the 'real world'. Pupils were originally transferred to the hostel at thir- teen or fourteen years of age so that they might attend ordinary school if they were considered ready to do so. On subsequently finding employment they could remain in the hostel as long as it was thought necessary.

After leaving Bodenham Wills gave considerable attention to the problem of after-care[62] and in 1965 he was asked by the National Association for Mental Health to become the warden of Reynolds House, Bromley, an experimental hostel for school-leavers in need of special care. Reynolds House was not a treatment centre but a place devoted to ensuring that the work done in therapeutic establish- ments should not be wasted because of a boy's inability to cope with the strains of returning home. The intention was to maintain a stable, and even stimulating, environment and support in time of difficulty. This Wills provided until his retirement in 1968.

Wills is the pioneer *par excellence* in that he led, often impetuously but always with conviction, along uncharted paths which others follow more cautiously. (The News Barns School, founded in

G

Gloucestershire in 1965, of which Wills is chairman of the governors, is perhaps the only example of a pioneering experiment being continued both consciously and directly into a second or third — counting the Little Commonwealth — generation.) Wills seems more interested in discovery than in settlement, more interested in practice than in consequent academic theorizing. What he pioneered was probably an art form rather than a scientific process.

At a recent conference of the Association of Workers for Maladjusted Children (of which, with Shaw, he was a founder member) he pleaded for two principles to be understood in therapeutic education. The first was that 'maladjustment' in the sense in which it means the application of individual energy in ways not always consistent with social norms, should be used and directed rather than eradicated (he pointed out how useful Churchill's socially maladaptive aggressive behaviour had eventually become). The second plea was for the worker with maladjusted children to be regarded as an artist rather than a scientist.

It might indeed be said of Wills what C. H. C. Osborne said of his mentor Homer Lane : '[He] was more the artist than the man of science. He claimed, it is true, a scientific justification for his theories [Wills's justification is largely pragmatic] . . . but his understanding of people and ideas was essentially intuitive.'

REFERENCES

CHAPTER 10: George Lyward

1 LYWARD, G. A. 'A Comment on Standards: particularly for Parents', *New Era*, **34** (7) *p* 122. 1953.
2 BURN, M. *Mr Lyward's Answer p* 38. Hamish Hamilton, London, 1956.
3 LYWARD, G. A. *New Era* (Ref. 1). *p* 119.
4 —————— The Residential Care of Disturbed Children: the proceedings of the 14th Inter-Clinic Conference of the N.A.M.H. 1958.
5 —————— Feeling Their Way Through. *New Era* **3** (7) *p* 116. 1938.
6 Ibid. *p* 115. *See also* DANBY, J. F. About Finchden Manor. *New Era*, **37** (3) *p* 168. 1956.
7 BARNES, K. C. About Finchden Manor (Ref. 6). *p* 169.
8 BURN, M. op. cit., *p* 227.
9 —————— op. cit., *p* 128.
10 LYWARD, G. A. In Conclusion, in *Problems of Child Development*. *p* 94. New Educational Fellowship, London, 1948.
11 —————— The Permanent Need for Discipline. Summing-up of annual conference of Home and School Council, 1948.
12 —————— In Conclusion (Ref. 10). *p* 94.
13 —————— *The Residential Care of Disturbed Children*. N.A.M.H., 1958.
14 —————— Loyalty to the Maladjusted Child, *New Era* **36** (3) *pp* 43 and 45. 1954.
15 —————— In Conclusion, (Ref. 10). *p* 93.
16 —————— Loving Children, *New Era* **4** (12) *p* 240. 1940.
17 —————— Loyalty to the Maladjusted Child, (Ref. 14). 1954.

CHAPTER 11: Otto Shaw.

18 SLAVSON, S. R. Group Therapy in Child Care and Child Guidance. *Jewish Social Services Quarterly* **XXV** (2) 1948.
19 SHAW, O. L. *Maladjusted Boys, pp* 62–64. Allen & Unwin, London, 1965.
20 BETTELHEIM, B. *Love is Not Enough, pp* 224/225. The Free Press of Glencoe, (Illinois). 1950.

21 FREUD, S. Analysis of a phobia of a five-year-old boy. *Collected Papers* III *p* 144ff. London, 1925.

22 SHAW, O. L. Report (unpublished) on After Histories, 1968.

23 ——— *Prisons of the Mind, p* 197. Allen & Unwin, London, 1969.

24 Ibid. *pp* 81-6.

25 Ibid. *p* 126.

26 SHAW, O. L. A brief study of re-educational factors in a progressive boarding school for delinquent children and adolescents (unpublished).

27 ——— *Prisons of the Mind* (Ref. 23). *p* 19.

28 Ibid. *p* 234.

29 BLOOM, L. Some Aspects of the Residential Psychotherapy of Maladjusted or Delinquent Children. *Br. J. Delinquency* VI (1) *p* 46. 1955.

30 SHAW, O. L. *Prisons of the Mind.* (Ref. 23) *p* 167.

31 HOLLAND, W. Appendix to *Maladjusted Boys*, (Ref. 19).

32 SHAW, O. L. Educational Report for the Year 1968 (unpublished).

33 ——— *Prisons of the Mind.* (Ref. 23). *p* 163.

34 ——— *Maladjusted Boys.* (Ref. 19).

35 KLEIN, M. The Early Development of Conscience. *Psychoanalysis Today.* Lorand, S. (ed). Allen & Unwin, London, 1948.

CHAPTER 12: David Wills

36 WILLS, W. D. *The Hawkspur Experiment.* Allen & Unwin, London, 1941 (republished 1967).

37 BAZELEY, E. T. *Homer Lane and the Little Commonwealth* Allen & Unwin, London, 1928.

38 AICHHORN, A. *Wayward Youth.* Imago, London, 1957.

39 FRANKLIN, M. E. (ed.), *Q Camp, p* 10. Planned Environmental Therapy Trust, London, 1966.

40 WILLS, W. D. Ibid., *pp* 22-3.

41 MANNHEIM, H. Ibid., *p* 61.

42 WILLS, W. D. *The Hawkspur Experiment* (Ref. 36) *p* 12.

43 FRANKLIN, M. E. op. cit., *pp* 19-21.

44 WILLS, W. D. *Q Camp* (Ref. 39) *pp* 39-51.

45 MANNHEIM, H. op. cit., *p* 61.

46 WILLS, W. D. Address (unpublished.) to A.W.M.C. Conference, 1968.

47 Ibid.

48 FERENCZI, S. Quoted by FRANKLIN, M. E. in *A.W.M.C. Newsletter No.* **10.** *p* 37. 1968.

49 WILLS, W. D. *The Hawkspur Experiment* (Ref. 36) *p* 18.

50 Ibid. *p* 25.

51 BARRON, A. T. *Q Camp*, (Ref. 39) *pp* 33-34.

52 WILLS, W. D. *Throw Away Thy Rod, p.* 77. Gollancz, London, 1960.

53 JONES, H. *Reluctant Rebels*, *p* 137. Tavistock, London, 1960.
54 WILLS, W. D. *The Hawkspur Experiment.* (Ref. 36) *p* 52.
55 Ibid. *p* 51.
56 WILLS, W. D. *The Barns Experiment*, Allen & Unwin, London, 1945.
57 ———— Ibid. *p* 14.
58 ———— Ibid. *pp* 22-3.
59 Ibid. *p* 11.
60 WILLS, W. D. Shared Responsibility, in *Problems of Child Development.* New Education Fellowship, 1948.
61 ———— *The Barns Experiment.* (Ref. 56) *pp* 65.
62 ———— After-care at Schools for Maladjusted Children. *A.W.M.C. Newsletter* (*6*), 1965.

PART SIX

War and Evacuation

13

Rethinking Child Care

In September, 1939, the family life of large numbers of parents and children in England and Scotland was voluntarily broken up. 750,000 school children, 542,000 mothers with young children, 12,000 expectant mothers, and 77,000 other persons left their homes and agreed to go wherever they were sent.[1]

The national traumatic experience of war and evacuation in 1939 naturally produced and revealed widespread neuroses of which many people became aware for the first time. Families deprived of fathers, mothers deprived of husbands and children, children deprived of parents, often reacted predictably.[2] Moreover the sudden shift of population from urban to rural areas revealed to some sections of society for the first time the deplorable conditions under which many urban children had been living and the inadequacy of our child care and educational system to provide for their needs. This was not without beneficial results for, after the first shock, the public conscience was aroused in a way which inspired the complete re-thinking of both systems. In child care the Curtis Report of 1946 was followed by the Children's Act of 1948; in education the famous 'Green Book' circulated, as is well known, 'in a blaze of secrecy' in 1941 was followed by the Education Act of 1944. Both major pieces of legislation, although having their faults, represented a fundamental reorganization inspired by humanitarian considerations of social justice in the light of the psychological notions of the day. Each recognized the special needs of disturbed children within the system for the first time.

Evacuation surveys conducted under different auspices—for example, the Cambridge Evacuation Survey, edited by Susan Isaacs and compiled by a team including John Bowlby and R. H. Thouless,[3] the Evacuation Survey, a report to the Fabian Society in 1940 by Padley and Cole,[4] and the report made by a group of psychologists

201

for the New Education Fellowship (*New Era,* May 1940)—revealed the extent of the problem and suggested 'ways and means of minimizing the inevitable anxieties and delinquencies due to the separation of parents and children',[5] some of far-reaching effect.

The Cambridge Evacuation Survey reports on a group of London schoolchildren. 'Omitting the children graded under the Personality Defect 1 (sixty-one children with mild neurotic and behavioural difficulties whose difficulties are such as are likely with reasonable treatment at home and in school to clear up themselves), the figures show that in the total of 656 children, eighty-seven, or 13 per cent, are in need of skilled therapeutic treatment, and, of these, twenty-seven, or 4 per cent, are cases of considerable severity.'[6]

Assessment of Difficulties found among 656 London Schoolchildren

GRADE	Personality Defect 1	Personality Defect 2	Personality Defect 3	Personality Defect 2 and 3
A Anxious and/or Depressed	34	23	13	36
B Shut in, withdrawn	3	2	3	5
C Quarrelsome, jealous	24	11	3	36
D Aggressive		14 } 30	3 } 6	
E 'Circular' alternating Moods		5		
F Delinquent, Affectionless, anti-social	—	5	5	10
Total No. with Difficulties	61	60	27	87

Such cases, magnified on a national scale, would clearly outstrip the resources of sufficiently sympathetic and knowledgeable foster-parents.

Burt, writing on 'The incidence of neurotic symptoms among evacuated school children', produced rather less depressing statistics

Conditions Observed	Estimated Sample of Population	
	Before	After
Anxiety states	4·2	6·3
Neurasthenia	2·4	1·2
Hysteria	0·7	2·2
Anger-neuroses	2·3	3·4
Incontinence	3·4	7·2
Other neurotic symptoms	4·1	5·0
TOTAL	17·1	25·3
Theft	1·5	1·7
Other Offences	0·7	1·2
TOTAL	2·2	7·9

While Burt claimed that 'there is no evidence to show that evacuation has greatly increased the amount of serious nervous disorder', his figures demonstrate an increase of about 20 per cent in milder neuroses particularly those like 'incontinence' and 'anger neuroses' most likely to cause difficulty with foster-parents and for children.[7]

Burt suggested that 'special hostels or camps should be established for those who in virtue of physical, mental or social disabilities are quite unsuitable for billeting in private houses . . . social workers with special training and experience in child psychology should be available in each area to give advice and assistance in respect of individual cases of maladjustment. Cases of exceptional difficulty should be referred by them to a fully qualified educational psychologist.'

The child-guidance service during this period was not so much expanded as spread. As trained workers were evacuated from urban centres with the children, and as psychological skills were increasingly called on to help both difficult children and those who were asked to deal with them, some areas of the country in which no previous provision existed acquired a nucleus of a child-guidance service. In some areas this might originally have been betokened by no more than a single psychologist or psychiatric social worker being called on for immediate aid, but by 1944, when the child-guidance committee of the newly constituted National Council for Mental Health was set up, there were more than seventy child-guidance centres in Britain, over half of which were wholly or partly maintained by local authorities.

Not all were fully constituted on the traditional 'team' pattern. Many under local education authorities, particularly those in Scotland, operated largely through single psychologists while the majority of clinics attached to hospitals were, according to the National Council of Mental Health report, 'without a fully qualified psychologist or psychiatric social worker'. Interest was however greatly stimulated and widely spread by wartime needs and activities and in the seven years following the war the number of child guidance centres doubled.[8] This increase was the result of the expansion both of child guidance clinics and of educationally based centres. In 1943 there were sixty-eight clinics, many based either on hospitals or on university departments of psychology or education. By 1950, this number had increased to 162. Of the 136 local authorities in the United Kingdom investigated by Fulton[9] only ten had appointed an educational psychologist by 1939, but this number had more than doubled by 1944 (twenty-three) and by 1949 had increased to fifty-eight. The latter increase was probably the result of the impetus given by wartime work, the increased availability of skilled workers after the war and the effect of the Education Act. In the words of the Chief Medical Officer of Health to the Ministry of Education in 1947, 'The past was for child guidance a period of growing pains which were accentuated by the pressing needs of war; the present shows its recovery and strengthening; the future unfolds a hopeful prospect for a full life.'[10]

EVACUATION AND MALADJUSTMENT

The most immediate and 'pressing' need in 1939 was the provision of hostels for those evacuees whom it was found undesirable or impossible to billet. The problem was daunting. Susan Isaacs and her co-workers estimated that 2 per cent of the children would be 'permanently unsuitable for foster homes on account of nervous symptoms or difficulties of behaviour'. This, in view of the figures quoted above, was a very conservative estimate but still exceeded 15,000 children of school age over the country as a whole.

Susan Isaacs thought that 'these types of children can best be cared for in small groups of ten or fifteen. If there were opportunities for taking over one or two small houses in different parts of a Borough, or in small towns in a country area, it would be better to open several small homes rather than one large one.'

'It may occasionally be possible to find local householders with special experience who would be competent to run homes of this type if they had the advice of an educational psychologist or a psychiatric social worker, but it will usually be necessary to make a special appointment.'[11] The difficulty was not in finding the 'one or two small houses' but in finding the 'local householders with special experience' or even those people who might be 'specially appointed'. Apart from the fact that the majority of suitable men were already in the Forces there was no fund of experience to draw on in considering the residential treatment of maladjusted children other than that of rather isolated and individualistic 'pioneers', and no training course, system or centre geared to the special needs of workers with maladjusted children in residential institutions. Nor was there any national agency through which this work could be performed, especially since it was not yet the legal liability of the Board of Education. Nevertheless 'hostels for "difficult children", that is for children who proved unbillettable, were set up as part of the Government evacuation scheme; and when a hostel was opened in an area in which a child guidance clinic was operating, there was usually close co-operation between clinic and hostel. As time went on, local authorities were allowed to place in hostels in their area any of their own children who needed residential care, provided that no evacuated children were thereby excluded.[12] Various regions developed schemes of their own for coping with this vast new problem. Some are of special interest. Possibly the most systematically organized group was that set up in South Wales under the direction of George Seth[13] who, since 1935, had been associated with the Cardiff L.E.A. child-guidance clinic while a member of the University College staff.

Seth's concern and the existence of the clinic were not the only factors which operated to make South Wales a particularly fruitful area for the development of provision for maladjusted children. The chief impetus was given by the magnitude of the problem and its concentration in a relatively small and well organized area containing considerable urban communities. Almost half of the 100,000 children evacuated to Wales were in the three counties of Glamorgan, Monmouthshire and Carmarthen and a further 10,000 were in the adjacent counties of Pembroke, Brecon and Radnorshire. This meant that, although the problems of billeting were immense, what services there were could operate more easily than in other areas where evacuees were more widely dispersed.

Children who, by virtue of their behaviour or nervous condition, were found to be unbilletable were, as in other areas, gathered together into special hostels. They were however more fortunate than others in that from mid-1940 they were assisted and supervised by a voluntary psychological service consisting in the main of Seth, Mrs M. E. Hollings, a P.S.W. appointed by the Board of Education to assist with evacuation and Mrs J. Rhees, another P.S.W. based in Swansea. In June, 1941, Seth and Mrs Hollings prepared a memorandum for the Welsh Board of Health urging the development of an official psychological service with special responsibility for difficult children whether in hostels or in ordinary billets.

This document set out the needs which the far-sighted authors perceived as giving support not only to children who had succumbed to the emotional and social stresses of evacuation but also to their hosts. It was, in particular, emphasized that the mere re-billeting of children who suffered from, and created, tension was no solution. Hostels, to be effective, needed to be more than 'dumping grounds' or isolation units for the unacceptable and it was suggested that, if properly and professionally organized and supervised, they offered 'an unparalleled opportunity for an attempt to develop a positive policy of child care and training which will have regard to something more than physical health and scholastic achievement'.

The solution proposed was an official psychological service staffed by a psychologist and psychiatric social workers acting as a 'peripatetic, partially decentralized psychological clinic' supported by the school medical authorities. The function of such a service would be not only the assessment and placement of 'difficult' evacuees and the supervision of hostels but also advising war-time foster-parents and receiving schools in the handling of children with more superficial or temporary difficulties.[14]

The recommendations were accepted and in October 1941 the Psychological Service for Difficult Children was established. The staff originally consisted of Seth, Mrs Hollings and Mrs Rhees but within two years had expanded to include also an assistant psychologist, two part-time psychiatrists and two more psychiatric social workers.

Although two thirds of the difficult children referred to the new service were not in the special hostels it was inevitable that a great deal of time and attention had to be given to hostel establishment and supervision. There were, by 1942, five such hostels systematically organized and specially staffed to cope with differentiated problems. One of these, the hostel of the Good Shepherd at Tredegar, had been in existence for eight years as an independent establishment with a reputation for dealing with difficult cases. As well as Tredegar, which was for senior boys, there were also hostels at Tonypandy for maladjusted girls, Pontardawe for junior boys, Abertillery for all-age boys and Usk for maladjusted and backward boys and girls. With the exception of the last, which was a residential school with a wardenteacher, all were hostels from which the children attended ordinary schools. Hostels were administered by the local authority and the general management and control of admissions and discharge was in the hands of the psychological service. They were regarded not as independent units but as links in a regional chain. This permitted a degree of specialization within the hostels which promoted flexibility of provision. Psychologists visited the hostels regularly largely for individual sessions with the children, and clinic sessions were also held in the urban centres. The efforts of the social workers were directed largely towards individual billets, schools and referring agencies to whom the work of child guidance was previously unknown.

With the exception of a hostel for disturbed adolescent girls established at Highfields, Newport, all the hostels remained in existence throughout the emergency with considerable success. Seth writes: 'It is perhaps noteworthy that I cannot remember a public "furore" about any maladjusted, delinquent, or subnormal child at any time during the existence of the Service.'[15] Roughly three-quarters of the children were in residence at the hostel for less than a year and there appears to have been little tendency for relapses to occur during adolescence.

Apart from those geographical factors which aided communication the success of this scheme can be attributed to a number of considerations. The service which was set up was professional, direct, varied, and well integrated. The fact that it was psychologically based promoted co-operation with schools and biased it towards social and educational readjustment rather than 'cure', a bias which was realistic in that most of the maladjustment was likely to have been the result of stressful circumstances rather than specific neurotic illnesses. Above all, the people concerned, who at one time had the assistance of Cyril Burt—evacuated with the Department of Psychology of University College, London, to Cardiganshire—appear to have had not only the necessary insight and expertise but also a practical approach to the many problems with which they were faced.

Another local authority evacuation scheme that attracted considerable attention was that promoted by Oxfordshire. This was not only of some importance in itself but also in that it engaged the interest and stimulated the ideas of Dr D. W. Winnicott, whose subsequent influence on the care and treatment of disturbed children has been considerable. Within this scheme hostels for disturbed and unbilletable evacuees were grouped together to ease communication and transfer, to make the therapeutic and supportive work of the psychiatrist more possible, and to allow the whole enterprise to be supervised by one psychiatric social worker. Hostels ranged in size from twelve to twenty-five children and differed in type largely on the basis of the wardens' interests and abilities. The aim was to create a loving, tolerant, but firmly structured 'home' environment within which the children could, with psychiatric support, work out not only their temporary but also many of their more deep-seated disturbances.[16] Results were inevitably uneven and crises frequent but both in Oxfordshire and in many other localities 'a really big collective experience had been gained'. Here was the beginning of a nation-wide system of care for the maladjusted and, however *ad hoc* the basis was in 1940, the potential of such hostels was realized. Winnicott, addressing a group of magistrates, said of these wartime hostels: 'Here, surely, is the place for the treatment of delinquency as an illness of the individual, and here, surely, is the place for research, and opportunity to gain experience. . . . In these hostels for the so-called maladjusted one is free to work with a therapeutic aim and this makes a lot of difference.'[17]

Organization apart, there remained the chief difficulty of finding those people of 'special experience', interest and ability who, in manning the hostels, were the key to the whole enterprise. Some were already on hand and, as has been seen, experienced workers such as Leila Rendel, Dr Dodd, Dr Fitch and David Wills readily adapted their practice to accommodate the new problem or assimilated it within their existing institutions. Many new people had to be found, however, from the depleted ranks of the experienced and mature.

Winnicott lists the previous occupations of the Oxfordshire wardens as 'elementary school teacher, social worker, trained church worker, commercial artist, instructor and matron in an approved school, master and matron at a remand home, worker in public assistance institution, prison welfare officer'.[18] Many had less apparently relevant qualifications and the work of the vast majority of these involved and dedicated people (as of those who were quite inadequate to face the work which they undertook), is unrecorded. Some, however, contributed notably to an understanding of the wider problems and continued their work after the 'emergency' had ended. To some of these it is possible to give further consideration and indeed, such was the impetus given to the recognition of the needs of the maladjusted by wartime conditions that there is little that is considerable in the subsequent history of this subject which does not stem from this period. The evolution of child care, of 'special' education, of therapy was vastly accelerated and indeed one wonders whether these new approaches would ever have become nationally accepted if war had not made maladjustment a national problem. There were few signs before the war that the lone voices of the pioneer individuals would ever be swelled to a national chorus.

Faced with new problems, and with little guidance and few precedents to assist them, individual workers continued to experiment with idiosyncratic techniques, some of which were later conceptualized. Hostels developed into schools, some remaining determinedly independent, others being absorbed into the State system.

BILL MALCOLM

The career of Bill Malcolm is, to some extent, typical. Through it we can see a development from pre-war models and the pre-war pattern of the dominant individual moulding an environment pragmatically; through the testing time of war towards attempts at conceptualization; and utimately, perhaps, to a sort of isolation as treatment became more systematized and organization was centralized.

Childscourt by John Coleman, Malcolm's biographer, although, like Burn's account of Lyward's work, unfailingly panegyric, gives a picture of a human being, often changeable and inconsistent, grappling with real problems with the power of conviction and in the light of insight. The interest lies not in a method, for there appears little capable of conceptualization, but in the way in which Malcolm's career highlights the difficulties of this transitional period.

In some ways Malcolm resembles Neill, his early mentor, in his dogmatism and in the way in which he constantly re-fights the battles of his youth, some of which have already been won. Even Coleman admits that Malcolm's early experiences in an unimaginative and tough Derbyshire council school 'left an image of what he is inclined to imagine all other schools are like today'. His apprenticeship in 'toughness' was continued during the depression when he emigrated to Australia for twelve years' experience on sheep stations and in the Sydney Sailors' Home.

Friends helped him to rethink his moral attitudes and he returned to Cornwall where, at the beginning of the war, he had his first successful contact with difficult evacuees in his own home. His interest in problem children grew after a period of work at Summerhill (then evacuated to Wales) in which he was introduced to ideas of freedom, self-government and child-centred education which, from this time onwards, seem to have fought a running battle with his personality.

His management of the Bryn Conway hostel, of which he became warden in 1942, is fairly typical. Initially a 'self-governing structure' was used as an instrument by which Malcolm, as chairman, could gain support for his authority, which was directed mainly towards the breaking down of gangs and power-seeking individuals, but gradually the children felt sufficiently secure to form an effective law-making and law-enforcing body meeting weekly to discuss the condition and structure of the hostel, the social behaviour both of children and staff and the use of the school fund (all personal money was pooled).

This appears to have had a good effect on the social and emotional adjustment of the children and a report by Dr D. E. Parry-Pritchard, the medical officer of health, on thirty-one very disturbed children who passed through the hostel indicates that of sixteen who were 'beyond control' all made satisfactory adjustment to hostel, school, home or work; of seven who were incontinent five became continent, and, of the whole thirty-one, whose conditions on admission varied from 'nervous instability' to epilepsy, only seven appear not to have progressed successfully in the years immediately following their stay in Bryn Conway and, of these, two were there while awaiting placement at an approved school, to which they went subsequently, one

was transferred to an epileptic school and two absconded from the
hostel after the Malcolms left.[19]

Interest in Bill Malcolm's success grew and he was asked to take
over the Regional Evacuation Hostel at Penybrin which was for the
most difficult evacuees in the six counties of North Wales. With the
assistance of a nucleus of staff and children from Bryn Conway he
instituted the same regime at Penybrin. Most of the children were
extremely socially deprived, emotionally disturbed and frequently
delinquent. The hostel was unpopular in the area and the children
scarcely popular in the local schools which they attended.

In 1945, however, it was possible for the clerk to the Gwyrfai
R.D.C. to write: 'The hostel has become a happy home and we
have had no trouble with any of the children.'[20] The children
appeared to progress very well at the local schools and to profit by
a great freedom to use the facilities which the countryside offered for
play and adventure. It is interesting to note that as the home became
more established hostel meetings and children's tribunals were
gradually replaced by a more family-based principle of community
interest. This may have been partly Malcolm's need for a more
realistic paternal role but it is, in fact, interesting to speculate how
far the machinery of 'shared responsibility', in a small community,
hinders the development of family relationships, and how much
more fundamental the latter are in residential establishments for
socially and emotionally deprived children, whose primary need is
a strong affective relationship with someone who is not only adult
but is perceived to be playing an adult role. This may have been
particularly true during, and immediately after, the war when many
children clearly suffered from the absence of any effective father-
figure. At Penybrin, Malcolm offered the 'ordered freedom' of a good
and liberal family in which, while decisions were based on the discussion of individual needs, there was no doubt where the ultimate
security rested.

To the very disturbed children with whom he came into contact
Malcolm offered a sympathetic home and his own insight and intuition which was his greatest strength, although perhaps at times relied
on too implicitly. A good example of his approach at its best is
given in a welfare worker's account of Malcolm's treatment of a boy
who had been sent to him by a local hospital after the boy had
threatened the staff with a carving knife: The boy 'was an uncouth
lad hating everything and everybody'. His first action was to smash

half a dozen windows and flatten a fireguard. Malcolm was patient and tolerant but

for about five months Dennis remained absolutely unapproachable, until one night his housemother complained that he had got into bed with his clothes on. About half an hour later terrific roars were heard coming from his bedroom. Mr Malcolm dashed in thinking that Dennis was attacking someone. In actual fact he was calling 'Bill' as Mr Malcolm was known to the children.

When he arrived in the room Dennis was lying in bed with clothes drawn up to his eyes. By the side of his bed was a heap of wool which had once been a jersey, picked into very small pieces. He had also cut his pyjamas into very small pieces with a pair of scissors. The bed was in a filthy state with mud off his own boots and covered with his own excrement. It was almost the lad's final act of aggressive resentment against a world which he felt did not want him. Mr Malcolm sensed this and remarked: 'Well, son, I bet it took you quite a while to make this mess, and I expect you feel quite satisfied. Now I will clean all this up and get you some clean sheets – you mucky so-and-so!' He then obtained some clean sheets from the airing cupboard, made Dennis comfortable and cleared up the mess round the bed. As he was turning away he said goodnight to Dennis who gazed up at him and murmured 'You silly old sod', but with a humorous twinkle in his eye which converted this phrase to a term of affection. This was the first time the child had shown any human feeling apart from hate.[21]

Malcolm's success in the comparatively limited hostel situation, both at Penybrin and after the war in a hostel for difficult delinquent boys at Maidenhead, brought him to the notice of Dr Marjorie Franklin and Children's Social Adjustment Limited who, in 1948, were endeavouring to found a school, Arlesford Place, on 'planned environmental therapy' lines (see Chapter 15). This conjunction of the pragmatic exponent of environmental therapy and the person most concerned with giving it a sound theoretical base seemed auspicious but proved fatal. Malcolm had no place in his scheme of things for psychological theorists, psychoanalytical interpretations or psychotherapeutic 'interference'. Dr Franklin was endeavouring to meet the criticism that had been levelled at earlier experiments, that they lacked a sound theoretical justification by conducting 'on-going' research, was herself of a Freudian persuasion and, as honorary psychiatrist, believed that psychotherapy was necessary for cure. The latter was also chairman of the management committee, which body had more members than it was intended there should be children in the school. At no point was there any fundamental agreement on policy. While Malcolm considered, as did Dr Fitch, that 'maladjusted' children were mainly normal children reacting to abnormal conditions, the psychiatrically orientated committee frequently sent him extremely emotionally disturbed children whom he admitted that he could neither understand nor treat.

When, in pursuit of their own expressed treatment policies, the committee encouraged psychiatric intervention and the appointment of psychologically trained staff Malcolm saw his authority threatened and his concept of a normal community centred round a normal school damaged. Inevitably, in this situation, the psychiatrists' visits were followed not only by what might be seen as therapeutically desirable regression of individuals but a regression in the life of the community. While Malcolm legitimately saw himself as able to do normal, if difficult, work with normal, if difficult, children, the managers, equally legitimately, saw the school as one in which specialized techniques were used to treat 'special' children.

At no point does there appear to have been a meeting of minds. Even 'environmental therapy' in its narrowest sense was an area of conflict. While the committee, still thinking to some extent in Q Camp terms, believed in the therapeutic value of the children converting impoverished surroundings to their own use, Malcolm believed in the importance of introducing a sense of luxury and superiority into the surroundings so that no child or parent should think of the school as inferior to others.

Again, while both sides believed in the value of 'shared responsibility', neither was really consistent in its use. The committee represented an authority which could radically affect the life of the community while not being responsible to it, the will of the school was, in the context, necessarily subordinate to the needs of psychotherapy, and Malcolm appears also to have continued his own inner struggle. He was always alert to threats which individuals or groups posed to the authority of the community. These he opposed with his own authority (ostensibly in the name of the community), sometimes by displays of force.

An example of this occurred when Malcolm returned to Arlesford Place after he had resigned in 1951 and had then been recalled when the school dissolved into chaos. Four large boys, accepted in his absence, challenged his authority by insisting on going out. 'In an instant Bill saw what they were doing and instinctively felt that the one thing they must not do on that afternoon was to go out. They were intent on attack. Bill attacked first and before they had time to think what was happening he'd knocked their spokesman flat on the ground. "What are you going to do about your bloody friend?" he asked in the same tone of voice as that in which they'd announced their intentions for the afternoon. "There are odd occasions when you have to step out of line and act against all your principles and if you don't all your work will be destroyed," said Bill afterwards. In his opinion that occasion was one of them and in fact it was mainly a matter of self-defence. "They were big, powerful boys intent on destroying me and the school. For a moment I felt like a cornered fox taking the only way out." '22

Such behaviour earned Malcolm the reputation of a 'muscle man' but, while opposing corporal punishment and retaining his pacifist views he rationalized these actions as the need to 'forcibly restrain badly disturbed children, who are in a primitive state of hate against the whole world and beyond reason, from being cruel to each other, or to animals, or interfering malignantly in the peaceful pastimes of their companions'.

With such an approach to the establishment of the security of the community and to the treatment of the most disturbed members in it, it is not surprising that Malcolm did not co-operate with psychiatrists of an analytical persuasion nor welcome the intervention of psychologically orientated staff and observers.

The failure of Arlesford should not obscure either the important principles involved in the unfortunate but inevitable conflict or the value of much of the work which was done. Considering that his role was mainly to help deprived children weather the normal storms and stresses of growing up, Malcolm continued to put his faith in the structure of 'shared responsibility', community life, in freedom from unnecessary social or moral pressures and in a wide and sympathetic tolerance—once described by a B.B.C. reporter as 'Christ-like'.

In school work, in which he battled constantly against that lack of concentration which is the maladjusted child's chief educational handicap, he demonstrated his belief that 'get rid of the pressures, and many of the standards which to them are meaningless and 90 per cent of them improve automatically'. He believed that in a free environment most of the children could 'cure themselves' with the support of other children. Mental health and educational progress would come largely by expecting it. In his discussions with children and with parents he stressed reality—the real capacity of the children, the real demands of society, so that the child's expectations on leaving Arlesford were not inflated by a feeling that since he was 'special' a 'special' position awaited him.

In 1960, Malcolm gave up the struggle at Arlesford, which closed shortly afterwards and, with the support of friends and admirers of his work, set up his own school—Childscourt—at Long Bredy in Dorset, moving to Lettiford House near Wincanton in 1963. His work here, in moulding the sort of community he desired, is not properly within the scope of this study but may be mentioned briefly as illustrative of the personality of an early worker in this field, who, like many others, was the centre of controversy, convinced of his own rightness but often inconsistent, developing round himself an extended family to whom he was at the same time elder brother, stern but loving father and, at times, God.

At Childscourt, Malcolm, although continuing the 'meetings', which John Danser considers might be more appropriately called 'grouse and trial sessions',[23] seems always to have been sensitive to any challenge to authority. He appears particularly to be sensitive to the threat of what he refers to as 'Nazi' gangs and also to the expressions of individual aggression. This threat was used as an explanation of such actions as physical assault, restrictions on camping, and the bulldozing of bushes around the school. His suspicion of doctors, and of psychiatrists in particular, did not diminish and, in fact, he was inclined to remark 'Ah, they're a nutty lot these people who go around prying into you', which could hardly have been helpful to those children who were still under treatment.

This attitude may have been partly an expression of his need to be the central character, a need to which at Childscourt he gave overt expression. In school plays he wrote, produced, and acted the leading role. In games he was automatically the captain of his football team (taking children away from other activities to play). He considered it necessary to the community that he should play the hero both to the boys and to the girls.

His attitude to the girls appears either suspicious or possessive. They are harangued on St Valentine's Day because they make a beeline for an attractive new boy: 'You're not going to turn this school into a bloody night-club, it's got to be a place where boys and girls can live together, normally.' Like Homer Lane, Malcolm also evolved a policy of retaining certain children as junior staff-members, thus continuing their dependence on the community.

In a more positive way Malcolm hopes to equip his children with a realistic and questioning attitude to life, a belief in their own worth, and as much educational attainment as is found consistent with the needs of emotional adjustment. The school work, which covers a full range of subjects for both boys and girls between five and fifteen with I.Q.s ranging from 80—130, and at various stages of emotional adjustment, is arranged into small groups of six or seven with a class teacher. Division is largely by two-year age groups. The ability to achieve in school work is seen as a necessary part of the child's personal and social adjustment and C.S.E. passes are sought after both as a boost to morale and as desirable equipment for re-entry into a competitive society.

From A. S. Neill, Malcolm has taken his rejection of religious and moral restraints although they reappear in his demand for conformity to the perceived social needs of the school. From Arlesford he has taken his rejection of the psychiatric approach as damaging to the idea both of a normal process of individual development and to social integration. It is from his wartime hostel experience that he has taken his most fundamental guideline, a belief in the importance of 'common sense' based on practical experience as superior to all theories and general principles.

ARTHUR BARRON

Another for whom wartime hostel experience was significant but who came to very different conclusions is Arthur Barron, whose career may illustrate, in another way, the nature of this transitional, or evolutionary, period. Barron, who is now a psychotherapist for the Greater London Council and a trustee of the Planned Environmental Therapy Trust, was not an originator but a person involved in many important aspects of this work who moved steadily towards a greater clarity of purpose and conceptualization of role. An account of this personal search may be of some importance to those who face similar problems in this field.

As a 'student helper' at the Hawkspur Camp he was, at the age of eighteen, one of the youngest members of that pioneering community, and having practical experience, he was appointed director of all constructional work. As we have seen (see Chapter 12) this work was regarded as an important part of the therapy, being a co-operative enterprise and an experiment in producing an environment in direct response to need.

From this experience he acquired a belief in work 'not just as something to do in order that the community will not strafe one: it is something essential to do if one is to be happy, or to gain or retain self-respect, or to develop one's character or to use one's powers'.[24] As the work became inevitably more complex and systematic, individual freedom had to be curtailed by more structured patterns of work and it had to be accepted that the experience of law and order was necessary not only for the continuance of the group but to individual happiness. This was possible within the framework of 'shared responsibility' but it was necessary for all to share and accept responsibility. This, in a community of disturbed delinquents, was not always easy to achieve. No one was instructed in doing a job unless, faced with a practical problem, he asked for advice, which was sometimes given in the form of a reference to a manual or a suggestion that he might observe the local builder at work.

From his experience at the Hawkspur Camp, therefore, Barron acquired certain fundamental beliefs about the treatment of disturbed youths. These may be briefly summarized as an understanding of the importance of freedom, of individual and corporate creative activity, of the value of responsible work and of the underlying principles of 'shared responsibility'.

In 1940 Wills was asked to transfer the members and staff of the Hawkspur Camp to Bicester in connection with a scheme to house unbilletable evacuees. He found that the accommodation offered for both members and children was a disused workhouse with ninety-five rooms, barely equipped and with most of the windows painted out. Faced with these conditions and official lack of acceptance of Q Camp principles Wills and his staff, including Barron, resigned. The problem of 'unbilletable evacuees', however, remained with them both.

Barron's next post was as a teacher at Rest Harrow Abbey School, established specifically as an experiment in the education of maladjusted children — junior boys and senior girls — under the direction of Dr Ida Saxby. Dr Saxby was a remarkable woman of German origin. An early graduate of Newnham College, Cambridge, in mathematics, she subsequently became interested in abnormal psychology and took a D.Sc. at London with a thesis on the connection between motivation and memory. Some of her work was supervised by Burt and she also kept in close touch with Freud and his followers. She was much influenced by J. C. Flugel and the 'British' school of psychoanalysis (dominated by Melanie Klein), with its emphasis on the central importance of the early mother-child relationship.[25] While a lecturer in the teacher training department of University College, Cardiff between 1915 and 1925 she published her book *The Education of Behaviour*,[26] in which she examined the inter-relation of personality and behaviour and explored the possibilities of various forms of environmental manipulation such as self-governing institutions. Her chief influence at this period was McDougall rather than Freud, although she regarded psychoanalysis as important both for the disturbed child and for increasing the teacher's own self-awareness. Motivation was seen as the key to action and the teacher's role as producing the right stimulus for motivation towards socially approved goals. Dr Saxby was also in close contact at this time with the staff of Glamorgan Mental Hospital, Bridgend, being particularly interested in the study of neuroses through the interpretation of dreams. In the 1930s, after leaving Cardiff, she studied medicine and at the beginning of the war undertook the headship of Rest Harrow Abbey School, near Haslemere.

The experiment was not a success. She was, by this time, elderly and lacking in effectiveness as a leader of a therapeutic community and of a staff whose interests and experience did not match her own. Although her ideas on organization and teaching were conventional she combined the roles of headmistress and therapist. Therapy, apart from some outside psychiatric assistance, was largely in terms of hour-long sessions 'on the couch', with Dr Saxby playing her role of psychoanalyst of a basically Kleinian persuasion.

The subsequent conflicts among the disturbed children (largely of upper-middle-class origin) explains, perhaps, Barron's dramatic introduction to maladjusted girls. Now in his early twenties he was about to take his first lesson with the senior girls when they all proceeded slowly to undress in front of him until he was faced with a class of naked young women. Barron attributed this phenomenon to the generally confused and repressive situation in which treatment was not applied to the whole child the whole of the time through the environment and he sought to get Dr Saxby to re-organize the school on lines more similar to those which he had experienced at Hawkspur.

The too rapid taking off of brakes when Barron was given authority as senior master, wartime shortages of adequate staff, a move from Haslemere to the woods of Grayshott and the arrival in the woods of a camp-full of Canadian soldiers proved disastrous. The school was closed amid chaos and scandal and Dr Saxby returned to the individual consultative work which was her *forte*.

Barron considers that Dr Saxby failed to understand that maladjustment is a condition of the whole child and not just something 'in addition to the child'. Despite her devotion and nobility of the spirit the confused educational and treatment situation and the complete absence of any comprehensive theory made failure inevitable.

After this further failure to realize his Hawkspur principles in action Barron served on an international commission for refugees and unbilletable evacuees at Lindwood, near Market Rasen. This also proved an unhappy experience. Barron was in charge of the children who were maladjusted but not of the hostel itself, for which there was no clear line of authority. The sixty or so children were of thirteen different nationalities and there was constant war between evacuees from the north and south of Britain. The children were supposed to attend local schools but because of language and other difficulties few were able to do so and very little provision could be made within the hostel. Barron ran an art class largely for therapeutic purposes.

The refugee children felt guilty because of those who had been left behind in occupied Europe and the staff felt guilty because they were lavishly equipped and fed by American and Canadian sympathizers in a way which Barron felt to be quite inconsistent with their role. Reacting to this Barron then took over a hostel for unbilletable enuretic evacuees run under the aegis of the Truro Rural District Council at Perranporth. This appeared to be run largely by the sanitary inspector's assistant and the local W.V.S. The sixty-five boys and three staff were in three separate houses overlooking the sea, and both the houses and the children were suffering from varying degrees of neglect. To reorganize the hostel, Barron stayed for five months, during which he had only three days in which he was, even for a time, away from the job. His newly married wife, who was matron, was in charge of another house and scarcely saw him. The turnover of children at times reached as many as fifteen a day.

In this experience he found an increasing concern with the needs of the disturbed child in care. He was convinced of the importance of fundamentally re-organizing the whole attitude of the State to such children and with youthful and characteristic zeal he proceeded to organize pressure groups. As a Special Correspondent of the *Times Educational Supplement* he publicized the inadequacy of the provision and supported Lady Allen of Hurtwood in her influential advocacy of the needs of the destitute and neglected and of the importance of the reform of child-care provision. Lady Allen perceived that: 'The social upheaval caused by the war has not only increased this army of unhappy children, but presents the opportunity for transforming their conditions.'[27] She urged a Government enquiry and such advocacy bore fruit in the appointment of the Curtis Committee in March, 1945. In her pamphlet *Whose Children*[28] Lady Allen roused the public conscience by citing many extreme examples of neglect which had been brought to her notice by such concerned workers as Arthur Barron, who after his experience at Perranporth had become warden of a hostel for unbilletable evacuees near Malmesbury.

Lady Allen, in her initial letter to *The Times* in 1944, had also stressed the importance of adequate staff and adequate training and support for the staff concerned with this most difficult area of child care. Here also Barron had recognized a need and with typical directness he looked first to organized self-help. At a refresher course for evacuee hostel staff in 1943, he, together with W. G. Sharman and John Elvidge, expressed the need for an association of workers engaged in dealing with maladjusted children in hostels. This was conceived as an informal body for mutual support but it was opposed by the Board of Education, who feared that it would become a channel of complaint. Barron was already well known for the forcefulness of his views. The proposal was withdrawn and it was eighteen years before such a body came into existence.

In 1944 Barron was appointed Camp Chief of Q Camp for boys in the original Q Camp buildings at Hawkspur. This he and his Q Camp advisers conceived as an enormous creative activity designed to counteract the violence and aggression so prevalent in children who had been deprived of their fathers during the war and who had learnt to identify with the heroes of war and destruction. Here again Barron's experience was illuminating not only to himself but to all thinking exponents of environmental therapy. Principles, as Barron had learnt, may be tested by apparent failure as well as by apparent success.

The plan at Hawkspur was to root the children in the community by encouraging them to create their own environment both physical and political. Although Barron had been convinced of the value of this policy at the original camp for senior delinquents he began to see it, as did David Wills and Hermann Mannheim, who resigned from the committee, as mistaken in this context with young adolescents. The disorder and physical hardship of the 'back to the earth' philosophy of the early Q Campers offered too little physical care to children in search of security after five years of war. Barron learnt that 'one cannot use a kid's neurosis as a basis for his education'. He illustrates this insight by the example of a boy who was a perpetual horse-thief. At Q Camp he was given a horse to look after. He neglected the horse. 'The worst thing one can do for anyone is to make their fantasies come real.'

The children were too young to create their own sociey with their own hands. The clearest example of this was when the adolescents at Q Camp refused to accept the 'shared responsibility' which was offered them and demanded to be looked after. The extent to which the democratic principle was rejected was seen when those who opposed shared responsibility were allowed to devise their own political system. They evolved an organization of 'slaves and masters' in which the roles were clearly delineated. This Barron took to represent a desire for a lost mother-child relationship, although it seems likely that the significant factor with these wartime children may well have been the absence of a satisfactory father-figure playing a strongly supportive, at times authoritarian, role—a conclusion which gains some support from Balbernie's recent analysis of the social needs of deprived children.[29] Both views may well be true since the range of conditions of disturbance and deprivation in such an institution are not satisfactorily discriminated, and what is appropriate for one condition may be quite inappropriate for another condition of which the presenting symptoms may be similar.

In any event Barron was convinced that the quality of child care was inadequate to meet the needs of these particular children and an attempt was made to move the camp into a building—Arlesford Place. The transition caused further chaos, and Barron and his staff resigned. This marked the end of Q Camps, although the concept still has its protagonists who hope for a resumption of the experiment.

This failure taught Barron, whose mind remained refreshingly open, a number of lessons. Its implication for the care of deprived and disturbed children within the general context of environmental therapy was that, in such a situation, children need a super-ego figure who does not avoid the responsibility which the children wish him to bear. The implication for Barron himself, who was not yet thirty, was that he was inadequate for this role without the support of a basic theoretical structure and a deeper knowledge of himself. This he found in Freudian psychoanalysis and Barron is not alone in his belief that without this process and structure an individual is unlikely to be of great use as a therapist with severely disturbed children since he will be unable either to understand the nature of the disturbance or his role in its treatment. Barron's rethinking of the nature of maladjustment—derived largely from the work of Anna Freud—and his important contributions to the understanding of the role of the worker with maladjusted children are considered elsewhere, but these insights, forged from experience, fundamentally altered his own course.

He entered into a lengthy period of analysis and training in psychotherapy and, while still a student, he became warden and psychotherapist in a Surrey County Council hostel for maladjusted children at Ripley (subsequently transferred to Starhurst, near Dorking). Here he was able to work in much greater depth than had been possible when he had been involved in the emergency situation imposed by the war, and his research work (together with Dorothy Burlingham), further convinced him of the need of a psychoanalytically orientated depth approach to the problems of seriously emotionally disturbed children if anything more was to be achieved than a superficial social adjustment.[30] In pursuance of this end he became psychotherapist to, and therapeutic adviser in, a number of schools for maladjusted children while continuing his research into delinquency and allied problems at the Hampstead Child Therapy Clinic.

As with many other workers with disturbed evacuees, his experience had been crucial. It emphasized to him the importance of the breakdown of the parent-child bond in the production of the most severe disturbance and the basic need to tackle this problem in treatment. During the war he had recognized his own inadequacy, and that of organizational manipulation, to deal with this problem and, in fact, had, despite much official opposition, worked hard to re-unite children with their parents, even at the risk of their death by bombing, before re-evacuating them after careful preparation for the separation. Although unable to collect reliable figures he 'formed a strong impression that this technique worked'.[31] In his subsequent work in residential institutions he put great emphasis on adequate preparation of the child to face the reality of the emotional situation and on work with the parents so that children, parents and members of staff could face the experience with less guilt or feeling of rejection. Without such preparation (rather than the usual interviews which are often superficial and based largely on 'selling' the school to the child) Barron considers that residential placement is not only likely to be ineffective but actually harmful leading, on all sides, to the building up of fantasy defences which inhibit the normal processes of the painful development towards independence.

The child, unable to find satisfaction in reality because he is separated from the now intensely desirable Mother, alters part of himself to be like her. Thus we have the situation that the child indentifies, with the whole strength of his personality, with that part of the environment from which we sought to spare him by placing him away from home. At the same time he takes a decisive step away from reality-based thinking towards fantasy thinking. The direction of his libido is reversed, from the normal gradual lessening of emotional ties with the parents to an intense desire for the closest unity with them. From the point of view of the school and society, the important factor is that these unconscious processes render the child inaccessible to environmental help or influence.[32]

The implication for work with maladjusted children, and in child care, of such a theoretical position is clear. To send a child into a residential institution, whether it be school or home or foster-family, without preparation and subsequent care by skilled psychotherapy is a recipe for disaster. The results, based largely on a chance 'transference' to someone who does not know the nature or the extent of the condition and who may unwittingly be drawn into the fantasy situation in a collusive relationship, are at best chancy and fraught with peril.

CHILD CARE

In these terms 'child care' in any form has a long way to go and, indeed, may be on the wrong road as it puts increasing emphasis on sociology and on organizational superstructure. Nevertheless the progress that has been made since Barron found children dying of neglect in wartime 'child-care' hostels has been considerable. The notorious case of Dennis O'Neill, who was taken into care for neglect, for which his parents were punished, and who subsequently died of neglect in 1945 in the foster-home in which he had been placed by a local authority highlighted the faults of the existing system.[33] Administrative confusion, individual incompetence, inadequate supervision all contributed to this tragedy and to others detailed in Lady Allen's pamphlet.[34]

The Curtis Committee and the Clyde Committee (Scotland) were set up in 1945 to examine the whole problem of children deprived of parental care and to recommend measures 'to ensure that these children are brought up under conditions best calculated to compensate them for the lack of parental care'.[35] The conclusions of the two committees were essentially similar.

A chaotic situation was uncovered by the Curtis Committee in which such deprived children received inadequate care and supervision from four different central authorities—Health, Home Office, Education and Pensions—or from local authorities or from largely unsupervised voluntary organizations. Many children over nine years of age, whether fostered or in voluntary homes, were completely unsupervised by the State.[36] In general the committee found that the quality of care, both short-term in workhouses and long-term in both large and small institutions, was inadequate in that it failed, almost completely, to consider the emotional needs of the individual child. While physical conditions were often adequate (although sometimes dreary, drab and over-regimentated) discipline, while seldom damagingly harsh or punitive, lacked imagination and warmth. The committee was shocked by a fairly general absence of sympathy for the child's need of individual self-expression or of the experience of a kindly, loving relationship.

As Lady Allen had suggested in 1944, the committee found that the majority of the staff in such homes were 'overworked, underpaid and untrained'; indeed no specific form of training existed and where good work was being done it was largely as a result of the presence of a worker of unusual insight and sympathy. There were too few such workers.

The committee, although critical of the lack of care in choosing, and subsequent supervision of, foster homes, clearly preferred this alternative to the large institution. Since the child 'in care' was primarily the child deprived of the experience of family life the foster-home clearly offered an opportunity for greater compensation. Bearing in mind the O'Neill case, the committee's enthusiasm was qualified. 'On the whole our judgement is that there is probably a greater risk of acute unhappiness in a foster-home, but that a happy foster-home is happier than life as generally lived in a large community.'[37]

The committee's general recommendations, the majority of which except those which referred to maladjusted children, were incorporated into the Children's Act of 1948, are detailed in the Report (Sections 423–515) and were greatly concerned with the reorganization of administration and the centralization of control (through the Home Office under the 1948 Act). The general emphasis was on recognizing the child's individual need for family life and on care in placement whether in 'small group' homes or foster-homes. This entailed a considerable and valuable increase in individual and family casework and in provision for training in child care. The urgency of the latter need was recognized immediately by the establishment in 1946 of the Central Training Council and the provision of child-care courses.

In this re-organization the needs of maladjusted deprived children were largely overlooked. Enquiries made by the Curtis Committee about the problem of the treatment of 'difficult' children in Public Assistance homes, voluntary organization homes and in remand homes were generally met with what seemed to be astonishing complacency, although the committee suggests rather a lack of awareness. Enuresis, pilfering, destructiveness and abscondings existed or occurred but were coped with within the usual disciplinary structure, whether severe or sympathetic, without any special regard to the disturbances of which these were symptoms. It was one exceptionally insightful matron who attributed the fact that children did not wet their beds so often when they were ill to the degree of individual attention which they were receiving.

Only in the more progressive of voluntary organization homes

H

was there 'an awareness of the need for special treatment of difficult children. As a general rule such children were considered "naughty" and were dealt with in the same way as the rest. In the worst homes such problems as enuresis were treated by punishment or accepted with a fatalistic attitude. . . . As in the local authority Homes the less noticeable symptoms of difficulty usually remained unrecognized. Pilfering (especially of food), destructiveness, secretiveness, fantasies, were all mentioned as examples of naughtiness and punished severely. . . . It was rare to find that use was made of Child Guidance Clinics or other specialist advice.'[38]

The committee recommended that there should be greater awareness of the emotional implications of such symptoms as enuresis and pilfering which should be dealt with by non-punitive means. It stressed the urgency of retaining those hostels for maladjusted children which had grown up during the war, both for the children's sake and to lessen the disruption of ordinary homes.

Its proposals for the establishment of homes specifically for maladjusted children are of particular interest, although their effect has been relatively slight.

While we recommend the small family unit as being, after adoption and boarding out in the best conditions, the most satisfactory method of meeting the needs of normal healthy children, we see a limited use for the larger Homes of say about thirty. Apart from special experiments by voluntary organisations under exceptionally able leadership, which we should be sorry to discourage, we think the larger community may be the more successful for the abnormal group. There will always be a need for temporary removal from its home of a maladjusted or difficult child, as evacuation experience has amply shown, and notable success with such children has been secured in Homes of the size of 20–30. The unstable child appears to be better in a community with many activities and friends to choose from, and with an expert in charge of the discipline. Our evidence indicates that what is required for such a Home is an exceptionally competent and sympathetic superintendent and matron, and visiting advisors qualified in the treatment of childish abnormalities. It would serve in a sense as a residential child guidance clinic. Our witnesses have not advised us that any special regime can be prescribed for such establishments. Remarkably successful results are achieved by dissimilar methods, given personal suitability and enthusiasm on the part of those in charge. . . . We should welcome research and experiment by local authorities on the best way of tackling the cases which, for some reason, are abnormal.[39]

In such recommendations the committee implicity recognized maladjustment as a form of handicap requiring special child-care treatment although recognizing that, under the Education Act 1944, the rehabilitation of such children 'is the responsibility of local education authorities, and we assume that "deprived" children, equally with those from normal homes, will enjoy the benefit of whatever remedial treatment is to be found the most effectual'. Thus the problem of problem children was placed largely in the hands of education authorities from whom, in the current reorganization, the child-care authorities are proposing to wrest them back.

The Child Care Act of 1948 made no explicit reference to maladjusted children. Presumably the view was taken that adequate provision for their needs would be made by the Ministry of Education and that local authorities would find sufficient scope in Section 12 (1), in which they were empowered to act in respect to the child 'so as to further his best interests, and to afford him opportunity for the proper development of his character and abilities' for the establishment of facilities or the placement of children in residential schools. In fact few homes such as those envisaged by the Curtis Committee were established under the aegis of the Child Care Department, although considerable use was made of boarding homes established by local education authorities (currently about forty catering for roughly 600 children).

There was also a specific recommendation that reception centres should be established in each area but the 'necessary facilities' were for observation of 'physical and mental condition' (Section 15 (2)). No mention was made of psychological or emotional need although the actual terms have, of course, been variously interpreted. In anticipation of a wide extension of available facilities the Curtis Committee had stressed the need for at least one reception centre in each area in which children taken into care could be placed while their physical, social and psychological needs could be assessed. The experimental reception centre established under the aegis of Leila Rendel was to some extent the model but, as has been seen, was immediately restricted in its aims by a tendency to have referred to it only children who had been through juvenile courts and, of course, by the absence of any real choice in placement. Of the few reception centres subsequently established, over a quarter had no special facilities for observation and assessment and many became at best containing units and at worst the first stage in what are still, in public regard, 'children's prisons'. This widespread public attitude was an unfortunate but inevitable side-effect of placing the child-care provision under the aegis of the Home Office. There would certainly be no general agreement that this choice was the appropriate one on the basis of the Home Office's 'historically progressive traditions in the case of homeless children'.[40] Whatever the expressed attitude of that department its association with the whole penal structure could only have an adverse effect, not only on the actual organization of provision but, perhaps more importantly, on public attitudes towards such provision.

APPROVED SCHOOLS

The wide discrepancy between official attitudes, current practice and public regard is nowhere more clearly illustrated than in the development of the approved-school system. A detailed study is not relevant here since, as has been pointed out, delinquents cannot necessarily be regarded as maladjusted, but, particularly in view of the current blurring of distinctions between 'approved' and 'special' schools[41] brief survey may be helpful.

Approved schools officially came into being in 1933 as places of care, detention and training for children committed to them by the juvenile courts. They were directly descended from the industrial and reformatory schools which had originated in the middle of the nineteenth-century in the altruistic efforts of the Philanthropic Society and of such individuals as Mary Carpenter (see Chapter 4). Industrial and reformatory schools were normally run by voluntary managers, largely co-opted from people of considerable means and social status and with strong religious and philanthropic views. The State, although empowered to do so in the Reformatory Schools Act, 1854, and the Industrial Schools Act, 1857, exercised little supervision and its own experiments in 'reformatory' work were tainted by the memory of the first State-directed reformatory school—Parkhurst—which Mary Carpenter vilified so roundly.[42] The absence of effective supervision was partly the result of the Government's reluctance to accept financial responsibility, partly of the resentment of the managers to interference with their voluntarily-accepted responsibilities and partly the result of extremely rapid growth. By 1861 there were forty-five reformatory and nineteen industrial schools and by 1914 there were 223 schools containing 25,357 children, industrial schools being largely designed for those under-fourteen thought to be in moral danger or in need of care, while the reformatory schools were for those juveniles over fourteen years of age who had been convicted of an offence punishable with penal servitude or imprisonment.

From the beginning the complexity of the problem and a general uncertainty as to aim urged managers and staff towards the security offered by uniformity and systematization. Economy also, in schools largely maintained by public subscription, suggested the advantages of large institutions, underpaid, overworked and often undervalued staff, bleak physical conditions, and work engaged in more for its financial than its educational value. Under such conditions the value that the reformers attached to individual care and family experience tended to be lost sight of and arrangements based on humanitarian principles of child care and reform were superseded by severe discipline, uniformly imposed, and by traditions of regimentation. This legacy was persistent and has been the main focus of attack both for those who sought to improve the system from within and the large body of liberal critics who are, even today, mainly responsible for the approved school's unfavourable public image.

It is ironic that, as the State acquired greater control of the system the Home Office, particularly in the persons of such notable chief inspectors as Sydney Turner (1857–76), J. G. Legge (1896–1906), C. E. B. Russell (1913–17) and A. H. Norris (1917–40)[43] became increasingly the instrument of enlightened and progressive reform, while the managers of the schools sought mutual protection in an entrenched conservatism. This may largely have been caused not only by the financial interests of the latter (*freedom and individualism are expensive and 'inefficient'*) but also because managerial bodies were predominantly composed of wealthy, aged and upper-class members of society who, for all their philanthropic interests, were more concerned with the schools' role in protecting society than in their role as agencies of individual rehabilitation and re-adjustment.

The many Acts of Parliament through which the State endeavoured to modify the system,[44] sometimes in the teeth of fierce opposition from the managers, could be effective only if accepted both by the individuals directly concerned with school management and by the general public, whose alienation from the schools became more acute as the 'certificated', later 'approved', schools retreated further into a defensive isolation reinforced by their customary geographical position in the depths of the country. In the era of 'enlightenment' which followed the First World War the population of industrial and reformatory schools fell rapidly and from the pre-war peak of 25,357 numbers declined and schools closed until in 1925 only 2.4 per cent of all children found guilty of offences were sent to reformatory schools.[45] Courts became increasingly reluctant to use schools which had such an unfavourable public image and the growth of the probation service offered an attractive alternative for 26 per cent of the children.

The effect of this trend was largely salutary not only for the children who were increasingly retained in their own families but also for the service which, by the elimination of many of the worst schools and by the response to pressure from such enlightened administrators as Norris, were able to do much to reform themselves. The Curtis Committee's assessment of the work of the remaining approved schools was on the whole favourable and a pamphlet issued by the Home Office in 1946, largely as an act of public relations, described many satisfactory aspects of existing schools in their slow move towards a more humanitarian ethos and a more meaningful concept of 'training'.[46]

Nevertheless it is in its concept of 'training' rather than 'treating' that the approved-school system appears most divorced from the emergent framework of schools for maladjusted children. The attitude of approved schools to 'training' is largely a product of their ambivalent position. They are expected both to protect society against delinquent individuals and also to restore the individual to society after a process of 'correction'. What this 'correction' consists of depends both on a clear statement of the problem in terms of a workable definition of delinquency and also on a recognition of specific aims. If delinquency is, as Mary Carpenter suggested, largely the result of social and emotional factors working within the family then the 'correction' must be in terms of the treatment of the emotional imbalance by the establishment of close individual relationships. If the delinquent behaviour is, on the other hand, the product of inappropriate learning experiences, there is some hope that by a process of retraining, with the reinforcement of systematically applied rewards and punishments, the child will learn a more socially acceptable pattern of behaviour.

One of the chief weaknesses of the reformatory school system is that it has tended (at least when pressed) to argue from the former position but to proceed from the latter. In *Making Citizens* (1946), for instance, the Home Office spokesman M. M. Simmons expresses the dilemma unconsciously but well: 'It has been emphasized that the main concern of the Approved Schools is the welfare of the individual child, that it sees its work as education, and that its method is to provide a lively and ordered community planned to meet the needs of the young people.'[47] What these needs are and what sort of community is required are areas of similar confusion. While recognizing that 'most of the boys in Approved Schools have arrived there because of emotional rather than physical disturbances'[48] Simmons considers that there are only 'a few Approved School boys and girls whose need for love has been denied', for whom he admits that little can be done in the approved-school context and suggests that only about thirty or forty children at any one time in the total approved-school population require skilled psychological or psychiatric treatment. Again, while accepting that much of the problem of delinquency lies in the child's inadequate experience within the family, he describes, with general approval, a system within which the attributes of a normal family are almost entirely lacking. The training offered is largely that designed to produce conformity to the pattern of a large and impersonal community, with very little opportunity for effective — or affective — individual relationships: a community for one sex only, usually housed in conditions and a locality completely alien to those to which the majority of children will return and one in which the freedom implicit in family life is usurped by continual organization of activities so that no part of the day or night is left unsupervised. The value of the experiences offered may also be doubted if the process is seen as a 'training for life'. Team games, farm work, maintenance of stately homes and gardens, extra-curricular pottery and puppetry bear little relation to the probable after-experience of the approved-school child, although they might be justified, or at least rationalized, if therapy was recognized as their aim.

If the aim is considered to be 'making citizens' the process also appears to be singularly ill-directed. Although, in more 'progressive' approved schools gestures towards 'shared responsibility' have been made in the form largely of consultative meetings of senior and conforming pupils with the headmaster, the children normally have no actual experience of political responsibility. As Simmons did, the Franklin Committee (1951)[49] also doubted whether it is either possible or desirable to have any form of self-government in a delinquent community and the examples of the Little Commonwealth, the Hawkspur Camp and other experimental establishments are almost totally ignored. The effectiveness of shared responsibility in schools for the maladjusted, e.g. Red Hill, is not of course conclusive argument for its viability in places of detention. Not only may the inmates be fundamentally dissimilar but also children in an approved school are there as the result of compulsion exercised on both themselves and their parents and there is little reason why they should identify with the aims of the school—one of which is, specifically, the limitation of their freedom to behave anti-socially.

Thus the only way of repossessing freedom is to conform to the standards of behaviour imposed largely by an alien authority. The effect of such imposed conformity is likely to be transitory and it is little wonder that, in a world increasingly conscious of the need for individual freedom, the success rate for approved schools is constantly falling.*

This complexity of aim and uncertainty of purpose has been reflected in the attitude of the Home Office to those who have used experimental methods to achieve what they consider to be primarily a therapeutic purpose. Although it is true that 'the Home Office has been responsible for more innovations, improvements and changes, than any or all generations of managers and heads of schools'[51] its attitude to individual pioneering enterprises has been ambivalent. There has been a tendency to accept and support work once established until something occurs which threatens the official role of representative of the public conscience. Thus the Home Office supported the Little Commonwealth despite, or because of, its originality, until a suspected weakness in Homer Lane himself presented a potential situation which it would have been impossible for the State to justify to the public. Similarly in withholding support from the Hawkspur Camp the Home Office represented the public's fear of the inability of a democratic organization to protect its security.

Other institutions, usually with longer traditions of success or less extreme methods, it has endeavoured to coax into its ambit (e.g. the

---

* Failure rate in terms of percentage reconvicted within three years: 1960, 57% (Boys) 15% (Girls); 1961, 60% (B) 17% (G); 1962 62% (B) 21% (G); 1963, 65% (B) 21% (G); 1964–7, 68% (B) 21% (G).[50]

Caldecott Community during the war) or has dealt with on an individual basis in which the responsibility and control (and therefore the freedom to experiment) has been retained by the individual experimenter (e.g. Lyward).

FATHER OWEN

An account of the work of Father Owen illustrates some of these points, and spans most areas of 'child care' work. As a young medical student in the 1920s he helped with the work of the 'Ragged School Union' in Lambeth, South London, and with a large camp for boys from the training ship 'Exmouth', run by the Metropolitan Asylums Board for boys who were either without families or in need of care and protection. He was ordained in 1932 and subsequently continued his social-work experience during the Depression as curate of St John's Church, in London's Waterloo Road. In 1936 he joined the Franciscan order and until the outbreak of war he worked as a friar with Brother Douglas's community for young 'wayfarers' at Cerne Abbas, in the buildings previously occupied by the Little Commonwealth. The inmates of what would now be known as a Rehabilitation Centre were mostly aged between eighteen and thirty and were the homeless unemployed who were often both maladjusted and of subnormal intelligence. They were fundamentally insecure and their chief characteristic was a 'touchiness' which caused them to 'walk out' of any situation—whether in the hostel or in employment—which imposed strain or responsibility on them.

Father Owen describes as typical one 'from a very broken home—violently broken—asthmatic and with a bad stammer' who after military service was 'in and out of prison most of the time. He is intelligent and witty and always writes me most amusing letters. He is now out and in a chest hospital.'[52] It is significant that this individual is regarded as a success in that he can maintain a meaningful and lasting personal relationship, for this was the chief objective of the friar's efforts with those pre-war 'drop-outs' during their three-to-six-month stay in the home.

At the beginning of the war the centre was taken over by evacuees from Southwark and between 1940 and 1945 Father Owen acquired his first experience with younger boys when the Dorsetshire County Council established a remand home. Following his natural bent,

Father Owen worked in one of the four houses which was set aside for the most disturbed boys. His efforts were sufficiently rewarded that attempts were made to place the school, which had developed within the remand home, on a more permanent footing. Although the value of the work done in both education and in the care of disturbed children could be measured against the almost universal inadequacy described in the Curtis Report (see Sections 313–324) both the Home Office and the Ministry of Health refused their support and the Board of Education advised delay until after the re-organization envisaged in the 1944 Act. Support was obtained from the Church National Society and a school was established at Hooke Court, in West Dorset, in 1946 (this including what was left of the original remand home). Father Owen saw as the ideal plan a small school with a large staff allowing for small-group work, near to a town to allow for the maximum of local contact, and supported by a chain of progressively graded hostels to allow for individual progress back into society.

In the event, the school was organized as one of forty-five boys grouped into three houses with the senior house — of boys between the ages of fourteen and sixteen — acting to some extent as a hostel, and having progressively greater contact with the local community.

The essence of the school was work in small groups, with close inter-personal relations between the boys and the large staff of lay-houseparents and teachers as well as members of the order. Father Owen, in addition to being responsible for the general direction, was in charge of the farm (at one time 200 acres) and gardens. There was a good deal of emphasis on practical and craft work, including pottery.

As well as providing a high staffing ratio the basis of the organiza-tion in the Franciscan order had certain other advantages. Hooke Court had a degree of permanence in its staff which few special schools have; it also had some financial stability — partly because the Brothers' salaries were paid into the funds of the school. (At one point it was suggested that Father Owen could not retire until his salary had paid off the mortgage on the gymnasium!) The Brothers' too, were always available in a way in which ordinary teachers — possibly with family commitments — were not. When the school was not in session great emphasis was placed on activities such as camp-ing, foreign travel, scouting and home visiting.

Above all, the religious basis gave the school its basic ethos. Father Owen says:

People ask whether the school [is] permissive. If by that they mean did we set out to run the school on permissive lines the answer is 'No'. The answer really is, I suppose, that all of us who started the school had a common aim of allegiance to serve our Lord to the best of our ability. We did not set out to call everyone by their Christian names; we just did naturally. The boys would be angry if called by their surnames by the staff. I did not say that they were to call me 'the Old Man' — it just happened quite naturally. These are small indications.

A better description would be mutual understanding and tolerance. The more important thing being tolerance, because understanding is a more difficult thing. There is a complaint current that the old do not understand the young and the young the old. But why should they? Do we really understand ourselves? If we do, then we can more likely understand each other, but my bet is we do not. So let us plump for mutual tolerance and respect.[53]

This tolerance and respect was extended also to the staff. Each was encouraged to work within the structure of his own personality and so considerable variety of approach prevailed and boys could identify and work with those people most sympathetic towards them. Discussion took place, advice and support were given, but there was no structure of shared responsibility, and the weekly meetings were concerned with the discussion of the personal needs of the individual and the collective needs of the community rather than the making of rules or the imposition of sanctions.

Individual contact was close (there was more consistency of purpose than in most special schools) but individuality was respected and individual idiosyncracy appreciated.

When a Brother who worked in an authoritarian manner in the workshop was threatened by a boy who took knives from the kitchen and went round smashing windows, he appealed to Father Owen: 'What do I do if I tell a boy to do something and he doesn't?' Father Owen's reply was 'Well, don't put yourself in that position in the first place' — which, however perfectionist it may sound, indicates the degree of flexibility of approach that is necessary with maladjusted children who are not capable of accepting the assumption of the adult world.

Social conformity was often seen as destructive of the individuality which was valued. 'I always thank God that there are many maladjusted—there are far too many people who are well adjusted to a society that should not be adjusted to. The so-called maladjusted are far better "material" because they question everything and, in my opinion, are more thoughtful than many of their age.' This paradox of maladjustment and the basic dilemma facing those who have undertaken 'adjustment' echoes Russell Hoare's faith in the delinquent and has recently been well expressed by Marshall McLuhan.

The poet, the artist, the sleuth — whoever sharpens our perceptions tends to be anti-social; rarely 'well adjusted', he cannot go along with currents and trends. A strange bond often exists between anti-social types in their power to see environments as they really are. This need to interfere, to confront environments with a certain anti-social power, is manifest in the famous story *The Emperor's New Clothes*. 'Well adjusted' courtiers, having vested interests, saw the Emperor as beautifully appointed. 'The 'anti-social' brat, unaccustomed to the old environment, clearly saw the Emperor 'ain't got nothin' on'. The new environment was clearly visible to him.[54]

One of the greatest strains of the many in working with maladjusted children is in ourselves adjusting to their different perceptions of the world which may make many workers with maladjusted children feel that they too 'ain't go nothin' on'. Father Owen endeavoured to preserve this individual vision within the context of a Christian community.

His early experience with 'wayfarers', many of whom he regarded as the 'un-treated maladjusted', had given him considerable insight into the individual problems of the socially and emotionally deprived. He had no comprehensive therapeutic policy, was largely unaffected by 'trends', he believed in the acquisition of personal responsibility (which, as at the Caldecott Community with which he had had contact during the war, was rewarded by privileges), but above all he appreciated the individual importance of the minutiae of human relations.

On one occasion travelling shortly after the war with an orphan of the Blitz he realized that although the welfare authorities had provided the boy with new clothes, luggage, money, and all long-term necessities they had failed to pack any food. Father Owen considers that in sharing his 'pop' and sandwiches with the boy he made a significant step forward in the boy's adjustment. He had re-established human contact—significantly enough, perhaps, in the breaking of bread.

Being essentially modest in his person and objectives Father Owen recognized that the unambitious structure and comparative 'lack of treatment' at Hooke Court was sometimes not helpful to the deeply disturbed boy and then, like Leila Rendel, with whom he has much in common, he was eager to seek help from other workers or from hospital units, but normally the boys were expected to stay until they were sixteen.

The problems of reintegration into ordinary life which had so concerned Father Owen and his colleague Anthony Lewis when they were working in the context of the remand home had not been forgotten. Contacts with the neighbourhood were sedulously culti-vated both by bringing people into the school on open days, for work in the school and for youth club activities, and by going out into the environs to help with church activities, to join in the work and play of local schools and youth clubs, by playing in 'pop' groups, competing in games, and visiting places of work and cultural interest.

Father Owen helped at local village churches, became a rural district councillor, talked to Women's Institutes and mothers' unions, and was eventually co-opted on to the Dorset County Council children's committee. He made a particular point of establishing friendly relations with the police. He tells how when he went to see a new chief constable about some boys who were in trouble he talked about their backgrounds and problems until the chief con-stable gave in with the wry admission that 'I have been warned about you'. The local police were encouraged to know the boys well, to help in running their cadet force and Duke of Edinburgh Award Scheme, to put police dogs through their paces at school fetes and generally to feel involved in the work. Eventually police cadets were encouraged to spend a week at a time at the school.

This approach not only helped to explain the school to the com-munity, and thus helped it to survive where many others have failed, but was a very important part of the social rehabilitation of the many anti-social disturbed boys who went to Hooke Court.

Nevertheless many boys left who had no homes of their own, no family and no contacts with society at large. Like many other workers with maladjusted children Father Owen saw that much of the work of the school would be wasted unless this transition were satisfac-torily accomplished. It was not, however, until he retired in 1966 that his ambition to solve this problem began to be realized in a small— but characteristic—way. He now occupies a small, photograph-festooned bed-sitter in Toynbee Hall, part of a flat which acts as a hostel for six former-pupils who are being carefully supported through the last stages of adjustment.

His work at Hooke Court continues and the manner of its continuance is also of importance in explaining its particular quality. When Father Owen indicated his intention to retire, his successor— Brother Anselm—was chosen for training. He was given a wide and varied experience in ordinary schools—from primary to a tough secondary modern. He was sent to the London Institute of Education to do the course for a diploma in the education of maladjusted children under Dr Oakeshott. He then spent some time at the Mulberry Bush School for severely maladjusted children, learning from Dockar-Drysdale and finally, before taking up his duties, he visited the homes of all the boys who would be in his care.

Thus, however far Hooke Court was an extension of Father Owen's personality, its continuance was assured under expert guidance. Other pioneer schools have died, and many may well continue to die in the future, with their founders.

The lessons to be learnt from Father Owen's experience with the deprived and disturbed are, above all, the importance of a continuing and direct individual relationship based on faith and of tolerance and mutual respect within a secure but dynamic structure in which the individual is unquestionably more important than the organization. It is this experience which most approved-school boys lack.

14

Rethinking Education

If we cannot move forward in our educational theory and practice, we are indeed a lost nation. – H.A.T. Child.[55]

As the First World War may be seen as the real beginning of pioneer work in therapeutic education so the Second World War may mark its end. During the latter's course the problem of re-educating maladjusted children was at last recognized as beyond the resources of private initiative and enterprise, the magnitude of the problem enforced a degree of conceptualization and generalization, and the State finally acknowledged its responsibility.

In conditions of wartime chaos independent experiment flourished to satisfy an overwhelming need but, although many of the experimental institutions survived and although independent schools continue to be an important part of the provision for maladjusted children, postwar economic and administrative pressure proscribed genuinely pioneering individual ventures. The State, being more directly subject to public opinion and more committed to academic educational objectives, while acknowledging and profiting by the exploratory work done in therapeutic education by private individuals, had little real sympathy for idiosyncratic experiment.

While the war lasted private schools flourished. Some, like Chaigeley, evolved from providing for the needs of 'difficult' evacuees; others, like Monkton Wyld and Wennington, provided for a more general need for boarding-school places for children separated from their homes and families by the war.

CHAIGELEY SCHOOL

In many ways typical of the almost accidental growth of private schools for the maladjusted during the early 1940s, Chaigeley School was sponsored by the Society of Friends as an evacuation centre.

239

became a school, found itself increasingly concerned with the re-education of maladjusted children, 'moved house' and was finally recognized by the Ministry of Education in 1944 as a residential special school for maladjusted children, in which capacity it still exists.

Its first warden was J. Edward Seel, who had been educated in Quaker schools and was, by profession, a teacher of art. In 1941 he was asked by the Friends' War Relief Service to take over Chaigeley Manor near Clitheroe as a hostel for schoolchildren evacuated from Liverpool after the Merseyside air raids. Dr J. D. Kershaw, Medical Officer of Health for Colchester, who was closely associated with the venture, said in 1966: 'Two people endured throughout the changes, Edward and Margaret Seel, in charge of the whole venture, and here again we were lucky; the unorthodox work and its unprecedented challenges needed faith, the sensitivity and flexible approach which comes with the temperament of the artist and it was these qualities, by no means divorced from practicality, which they brought to the task.'

It was a difficult task not only because the Liverpool children were in a poor state both physically and psychologically—many of them having been 'running wild' in Liverpool for weeks or months after their homes had been destroyed and parents and relatives killed—but also because the manor was the site of the Accrington and District Children's Convalescent Home and, although Accrington could no longer staff it, it was insisted that Accrington children should continue to be received at Chaigeley for three-week periods of convalescence all the year round.

The 'convalescence' could hardly have been regarded as a peaceful, inactive period as the small groups of Accrington children, aged between four-and-a-half and fourteen, found themselves bitterly resented in their own 'home' by the permanent Liverpudlian residents. Mr Seel reports (in documents relating to this period which he has kindly allowed me to use), that 'The staff of ten found themselves at first in a no man's land of flying stones' in the war between the 'Accies' and the 'Vaccies' but that by 1943 'active hostility between the groups had become . . . a sympathetic toleration'.

It was not surprising that the original Liverpool evacuees should have been resentful and intolerant of the Accrington children, who were having a pleasant holiday separated for a brief while from their safe homes and loving parents. Many of the Liverpool children had neither homes nor parents and, of those who had, most had little contact with them. The original group of twenty boys and girls between the ages of nine and fifteen had been selected by the Child Welfare Association on the basis of need and where homes existed they tended to be destitute, broken or unhappy. Nevertheless the 'vaccies' resented the substitution of Chaigeley for their homes and of foster-parents for parents, however inadequate the originals may have been, and had feelings of resentment at being 'turned out' by parents by whom they felt they were not wanted.

From the beginning, therefore, Chaigeley had to adapt itself to deal with very disturbed children. The environment was beautiful, the staff sympathetic, affectionate and tolerant. There was sufficient organization to give a feeling of security, sufficient freedom to allow the disturbed child to find itself.

A system of 'shared responsibility' evolved; Seel was in touch with David Wills, who at this time was in Peebles. Initially weekly meetings of a committee took place under Seel's chairmanship, largely to arrange the routine of the hostel but, as the school developed, a weekly general meeting was given increasing responsibility.

In 1942 the hostel became also the school for its own children, many of whom had been found to be too disturbed to be managed in the village school two miles away. Then began one of the most interesting stages of the evolution of Chaigeley.

The children ranged in I.Q. from about 86 to 116 but many of these were by virtue of 'bad schooling, lack of schooling, ill health, emotional disturbances and home conditions' seriously retarded. Four of the original ten- and eleven-year-olds were unable to read. On the other hand, formal education was for most of them, at first, the only framework within which they felt secure. Gradually a system evolved in which the day was divided into a morning of more or less academic work in small groups followed by an afternoon of either practical classes or free activity and an evening of individual 'night school' or club activities. The children had to choose daily which period of the day they would spend in work groups. This improved the attitude to all school work, kept groups small, and maintained close and friendly contact between staff and pupils at all times.

After nearly two years (*Report*, April 1943) Seel was able to make out a profit and loss account (slightly amended) thus: Advantages.

They will have:

1 A sound diet.
2 Healthy surroundings.
3 Regular daily routine.
4 A natural and affectionate relationship with adults.
5 A variety of activities in school, not always available for all in elementary schools (e.g. cookery, woodwork, dancing for boys and girls alike).
6 Individual care, e.g. a psychologist makes visits at regular intervals and interviews each child.
7 A Christian community in which to live.

On the other hand the disadvantages for the children are real and clear. Three major ones are these (summarized):

1 Our lack of experience, particularly when mistakes become ingrowing and lead to, and spring from, lack of outward vision.
2 The almost total separation of the children and of ourselves from their mothers and fathers.
3 The contrast of conditions at Chaigeley with those in Liverpool, which may well add to difficulties of readjustment.

These last two problems still persist in many schools for the maladjusted but were acutely present in the pioneer schools facing wartime problems with, as Seel modestly admits, insufficient experience or reliable precedents. As the staff became less changing and more confident and contact was established with parents, largely through the Society of Friends, the disadvantages lessened and fewer children returned home.

In 1944 the evolution of Chaigeley into a school which specialized in dealing with maladjusted children was recognized officially and 'although technically linked up with the evacuation scheme it had become accepted as an informal auxiliary to the Liverpool School Medical Service and the selection of children was primarily made on the grounds of maladjustment'. In April 1944 Seel reported that 'We have twenty-one children from Liverpool in the hostel: four came through probation officers, six from homes with serious husband-wife difficulties, six have one, or neither, parent alive, five were illiterate on arrival. All have come suffering from different degrees of maladjustment. . . . All twenty-one children come from homes which are unfavourable to normal development.'

The impact which Chaigeley, together with other pioneer schools in the treatment of maladjusted children, was beginning to have on the public mind is suggested by a correspondence which took place in October of that year in *The Manchester Guardian*. This was in response to a letter published on September 2nd from a Miss Blackburn appealing for action to be taken before children reached the juvenile courts. This correspondence, under the heading *The Anti-Social Child*, included a letter from the teacher in charge of Chaigeley, E. Firth-Barlow, urging the foundation of more residential schools on the same pattern on the grounds that:

1 The normal curriculum is not good enough for abnormal children.
2 The delinquent and the pre-delinquent child are both suffering from only different degrees of maladjustment.
3 There is real advantage in a small combined hostel and school which removes the customary confusion of a double standard of discipline and behaviour—that of 'home and school'.
4 Some maladjusted children need to be away but not cut off from influence of home and parents.

He urged that: 'Schemes such as ours, supported by emergency funds to meet an emergency, are in danger of being closed down all over the country. The war will end but the emergency will remain.' He was supported by, among others, W. Hirst Bateman, chairman of Rochdale Juvenile Court, who recommended day/boarding schools in attractive environments 'not too far away from the children's home', and by Frank Mathews, honorary secretary of Birmingham Society for the Care of Invalid and Nervous Children, who recommended residential units of not more than twenty-four to thirty children. (He saw the chief difficulty of establishing such homes as being that the cost for twenty-four to thirty children 'works out at not less than £3,000 a year'!)

The cost of maintaining Chaigeley had so far been borne largely by the Quakers. In the latter part of 1944 the Friends Relief Service (which was primarily concerned with evacuation) gave way in running Chaigeley to 'an independent committee of persons connected with educational medical and psychiatric work in Lancashire', and the Board of Education recognized the school under Section 80 of the Education Act of 1921, so that it became possible for L.E.A.s to send and maintain children directly.

The demand for places increased rapidly and it was decided to move to a larger building at Thelwall, near Lymm, Cheshire, and it became the first school to be recognized as a school for maladjusted children under the 1944 Act.

Prophetically the prospectus of 1945 says: 'While proud of the pioneer work which it has done in the making of a type of educational provision for which all those who have been associated with Child Guidance work have long felt the need, the school realizes that its development is by no means finished. The very nature of this work makes it clear that the education of the maladjusted child is something which will be the subject of continued experiment for many years to come'. Indeed after 1945 and before 1950, when Edward Seel retired, Chaigeley was the venue of that exciting experiment in education which Howard Jones reports in *Reluctant Rebels*.[56]

Jones examines the rationale of a method not very dissimilar from, and to some extent consciously based on, that of Wills, in terms of group therapy. The group, whether it is the general meeting, watch committee, court or psycho-drama session, becomes not merely the basic means of government and organization but, under the control of insightful adults, the basic means of treatment. The apparently endless inter-analysis of personal and social problems, the 'transference' of attitude to the institutions, the group and the individual, the inevitable 'abreaction', constitute the basis for a living therapy which, if Jones's conclusions are valid, is particularly appropriate not only for maladjusted children, with their powerful urge to 'belong' and to feel accepted by others, but for residential institutions in particular. This practice is urged not only for those reasons which Wills gives in justification of shared responsibility (see Chapter 12) but also on the purely practical ground that not only is individual analysis clearly not possible but, as Jones points out, 'it is not always necessary, for the achievement of social adjustment, to penetrate the lower reaches of the unconscious'. The delinquent may be faced with the reality of his behaviour and the maladjusted child 'may not always need to understand clearly the Oedipal conflicts that form the basis of his hostility towards authority, if the process of projection by which he justifies it is analysed and made clear to him in the group. Self-knowledge could then lead to sublimation and self-control'.[57]

During this period, therefore, an elaborate structure grew up based on the weekly general meeting as the basic legislative and administrative unit. A cabinet, under the chairmanship of Edward Seel, eventually evolved to act as the primary executive unit, and a children's court, the watch committee, provided the judicature. The watch committee met daily and consisted of both child and adult members elected at the general meeting. Complaints for the attention of the watch committee could be raised after every mealtime and discussion could also be initiated then on any matter too urgent to be left to the next general meeting.

'Besides the Watch Committee, other officials were elected by the General Meeting, as the community felt the need for them. They usually included a Chairman and Deputy Chairman of the General Meeting, a Treasurer and Finance Committee, a Secretary, a Chairman and Deputy Chairman of the Dining Room and a Librarian. At various times there were also Games Secretaries, Supervisors of Work (to control those given work punishments for misbehaviour in the dining room), Keepers (to keep recalcitrant smaller boys out of trouble), and a host of *ad hoc* camp committees, commissions of inquiry and the like, as situations calling for them arose'.[58]

It will not surprise anyone who has worked within this sort of framework with maladjusted children that considerable tensions were produced in the community and an appearance of complete disorder often prevailed. This is valuable in that tensions can only be relieved if they appear and it is assumed that a desire for structure and discipline arise naturally and without resentment from an appearance of disorder. Great demands, however, are made on the tolerance of the staff, who must accept both the reality and responsibility of what must often seem very immature and arbitary law-making. Jones says: 'Radical experiments in institutions for problem children have been comparatively few, presumably because they call for more than ability and imagination. Great courage is also needed, for the innovator has to be willing to take risks, as well as to face the hostility of a fearful and insecure general public.'

In the wake of the uncomprehending general public came His Majesty's inspectors. Dr Kershaw recalls that the first blow came in 1948 when a 'snap visit to the school, in the absence of the headmaster and half the children, of an inspector who had no experience or knowledge of the kind of work we were trying to do' resulted in 'a report in which ignorance led to gross injustice and misinterpretation'. Mr James Lumsden, then Chief Inspector of Special Schools, admits that the critical inspection was undertaken by a district inspector with little knowledge of special schools who visited Chaigeley in the absence of both Seel and himself and subsequently made much of photographs of graffiti etc. in his adverse report. Lumsden suggests, however, that this report merely reinforced the impression which the Ministry already had that it was impossible to reconcile the school's aims and methods (particularly with regard to coeducation) with the ethos of the local community and the current attitudes of the administration.[59] The school was threatened with closure unless it became an all-boys school — a blunder which Ministry officials, concerned more with appearances than with the social re-education of maladjusted children, had, and have, repeated on many occasions.

Ministry attention, once attracted, proceeded to destroy the very promising experiment in group therapy then developing. Jones writes bitterly:

Recognition brought with it lavish Government grants, but also, unfortunately, a good deal of interference from the Ministry of Education. Because of their resistance to psychiatric principles ... this interference was uniformly disastrous in its effects.... Official insistence upon the maintenance of certain outward forms of order administered a death-blow to the group-therapy approach in the school: the apparent turmoil which this approach brought with it was not to be tolerated, whatever its value to the children.

It indicates one at least of the more important limitations of a state controlled educational system that, from Homer Lane down to Hawkspur Camp and Woodmarsh [Chaigeley], the greatest opponents of radical experiments in education in Britain have been the officials of the ministries concerned. And their power is such that the timidity and lack of insight of some of them can hamper and even kill the creative departures inspired by the genius of greater men.[60]

WARTIME L.E.A. SCHOOLS

Although the Board of Education was greatly concerned not only with the mass evacuation of urban children but also with the placement of misfits in special hostels it made little contribution to the evolution of special educational provision during the wartime period. It was, possibly, too concerned with the immense problem of maintaining ordinary education to concern itself with experiments with minority groups. A few local authorities made varying attempts to deal with the problem by establishing hostel schools which relieved reception areas of some of the intractable problems caused by disturbed evacuees placed in overcrowded village schools. Normally, however, even where special hostels existed, the maladjusted children went out to school.

It appears that the Perranporth Sands Hotel School might claim to be the first local authority boarding school in England for maladjusted children. Established by the London County Council in 1941 in a disused hotel in a 'select' seaside resort, this school accepted about fifty of the most difficult evacuees from London, Bristol and Plymouth. The boys were mainly very disturbed and aggressive adolescents whom it had been found impossible to place in ordinary foster-homes, hostels or schools. The staff normally consisted of Mr Murphy, the headmaster, and two or three other teachers. None was specifically trained to do this most exacting work. What precedents there were were derived largely from approved schools. There was little direct therapy, although there was occasional supervision by a visiting psychiatrist, and, although in theory the regime was non-punitive, great emphasis was placed on discipline and order particularly when the boys came into contact with the hostile and suspicious local inhabitants. Attempts were made to channel aggressive feelings into sports activities—including boxing! One interesting feature of the school, in that it was the reverse of the usual procedure, was that some boys who lived in ordinary hostels but who were difficult in ordinary schools attended Perranporth Sands Hotel School as day pupils. The school closed after about two years when Mr Murphy returned to London. It left no legacy of example for subsequent State schools.

Many independent schools had similarly brief and unremarkable careers in these troubled times. Many failed because, like the Perranporth school, they had no consistent organization or ideal to sustain them. They had, however, the advantage that they possessed, on the whole, more stable membership and were under less administrative pressure. Those few which survived the 'emergency', the return of the evacuees, and the inevitable strains of dealing with unprecedented problems without any established guide-lines were often sustained by the outstanding personality of their founders.

One local authority school which survived the war and which

still exists as a special school for maladjusted boys was Hill Orchard School, Meriden, Warwickshire (in 1953 moved to Henley in Arden as River House School). Its first headmaster, Walter George Sharman was by profession a soldier and, in an earlier tradition, his entry into social work had been largely through the Boy Scout movement. Like Homer Lane, whose work he admired, he was largely self-educated (a process which he continued energetically until his death in 1961). Also like Homer Lane, he set great store by craft work, of which he had been a teacher, and his school included many farming activities. One of his former colleagues remembers a typical classroom scene in which Sharman would be simultaneously teaching, cutting a boy's hair, and giving instructions to others about chasing the hens out of the garden.

Many small schools at this time did, of course, include some husbandry not only as an extension of education but also as a way of supplementing war-time diet. It is difficult to evaluate its effect which may have been caused as much by improved physical health as by opportunities for communing with nature.

Although Sharman was aware of psychological developments it would appear that his school owed more to the influence of Baden-Powell than to Freud. While aiming at 'unconditional acceptance' as an ideal he wished to reach a sympathetic understanding of the problems of children unable to 'stand up to' social pressures without his becoming too emotionally involved. His administration was paternal, liberal and sympathetic but he believed that retraining was the essence of the re-adjustment process. Thus the school contained as much 'structure' as the emotional needs of the children, chronic under-staffing and the chaos of wartime conditions allowed.

PRIVATE 'PROGRESSIVES'

As Weaver points out,[61] another incidental product of the world crisis which had a significant effect on both the practice and theory of therapeutic education, in its widest sense, was the arrival in this country of many Continental refugees from Nazi oppression. Many of these, like Kris, Friedlander, Lennhoff, Lowenfeld and Anna Freud herself, were not only distinguished Freudians or neo-Freudians but were also involved, or involved themselves, with work with children. As stateless aliens they frequently found jobs associated with schools, hostels, nurseries or clinics, sometimes without pay. The work of Anna Freud at the Hampstead Nursery is well known (see Chapter 15) and F. C. Lennhoff, although in some ways representing what was rapidly becoming a rather old-fashioned patriarchal approach to residential treatment, brought to it a wealth of experience and knowledge derived not only from Freud himself but also from a close acquaintance with the work of Aichhorn. Lennhoff's own 'pioneering' was done mainly before he came to this country and his school, Shotton Hall, was a postwar foundation, but although, as Ernest Glover points out, his policies were 'based on ideas that have been current in child-therapy and a few of our more enlightened schools for some considerable time',[62] his personal significance is considerable.

Many people, as well as the children in his care, have benefited from his insight into the problems of seriously disturbed children. Shotton Hall remains a centre for research and training and conferences are held annually; his book *Exceptional Children* describes his own personal exercise in therapeutic education. Shotton Hall aims, above all, to be a home in which boys can relax and be themselves, can learn from living in a small community and can profit by individual and group therapy in an environment structured to their needs.

The schools which appear to have profited most from the influx of trained and skilled therapists and teachers during the war were not, in fact, the few 'special' schools. Many such exiles found jobs in the small private progressive schools which proliferated during this period—schools such as Beltane, Burgess Hill, Hurtwood, Kilquhanity, Monkton Wyld and Wennington. Such schools, while not 'special' schools, shared the same problems. Many of their children, too, were disturbed by the disruption of family life, traumatic experiences of war, the emotional strains of separation common to all evacuees. Staffing was difficult and increasingly dependent on a limited supply of pacifists and aliens often with extremely unorthodox and radical views of education. The effect was often exciting, dynamic and experimental and 'progressive education' entered a new era derived from Freud and Marx rather than Froebel and Dewey.

In such an atmosphere, and with such staff, greater attention was paid to the therapeutic function of education not only through new approaches to such creative subjects as drama, painting and dance but also directly. 'The appointment of a child psychologist was not, in fact, uncommon. His work in enlightening the staff on the meaning of their observations and interpreting the unconscious origins of the children's (and their own) behaviour may be said to have forerun that of the psychiatric teams in special schools a dozen years later.'[63]

MONKTON WYLD

How far therapeutic education was conscious and how far it might be considered incidental to the progressive techniques used varied from school to school. It is interesting, for instance, that Eleanor Urban, in her account of Monkton Wyld,[64] lays no special claim for the school as a therapeutic establishment and indeed some such schools explicitly denied that they had such a function, possibly in order to prevent an over-balance of disturbed pupils.

The emphasis at Monkton Wyld was on community life, an implicit belief in the value of co-education, and on an educational process which stemmed essentially from the needs and interests of individuals. The community, including the staff who owned and governed the school in a co-operative enterprise, originally without pay, created their own environment for living and learning. When the school began, near Charmouth in 1940, all labour was shared in the school and on the small farm. Co-operation was seen as the most important principle here, as in education. Children of many differing abilities, backgrounds and degrees of personal adjustment learnt to value one another and themselves. Many of the difficulties were seen as the result of previous unfortunate learning experiences which had engendered feelings of inadequacy and hopelessness. A modified Dalton Plan allowed children to work at their own speed with the attention of individual members of staff. Weekly work meetings were the opportunity for the discussion of problems and the encouragement of the children by opportunities to display their work to others. Other meetings arranged the complicated timetable to allow for the pursuit of individual interests, ironed out personal difficulties and discussed practical day-to-day problems. One interesting feature of these meetings was that there was seldom recourse to majority votes. Discussion was continued until a generally satisfactory course was agreed on.

Education for leisure was considered very important and there was an exceptionally wide range of art and craft activities for such a small school (not more than sixty children). The importance of both individual freedom from being organized and of the need for 'the sublimation of destructive impulses' was recognized.

One problem of great difficulty and significance in small boarding schools was successfully overcome with an efficiency which many special schools might envy. The staff, beginning with the small group of friends who were the founder-teachers, was unusually without conflict and division. Although there was a nominal headmaster and headmistress the staff was regarded as a body of equals. Co-operation and consultation at all levels ensured that what was done was done by agreement. Again no contrived majority decision was found necessary. Perhaps this, more than any other single factor, made Monkton Wyld a truly therapeutic environment by guaranteeing security without coercion.

WENNINGTON

Kenneth Barnes, founder and until recently headmaster of Wennington School, links together several 'pioneer' sources in that he was educated at Emanuel School, Wandsworth, London, between 1914 and 1921, at which time George Lyward was on the staff, and he later taught for ten years under J. H. Badley at Bedales, which school served him as the model for Wennington in 1940. The school also unites the traditions of the 'old' New Education 'progressive' schools with many of the characteristics of the new 'progressives' formed under the pressures of the Second World War and in the chaos produced by evacuation.

In such schools the jingoism of Rennie or Devine was replaced by a convinced pacifism; the intellectual middle-class base was widened to include children from all social classes; intellectual idealism was frequently less important than moral idealism and new academic methods were often less marked than new approaches to what may loosely be called therapy. Nevertheless, they retained from earlier 'progressive' principles and practices a dynamic and experimental approach to education, an emphasis on sound social relationships based on mutual respect and co-operation between staff and pupils and boys and girls, a belief in the importance of the arts and an ultimate aim of a healthy individual rather than an approved social product.

It was not surprising, therefore, that they were believed to be particularly appropriate for disturbed or poorly adjusted children with a need to 'find themselves' in a tolerant, sympathetic and individually supportive environment. In schools such as Monkton Wyld and Wennington this belief has often been justified, although they have never claimed or sought a 'special' role.

In its early years there was much in Wennington which resembles the early experiences of the Hawkspur Camp. While not in quite such primitive conditions the staff and pupils, led by a convinced Quaker with a strong faith in the importance of the enterprise, had to work together to create a community. Resources were few and the staff worked without pay not only to teach but to create the physical structure of a school from the guest-house — Wennington Hall — which was offered them. 'Personal responsibility, full co-operation in the life of the community, the sharing in every kind of work, domestic, agricultural, constructional — these were not merely ideals but rooted in necessity.'[65] But they *were* ideals, and although 'educationally' rather than 'psychologically' derived they had most of those therapeutic values which are claimed when such experiences are described as 'ergo-therapy'. As Wills and Barron had found at Hawkspur, they not only contributed to social cohesion but also to the growth of personal self-respect and an appreciation of the needs and value of others.

Barnes also experimented at the beginning with self-government but found his heterogeneous and often disturbed pupils unready for the experience. A 'benevolent dictatorship' was established which was increasingly broadened by discussion in meetings of the whole school. As the school grew the system was again modified to vest the executive power in a senate of mature pupils.[66]

Barnes' aim was not to promote any new system or perpetuate an old one. 'The children themselves and the relationships in the community are more important than principles or methods or systems.' Nor was it considered necessary to have any special treatment for maladjusted children within the framework of a school the principle of which was to promote 'the energy and joy of its pupils'. Indeed, although adolescent disturbance was recognized it was also valued.

Barnes writes: 'Nearly all children in their teens go through disturbances of feeling and impulse, moods and rejections, and our handling of them must never be so strict and demanding as to prevent
their being successfully worked through. Too great pressure will also
destroy originality and fertility of thought.' Nevertheless, an unchal-
lenging permissivism such as that offered at Summerhill is seen as
neglecting the necessities of personal growth. 'Life in its very nature
is tough and reality is obdurate, not to be bent to our will. Co-operation in creative work does not come out of a slick fitting together of
human beings into a pattern; it comes out of a struggle in which
each person is challenged by others, and has to dig into himself and
face his own inadequacy as well as discover his own ability.'

Individuals are valued not for their balance and harmony and
adjustment but for their diversity. The capacity for loving and being
loved is valued above careful adjustment to the complicated patterns
of social demands. The 'abundant life' which Barnes stresses as
his objective may be 'surprisingly different to anything to which we
are accustomed'. Barnes does not see the end product as a child
thoroughly adjusted to the demands of an affluent and aggressive
society in the outside world. 'It would mean that our education was
a total failure. The important question to ask is whether the difficulty
stimulates from them a vigorous, discriminating and constructive
response.' Nevertheless, it is recognized that children may be frustrated in their enjoyment of abundant life by fear of their own
inadequacy in the face of experience, by jealousy or by feelings of
guilt. The necessary assistance is seen as coming from a trustful and
intimate contact with individuals within the community, the mature
members of which must be prepared to accept the hate and
rejection which the child may display in working through his
problems which are preventing him from living.

Such a school, as has often been recognized, offers many advantages to a maladjusted child who is not in need of the specialist
resources of a small therapeutic unit. It has no stigma of 'special'
attached to it; it is large enough to be both economically and educationally viable, it contains a majority of 'normal' children as a
contributory part of its therapeutic environment, and its independence outside the State system and outside the framework of 'special
education' allows it a freedom of action within which it can remain
dynamic.

LUCY FRANCIS

It might, perhaps, be appropriate in concluding an account of this last phase of individualistic 'pioneering' ventures to consider the career of Lucy Francis, principal of Kingsmuir School, West Hoathly, until her death on September 30 1969. Her work may never have been of major importance, except to the children who profited by it, but her life spans the period and is concerned with the personalities and influences of significance in therapeutic education. She may be seen as typical of the untypical individual from whom most work with disturbed children stems.[67]

Of middle-class South African origin, she followed her mother into the teaching profession. Her training she found unimaginative and depressing and of little assistance in her first job, in which she was given a class of children all of whom she considered 'maladjusted'. Inspired by reading A. S. Neill's early 'Dominie' books, she tried to teach in a way utterly at variance with the spirit of the school and the instructions of her bullying autocratic headmaster. The latter thrashed pupils who spoke to Lucy Francis freely on the basis of the trust she engendered and, on one occasion, insisted that she should cane two girls accused of cheating in her class. She refused, but eventually complied in a token fashion after the girls themselves had asked her to. She found that she could teach in her own way only by holding classes out of school.

At the same time she was struggling with her own problems of personal adjustment, which she solved largely by a complete rejection of her own restrictive and religious middle-class background. After the First World War she came to England and bought a run-down coffee-stall in London, near St Pancras. This she made a centre for down-and-outs, for whom she provided blankets and coats so that they could sleep near the stall. She was constantly warned of the dangers of her position, but she discovered that the chief danger to her health came not from her increasing family of 'drop-outs' but from an almost total lack of sleep, since she found that London in the daytime (when her stall was closed) had a life too fascinating to sleep through. Worn out by this routine she took several jobs, the most significant of which, for her, was one in which she discovered how 'deprived' upper-class children could be. She was appointed 'watch-dog' to two children of a wealthy divorcee and.

despite the opposition of their conventional and authoritarian grand-parents, she introduced the children to the joys of Woolworths and riding on buses—and encouraged them to speak at table. She lost her job.

Attracted by the principles of 'New Education' she accepted a job in the junior department of Bedales, of which she said: 'Bedales sounded like a free school and then was so awful'. She admired Badley but found the regime in the junior school under Mrs Fish 'terrible'. Still fighting hard against her own background (in a way strongly reminiscent of A. S. Neill at King Alfred's) she was con-stantly frustrated by Mrs Fish's desire to maintain 'dignity'. This conflicted with Lucy Francis's desire to deal with the disturbed children in her class by close and understanding contact. She also found that contact was difficult to establish with the majority of the largely upper-middle-class children. ('If they saw you they would always say... "Please".') Her particular insight and interest was, however, recognized and she was eventually given sole charge of one very disturbed and violently aggressive Indian boy. She began their relationship by saying: 'If you are angry you can come and do something to me'.

She then took a course with Dottoressa Montessori, whom she regarded as a 'frightful boss—terrible to her students'. As had Leila Rendel, she found Montessori's use of her material over-rigid and insufficiently stimulating to intelligent children. Thus when she sub-sequently started her own primary school at Hemel Hempstead the Montessori principles were very much modified. The school began with the four great-grandchildren of Lady d'Arcy Osbourne, a wealthy eccentric who cut off her own dresses when she arrived home late in order not to disturb her maid and who translated Gibbon's *Decline and Fall of the Roman Empire* into braille at the age of ninety-six.

Lucy Francis's ability as a teacher of disturbed children was soon recognized and the school expanded, but she still wished to live in London and so left the school to become secretary for the Golden Cockerel Press. When the Press collapsed during the Depression she went to Summerhill to work with A. S. Neill who, for so long, had inspired her.

When Neill had been working in Austria Lucy Francis had wished to visit him but she had been too afraid of being disillusioned to go. She did, however, visit him at Lyme Regis and was not disillusioned.

At Summerhill Neill acknowledged her skill by giving her a separate house with about a dozen of the more disturbed children. When the school was evacuated to Wales this arrangement continued in an abandoned and semi-derelict school which she restored with the assistance of Olive Lane, Homer Lane's adopted daughter. Her houses were known as 'junk'.

Although her admiration for Neill was unabated and although Summerhill provided an atmosphere in which she could work as she wished, Lucy Francis had certain reservations about Neill's work. In particular she felt that there were many children in the 1930s who were of a different sort from the earlier more disturbed children and who, stimulated by interested parents, wished to work and wanted to learn and that these were frustrated by Neill's inveterate prejudice against education. John Walmsley quotes her as saying: 'The only thing I used to get annoyed about with Neill was that he'd come round and talk to them and say Hello, and they'd say "Show Neill what we've done in lessons", and he wouldn't look at it. And I'd say "Oh Neill! I wish you'd be interested in what they're doing. You seem to think that all children hate lessons!" But then he'd tell them a story. They were always about themselves, you know, these stories. He would use them psychologically but not at all in a heavy way; and they would have the most wonderful adventures. He'd say: "And then Johnny said, 'No, I won't, I won't go up in that aeroplane. It isn't safe, I'm frightened!' And the child would say, 'I never said that! I would go! I . . . I went'!" '[68]

She saw Neill as a marvellous 'natural' analyst who always knew what was happening to a child.

Ill-health forced Lucy Francis to leave Wales and in 1944 she opened her own branch of Summerhill—Kingsmuir (named after Neill's birthplace) in Essex, moving in 1959 to her present school in Sussex. This she started with a capital of £5 and had to rely heavily on Local Education Authority children, but when it became clear that Lucy Francis put therapy first, even to the extent of considering lessons irrelevant to very disturbed children, L.E.A.s threatened to withdraw support. When they were faced with the alternative of leaving the school or of having compulsory lessons the L.E.A. pupils accepted the latter if Lucy Francis agreed to instruct them. Many of her private, and very disturbed pupils a colleague described as 'the ones Summerhill can't cope with'.

Her school, which eventually closed in December 1970, was an all-age, co-educational boarding school—although she clearly felt that she had a special responsibility to the maladjusted adolescent girls for whom there were so few places elsewhere. It was run basically on 'Summerhill' lines with the maximum of freedom of choice and self-determination as expressed through the school councils. Although therapy was paramount school work was recognized as valuable, but its direction and effectiveness was frequently dictated by the interests and abilities of a very unorthodox staff. Art was seen as of particular value and some work was remarkable.

Therapy was both direct and indirect. The children received regular treatment from a psychiatrist and a psychotherapist and the school was regarded as a therapeutic rather than an educational unit. Lucy Francis considered that maladjusted children are basically 'children who are frightened' and her first principle in dealing with them was that 'they must never be afraid'. Their relationships with the staff must be those of absolute trust. This, Lucy Francis suggested, implied the acceptance of the security of a certain degree of structure without which the fearful and anxious maladjusted child cannot be helped to help herself.

Thus Lucy Francis did not absolve herself of responsibility for the process even when in recent years she had to conduct the school from her bed. She recognized, honestly, the effect of her personality and laid no claim to theory. It may be true of her that it is only by looking at her life that one may perceive her effect. Of her whole career she said what is, perhaps, a fitting epitaph for many pioneer workers: 'I didn't work it out; I just did it.'

I

REFERENCES

CHAPTER 13: Rethinking Child Care

1 PADLEY, R. and COLE, M. *The Evacuation Survey*, *p* 42. Report to Fabian Society, Routledge, London, 1940.
2 ISAACS, S. Fatherless Children, in *Problems of Child Development*, *pp* 3-15 New Education Fellowship, London, 1948.
3 ISAACS, S. (ed). *The Cambridge Evacuation Survey*. Methuen, London, 1941.
4 PADLEY, R. and COLE, M. op. cit.
5 BOYD, W. and RAWSON, W. *The Story of the New Education*, *p* 115. Heinemann, London, 1965.
6 ISAACS, S. (ed.) op. cit., *pp* 96–7.
7 HENSHAW, E. M. Some Psychological Difficulties of Evacuation, *Mental Health* (1) *p* 6. 1940.
8 KEIR, G. A History of Child Guidance, *Br. J. Ed. Psych.* **xxii** (1) *pp* 25–6. 1952.
9 FULTON, J. F. Factors Influencing the Growth and Pattern of the Child Guidance Services, etc. M. A. Thesis, (unpublished) *pp* 143–4. Queen's University, Belfast, 1964.
10 MINISTRY OF EDUCATION, The Health of the School Child. Report of the C.M.O., *p* 64. H.M.S.O., London, 1947.
11 ISAACS, S. (ed.) op. cit., *p* 201.
12 UNDERWOOD REPORT, Section 47, H.M.S.O. London, 1955.
13 SETH, G. now Professor of Psychology, Queen's University, Belfast. (to whom I am indebted for much information about the expansion of psychological services in Wales.)
14 SETH, G. Memorandum on the Provision of a Psychological Service for the Evacuated Population in North Wales, (unpublished). 18 June, 1941.
15 PERSONAL COMMUNICATION.
16 WINNICOTT, D. W. and BRITTON, C. The Problem of Homeless Children in *Problems of Child Development*, *pp* 65-73. New Education Fellowship, London, 1948.
17 WINNICOTT, D. W., quoted in Shields, R. W. *A Cure of Delinquents*, *p* 151. Heinemann, London, 1962.
18 WINNICOTT, D. W. and BRITTON, C. op. cit., *p* 67.

19 COLEMAN, J. *Childscourt, pp* 30-32. Macdonald, London, 1967.
20 Ibid. *p* 46.
21 Ibid. *pp* 47-8.
22 Ibid. *p* 65.
23 DANSER, J. Review of Childscourt in *Therapeutic Education, pp* 21-23. January, 1969.
24 BARRON, A. T. in *Q Camp.* Planned Environmental Therapy Trust, *p* 36. December, 1966. (I am also indebted to Arthur Barron for much information about his career.)
25 FLUGEL, J. C. *The Psychoanalytic Study of the Family.* Hogarth, London, 1948.
26 SAXBY, I. B. *The Education of Behaviour.* University of London Press, London, 1921.
27 ALLEN, LADY MARJORIE, *The Times,* 15 July, 1944.
28 ALLEN, LADY MARJORIE, *Whose Children.* Favill, 1945.
29 BALBERNIE, R. *Residential Work with Children.* Pergamon, Oxford, 1966.
30 BURLINGHAM, D. & BARRON, A. T. A Study of Identical Twins, in *The Psycho-analytical Study of the Child.* **xxiii**, *pp* 367-423. 1963.
31 BARRON, A. T. Preparing a Child for Placement *New Era* **43** (2). *p* 31. 1962.
32 Ibid. *p* 32.
33 MONKTON, SIR W. *Report on the circumstances which led to the boarding out of Dennis and Terence O'Neill at Bank Farm, Ministerly, and the steps taken to supervise their welfare. Cmd. 6636, H.M.S.O.* London, 1945.
34 ALLEN, LADY MARJORIE, op. cit.
35 THE HOME OFFICE. *Report of the Care of Children Committee, (The Curtiss Report).* Cmd. 6922, Section 1. H.M.S.O., London, 1946.
36 Ibid. Sections 98 & 99.
37 Ibid. Sections 415-422.
38 Ibid. Sections, 265-266.
39 Ibid. Section 494.
40 HEYWOOD, J. S. *Children in Care, p* 144. Routledge & Kegan Paul, London, 1959.
41 THE HOME OFFICE. *Children in Trouble.* Cmnd. 3601, H.M.S.O., London, 1968.
42 For a critical re-assessment of Parkhurst and Mary Carpenter *see* Carlebach, J. *Caring for Children in Trouble, pp* 25-59. Routledge & Kegan Paul, London, 1970.
43 CARLEBACH, J., Ibid., *pp* 126-133.
44 *See* Appendix, also historical accounts in Hinde, R. S. E. *The British Penal System 1773–1950.* Duckworth, London, 1951; Rose, G. *Schools for Young Offenders.* Tavistock, London, 1967; and Carlebach, J., op. cit.

45 HOME OFFICE. *Treatment of Young Offenders. Departmental Committee Report*, Cmd. 2831. H.M.S.O., 1927.
46 HOME OFFICE. *Making Citizens.* H.M.S.O. London, 1946.
47 Ibid. *p* 50.
48 Ibid. *p* 23.
49 HOME OFFICE. *Report of a Committee to Review Punishments in Prisons, Borstal Institutions, Approved Schools and Remand Homes*, H.M.S.O., Parts III & IV. London, 1951.
50 HOME OFFICE. *Statistics relating to approved schools, remand homes and attendance centres, in England and Wales*, 1967. H.M.S.O., London, 1968.
51 CARLEBACH, J. op. cit., *p* 113.
52 Talk given by Father Owen at Spode House, (unpublished). Rugeley, 22 March 1969.
53 Ibid.
54 MCLUCHAN, M. & FIORE, Q. *The Medium is the Massage, p* 88. Allen Lane, Penguin Press 1967.

CHAPTER 14: Rethinking Education

55 CHILD, H. A. T. (ed.) *The Independent Progressive School, p* 8. Hutchinson, London, 1962.
56 JONES, H. *Reluctant Rebels*, Tavistock, London, 1960.
57 Ibid. *p* 141.
58 Ibid. *p* 75.
59 LUMSDEN, J., personal communication.
60 JONES, H., op. cit., *pp* 72-3.
61 WEAVER, A. The Treatment of Maladjusted Children within the Educational System of England. Ph.D. Thesis (unpublished), Oxford University, 1969.
62 GLOVER, E. introduction to Lennhoff F. C. *Exceptional Children.* Allen & Unwin, (London) 1960.
63 WEAVER, A. op. cit., *p* 24.
64 URBAN, E., in Child, H. A. T. op. cit., *pp* 108-123.
65 BARNES, K., in Child, H. A. T. op. cit., *pp* 156-168 (Information also from personal communication).
66 BARNES, K. *The First Four Years.* Pamphlet, 1944.
67 Material largely from interview with Lucy Francis and from her colleagues.
68 WALMSLEY, J. *Neill and Summerhill*, Penguin, London, 1969.

PART SEVEN

Conceptualization and Generalization

15

Some Theories of Therapeutic Education

So many charlatans have claimed to be therapeutic educators and have got away with it because the concepts are complicated and difficult and cannot be readily checked and assessed in the way in which a training approach can be assessed, that we are in danger of associating a therapeutic approach with woolliness of thought, laziness of practice and an irresponsibility towards the seriousness of our children's disorders. — A.T. Barron.[1]

It may be argued that before anyone can be regarded as a 'pioneer' he must not only do something which is original but he must point a way that others may follow. His individual practice must lead to theory, or some body of practical directions, which can be generalized from and which serve as a guide to others in similar but different situations. The link will normally be some degree of conceptualization. In therapeutic education 'experiments' are many and concepts few. Nevertheless some do exist. Some have been derived from apparently successful practice; a few have preceded practice; and others have developed in conjuction with practice.

'Planned environmental therapy' is of the last-named type. It is the most generally acknowledged theoretical base for work done with maladjusted children in this country, although interpretations of its principles have been wide, various and frequently far from legitimate. It represents an attempt to conceptualize the practice of people such as Aichhorn, Lane, Lyward, Wills and Shaw, within a general theoretical framework derived from a mixture of social psychology and post-Freudian psychoanalysis. Its chief exponent is Dr Marjorie Franklin.[2]

Dr Franklin, as a young junior medical officer in the Portsmouth Borough Mental Hospital in the early 1920s, became intensely interested in the relationship between mental illness and the patients' environment. She observed not only the often-noted improvements that occurred in response to a cheerful, encouraging environment and sympathetic nursing but also, in some cases, the dramatic improvement of the psychotic condition with the onset of severe physical illness. The latter phenomenon she attributed not only to a change in the location of the cathexis but also to the greatly increased attention and care which the ill patient received. The improvement was seldom maintained but Dr Franklin considered that with skilful psycho-analytical intervention and support it might have been.[3]

These experiences were very germane to her later understanding and they were strengthened by her subsequent psychiatric training in the United States and by her course of psychoanalysis with Freud's pupil and colleague Ferenczi. Through work with the Howard League and the Institute for the Scientific Treatment of Delinquency she involved herself in the problems of adult delinquency and established contact with Norman Glaister and Cuthbert Rutter (a former 'progressive' Borstal housemaster and then headmaster of the Forest School). The idea of Q Camps as an experiment in therapeutic community-living subsequently brought Dr Franklin in touch with David Wills, whose own ideas, forged from a very different experience, were so complementary to her own. The Hawkspur Camp was founded as the first practical experiment in planned environmental therapy (see Chapter 12).

The war brought an end to direct experiment but many of the ventures in caring for disturbed evacuees described in earlier chapters led to a closer study of the needs of maladjusted children and some modification of those principles which had been evolved with young adult delinquents. After the failure of the junior Q Camp under Barron (see Chapter 13), an attempt was made to launch an experiment in planned environmental therapy under the auspices of The Children's Social Adjustment Society, at Arlesford Place. Some of the practical difficulties of this venture have been described in considering the work of Bill Malcolm, but the principles invite further study.

Arlesford Place was planned as an 'on-going' experiment in that it was intended to measure, by testing and observation, the effect of a particular method of re-education on maladjusted children. The 'experiment' was to be conducted by psychiatrists, who were largely responsible for selecting the children and organizing the treatment policy, wardens and other staff responsible for constructing and maintaining the environment, and psychologists both inside and outside the establishment who were to assess the results.

The subjects were a group of thirty to forty, all-age, boys and girls with I.Q.s ranging from 87 to 167. They were all suffering from some failure to adjust socially, emotionally or educationally. The aim of the experiment was to test the effect of a specific therapeutic approach in terms of individual adjustment.

The methods to be used were specified and, in theory, contact was maintained between psychiatrists, school-staff and psychologists so that a specific policy could be adhered to.

In general terms, social adjustment was to be achieved by a creative use of the environment, which was an elegant mansion house near Winchester, and by the experience of 'shared responsibility' within the school council, which was a legislative and judicial body of which all staff and pupils were members.

Educational adjustment was to be achieved through improving motivation by making lessons voluntary, by the use of arts and crafts as creative outlets for tension, and by individual remedial teaching.

Emotional adjustment was to be achieved through close and loving personal relationships with adult members of the community and by individual psychotherapy. The warden, Bill Malcolm, saw the process as a three-stage one. 'First, sometimes after a brief period of distrust, a strong attachment to an adult; these attachments are treated with respect and care and then when this friendship has brought a feeling of security, an interest in other children will develop. Once accepted by them the third phase is reached, of interest in the government of the place. By this time the child has become less dependent on his grown up friends'.[4] It will be noted that this is largely a social interpretation. A direct attack on the emotional problem was to be made psychotherapeutically by the honorary psychiatrists, who visited fortnightly to talk to the children and discuss treatment policies with the warden. 'By this means', it was suggested, 'there is a close inter-relation between, on the one hand, the influence of adults in daily association with the children, who are responsible for maintaining the environment, and on the other hand, a more scientific and detached approach'.[5]

It was hoped that 'apart from . . . successful therapy the scientific experiment of which it is the result may eventually give Arlesford a value beyond its immediate aim'.

That Arlesford failed both as a school and as an experiment did not invalidate the theory of planned environmental therapy; rather it was the inevitable result of the nature of the research design.

In any educational research project the number of uncontrollable extraneous variables in a human and dynamic situation make anything like real experiment difficult if not impossible, however limited the scope of the enquiry. This piece of 'action-research' was endeavouring to measure changes in emotional adjustment (an exact evaluation of which is always impossible) occurring as the result of a number of widely different processes, variously interpreted and never clearly specified. The people concerned in the process consisted of a large number of subjects of widely differing ages, abilities, symptoms and degrees of adjustment and of observers of different, and frequently conflicting, disciplines, aims and personal attitudes. The warden, who was essentially concerned with the maintenance of the environment, appears to have been opposed to psychological investigation and psychiatric methods and interpretations. He did not accept the desirability of unnecessarily primitive conditions and his approach to 'shared responsibility' involved the exercise of a good deal of guidance. His periodic reports on children's progress can hardly have been helpful to people thinking in entirely different terms. It was inevitable that both professional and personal rivalries and jealousies would disrupt the work, particularly since its nature involved close personal and effective ties between staff and children.

In such an atmosphere any objective evaluation of the results or the drawing of any valid conclusions from them were clearly impossible. The failure of the Arlesford Place 'experiment' in 1962, however, did not unduly discourage the supporters of 'planned environmental therapy' who, by this time, had been joined by many eminent practitioners in both independent and State schools (whether as headmasters, wardens, psychiatrists or psychotherapists). In January 1963 a 'planned environmental therapy discussion group' was formed under the leadership of Dr Franklin, in whose house members met monthly 'to talk together about the theoretical and clinical aspects of treating people (of all ages) with emotional and/or behavioural problems by means of a therapeutically planned environment (residential or otherwise) of various patterns within the framework of methods loosely described as progressive or evolutionary (non repressive)'.[6] This sort of discussion both widened the context and clarified the common aims of various forms of environmental therapy and in 1966 the Planned Environmental Therapy Trust was formed to promote 'the serious clinical study of the use of the environment as a means of correcting asocial and other related character deficiencies'.

Dr Franklin claims that ' "planned environmental therapy" has long ago reached the stage of a serious branch of psychotherapy' and Barron describes it as 'the only method I know that provides a viable method and approach to the residential care and treatment of the maladjusted'.[7] Its terms of reference are very wide but there are certain principles of organization and certain ideas of therapy which appear, if not fundamental, at least customary.

Environmental therapists must initially have a concept of 'maladjustment' which lays stress on the environmental causes of the disturbance. The 'environment' may be widely interpreted to include the whole life experience, but particular emphasis has usually been placed on experience within the family. The maladjustment may be largely the product of social factors, which can be dealt with by the experience of living together in a tolerant and sympathetic community, or may be of more deep-seated emotional origin related to the quality of love which the child has received. Theoretical support for this position has been drawn from the work of Suttie,[8] D. W. Winnicott, Anna Freud and others, who stress the importance of loving relationships within the family as the prerequisite of mental health.

A planned therapeutic environment, therefore, must include provision not only for a new social experience but also for the rediscovery of the healing power of love. Therapy is based on the assumption that there is an 'inherent impulse towards health' which the therapist must encourage and assist. In performing this task the therapist will be aided by an environment free from unnecessary frustrations, but skill and insight will be needed to find the appropriate techniques and time to remove the harmful defences which the individual has constructed to insulate himself from hurt, fear and guilt. The aim is not to change habits of behaviour but to rebuild and strengthen the ego so that a healthy individual may be free to live his own life within society.

The therapist, whether psychiatrist, teacher or other staff member, is the key to the process. By identification with him and transference to him of the feelings of love and hate which have not found adequate expression within the family the child will be able to regress and recapitulate his experience and so find security and relief from guilt. At the same time the environment will give him challenging opportunities for building self-respect and sublimating his impulses and his energies in socially acceptable ways.

If this process is to succeed, certain characteristics are posited for the environment itself. Identification and transference will occur only if it is possible for the child to establish close personal relationships with adults who are mature enough to accept the child and his problems without reserve but without forming collusive relationships through which their own problems can be projected on to the disturbed child. Security will be the product not of organization but of mutual trust in an environment free of authoritarian coercion and discipline based on punishment. Punishment, in the traditional sense, is not only viewed as unconstructive but as positively damaging to therapy, destructive of human relationships and productive only of a moral code based on the idea that if what is punishable is wrong what is not punishable must be right.[9] The relief of guilt which punishment sometimes affords is seen as an inducement to delinquency. Guilt must be relieved by psychotherapy reinforced by opportunities to rebuild self-respect within the community.

Such opportunities are to be found in the experience of co-operation in creative activities and particularly in the creation of both the physical and political structure. Homer Lane, Makarenko, Wills, Barron, Marjorie Franklin and indeed many 'progressive' educationalists working with normal children have stressed the value of 'pioneering' experience through which children create and structure their own environment for living. This experience is thought to produce both individual self-esteem and respect for others and for the community. Where the physical circumstances have initially been adequate emphasis has been placed on estate work, building and crafts.

The principle of shared responsibility is also seen as a fundamental part of the re-educative process. By sharing together with the staff the full responsibility of the management of their community, children are thought to share in something much more than exercises in decision making. They learn to be responsible both for and to others, to accept the natural consequences of their own acts, and to value themselves as people who have something to contribute to the general good.[10]

In that the general purpose of planned environmental therapy is to create that experience of good family life of which the majority of maladjusted children are considered to be deprived, it follows that coeducation is considered important.

Although there are many variations, produced largely by the

personalities of those actually involved, the 'planned environmental therapy' establishment would therefore have certain determining characteristics. It will be, ideally, a coeducational community in which human relations are based on unconditional love and acceptance. It will be based on a belief in equality and trust and will be essentially non-punitive. Individual difficulties and disturbances will be treated by psychotherapy both direct and specialized and also indirect and non-specialist. The life of the community will be based on hard, co-operative work, and on shared responsibility in management. Cultural and educational opportunities will be geared to the needs of the individual. This is, perhaps, not so much a theory as a plan of action forged from experience.

ANNA FREUD

The most extensive single body of theory related to the needs of therapeutic education is that of psychoanalysis. The significance of such theory to the needs of individuals developing through childhood, particularly to those with severe problems of adjustment, was realized and variously interpreted by pioneer workers. Lane moved from Freud and Jung in an attempt to justify his idiosyncratic practice. Neill proceeded from Freud to Reich to put a conceptual gloss on his own ideas about freedom.[11] Shaw found Melanie Klein's interpretation of psychoanalysis most useful in interpreting the disturbances of adolescent boys. But despite the brief but important work of Susan Isaacs at the Malting House School psychoanalytic concepts percolated very slowly through education and even pioneers such as Lyward, Wills and Dr Fitch, although acknowledging the theoretical value of psychoanalysis, and sometimes using its terminology, subscribed to the convention that in their institutions 'psychoanalysis was not done but lived'.

As in so many other things the rapid development of psychoanalytically-based child psychology and its application to psychotherapy and therapeutic education was largely a product of the experiences of the Second World War. Before the problem of coping with the disturbed child within a disintegrating and inadequate educational structure became a national concern, teachers were able to reject Freudian concepts as repulsive, alien, impracticable ideas promoted only by foreigners and 'cranks'. This position was reinforced by the Freudians themselves since they tended to develop exclusive cults and mystiques into which only believers were fully initiated.

The advent of war not only generalized the problem but helped to disseminate information of psychoanalytical theory and practice with the arrival in this country of a large number of important Continental Freudians. Of these the most significant for education was clearly Anna Freud herself.

Since the 1920s Anna Freud had endeavoured to demonstrate to teachers the application of psychoanalytical theories to 'pedagogics, or the science of upbringing and education'.[12] While admitting that 'psychoanalysis, whenever it has come into contact with pedagogy, has always expressed the wish to limit education'[13] by loosening the control imposed by educators over normal child development, she sought to increase understanding and to expand the role of the teacher to include therapy. The task of the teacher was 'to allow to each stage in the child's life the right proportion of instinct-gratification and instinct-restriction'. This was no plea for unrestricted permissivism but its success did depend on the teacher recognizing the importance of the individual and also the general psychodynamic framework of child development.

Anna Freud saw psychoanalysis as doing these things for pedagogics: 'In the first place it is well qualified to offer a criticism of existing educational methods. In the second place, the teacher's knowledge of human beings is extended, and his understanding of the complicated relations between the child and the educator is sharpened by psychoanalysis, which gives us a scientific theory of the instincts, of the Unconscious and of the Libido. Finally, as a method of practical treatment, in the analysis of children, it endeavours to repair the injuries which are inflicted upon the child during the process of education'.[14]

Another way in which Anna Freud's work made psychoanalytical procedures more available for use in therapeutic education lay in the emphasis which she put on the 'ego' and its development rather than on the unconscious working of the 'id'. She directed attention to the actual behaviour of the child (rather than to analysis of concealed dream symbolism) and to the recognition of the existence and effect of defence-mechanisms, (such as phantasy, denial and indentification,) in overt acts.[15] This approach was partly the result of the obvious difficulties of applying the normal techniques of psychoanalysis to small children but it had the satisfactory effect of making psychoanalytical theory more communicable and more relevant to teachers.

Nevertheless, had Anna Freud stayed in Austria she might have tried in vain to communicate her message to English teachers resistant to the name of Freud and generally unsympathetic to psychological formulations. Her practical work during the war at the Hampstead Nurseries gave her opportunity for close study, disseminated her views and demonstrated her practice. It was, therefore, an event of great importance in therapeutic education in England and indeed in the whole sphere of the education of young children in this country.

The Children's Rest Centre in Hampstead was set up largely by a group of highly trained Continental refugees with four main aims: to repair both physical and psychological damage done to children by the Blitz, to prevent further harm, to do intensive research on the psychological effects of violence and separation, and 'to instruct people interested in the forms of education based on psychological knowledge of the child; and generally to work out a pattern of nursery life which can serve as a model for peacetime education'.[16]

The three nurseries (two residential, one day) provided a unique opportunity for the study of children under stress. The 138 children, ranging in age from one week to ten years, reported on in *'Young Children in Wartime'*, 1942, were selected only by circumstance, had suffered varying experiences of separation and deprivation, and were under the care and intensive observation of a staff consisting of 'highly trained workers in the field of medicine, psychology, education, nursing and domestic science'. The report which emerged was brief, objective, lucid and free from jargon. It makes no direct reference to psychoanalytical theory. Its impact was, therefore, very direct.

Anna Freud's main observation was that disturbance in the child was seldom derived directly from environmental causes such as bombing, living in shelters or being injured. As long as Mother was present the young child scarcely appeared to notice such events, which produced anxiety only if they caused anxiety in others or were used as symbolic representations of the child's own inner fears, e.g. of punishment for guilt. On the other hand although being trapped under a heap of rubble in a burning building might not be traumatic, a comparatively brief separation from Mother frequently was.

Many of the children at the Hampstead nurseries were the casualties not of war but of evacuation. For many, placement at Hampstead (although still in London) was their first experience of evacuation and separation from Mother. Observation of the children's reactions in these unique circumstances enabled Anna Freud and her co-workers to base their theories of child development firmly on experience. In the first few months of life the baby, although utterly dependent on a mother-figure, did not appear to require a particular individual to fulfil that function and rapidly re-adjusted after separation. After this period and until about three years of age the effect of separation was found to be particularly traumatic. Mother had become a personal love object, sole provider of pleasure and pain without whom the child became lost. He was, perhaps, plunged into a period of 'mourning' in which he became depressed, non-communicative and frequently physically unwell. If the separation occurred after about three years of age the children were more capable of understanding and externalizing their grief, could more easily identify with parent substitutes but were also at a stage when negative feelings towards apparently rejecting parents could either be strongly expressed in a reciprocal rejection or internalized as strong feelings of guilt. The observed effects of 'maternal deprivation' have been too well documented to require further elaboration[17] but the significance of Anna Freud's evidence has seldom been given its full weight. Her 'sample' was composed of 'normal' children, fairly randomly selected by the hand of war, a large group expertly observed. Her evidence did not rest on institutionalized children or on laboratory animals and her endeavour was to describe what happened rather than to advance any particular viewpoint at this stage.

Her study was, however, more than an account of the problems arising from a temporary wartime situation and was important to subsequent therapeutic education in that it gave a theoretical framework of use to those working with children deprived of maternal love by other forms of separation and rejection. As was consistent with her general approach Anna Freud worked from a study of overt behaviour towards an understanding of its origin. She observed the mechanisms by which children either expressed, or defended themselves against, the pain of separation. Some found relief in speech, often after considerable periods of silence. For others play was a more available form of expression and of therapy. Many, more seriously disturbed, expressed their maladjustment in bizarre behaviour or in neurotic regression to more infantile modes. Enuresis, compulsive eating, destructive aggression, autoerotic forms of gratification and temper tantrums all expressed a rejection of a society from which love had been withdrawn. Of particular interest in our present stage of concern with the condition known as autism is Anna Freud's observation of children whose reaction to separation and rejection was 'abnormal withdrawal of emotional interest from the outside world'. She describes one girl who, although she had no experience of air-raids, was moved into six different temporary homes between the age of two and three. She was hysterical and impossible to handle. 'She would not go to bed, could not sleep, would not eat, fought against being bathed, washed, dressed or undressed. She had fear of going downstairs, of leaving the house, of entering again through the front door. Sometimes she would like to play with other children, at other times she screamed with fear when they approached her.' Eventually she developed an undiagnosable neurotic illness. 'Hysterical symptoms alternate with phobic behaviour and compulsive mechanisms. The main feature is her withdrawal from the interests of the real outer world. Her expression is always worried, her glance fixed and stony.'[18]

On the basis of her experience Anna Freud stressed the importance of the careful planning of necessary separation, of preliminary experience in day nurseries, the rejection of the popular idea that children should not be visited for the first fortnight after evacuation, and above all the necessity of involving parents as closely, fully and continually as possible.

The effect of Anna Freud's wartime work, her subsequent publications, and her continuing influence as a great teacher of teachers and therapists is incalculable. The effect on certain practitioners of therapeutic education was immediate.

BARBARA DOCKAR-DRYSDALE

Perhaps the most important of these, both in practice and in her advancement of the theory of therapeutic education, is Barbara Dockar-Drysdale.[19] Much of her work is derived not directly from Anna Freud but from her mentor for many years, Dr D. W. Winnicott, whose own important contributions to the development of child psychology and psychiatry stem not only from his experience of wartime hostels but also from the theories of both Anna Freud and Melanie Klein. Like Winnicott, who describes her as 'a sophisticated therapist and conceptualizer', Dockar-Drysdale attached more importance to the earliest period of infancy than did Anna Freud. The period of basic unity in which the child is unable to distinguish between inner and outer reality and in which he is utterly dependent on the mother for the satisfaction of his instinctual needs is seen as crucial. This is the essential 'primary experience' which if inadequate or interrupted will lead to maladjustment.[20]

It is within this concept that Dockar-Drysdale has done her most important work in seeking to explain the nature and needs of the 'frozen' or psychopathic child. The emotionally deprived child is seen as 'pre-neurotic' since the child has to exist as an individual before neurotic defences can form. The extent to which there has been traumatic interruption of the 'primary experience' decides the form of the disturbance. A child separated at this primitive stage is, therefore, in a perpetual state of defence against the hostile 'outer world' into which he has been jettisoned inadequately prepared. Reality is, for him, incomplete in that he has been 'thrown back for all pleasure-pain experience on his limited part of the unity ... the desperate dread of self-destruction and the frantic hope of self-preservation being the deciding factors in the subsequent history of such a child'.[21] These children remain 'frozen' in a symbiotic state 'without boundaries to personality, merged with their environment, and unable to make any real object relations or feel the need of them'. They remain totally egocentric, using others for their own purposes. Since there is no past to regret and no future to consider they live for the moment without fear or remorse. They are often charming, subject to violent changes of mood and are invariably delinquent. Any relations which they appear to establish are merely a means to an end and will break down at the imposition of the slightest frustration which will lead to fury and the destruction of the frustrating environment. 'There is no gap between the instinctual need and the satisfaction of that need'.

Such a child, if untreated, is the prototype of the psychopath and the treatment is arduous, always doubtful of success, and dependent on the establishment of unity with the therapist so that the child may re-establish the primary state of dependency in order to experience the reality of separation.

Other children requiring essentially the same treatment are those which Dockar-Drysdale calls 'archipelago children'. These have suffered separation after the first steps of integration. They have, therefore, some 'ego areas' without any total personality. Their behaviour is consequently erratic and bizarre but they have some capacity for symbolization, which aids therapeutic contact. Others have become fixated at some point and have protected their 'embryo egos' by 'caretaker selves' which are set up as real. Regression is essential to allow a return to the point where the creation of the 'false self' became necessary.

The therapist's task in all cases is to give the child 'complete experience' so that he can find first unity then individuality. For the most difficult 'frozen' child the treatment begins by a process of 'interruption' in which he is made conscious of the reality of himself as a unit in the world. His behaviour is carefully observed and anticipated so that acts are made consciously, with an awareness of the consequences. If the child fails to close the gap in his defences he is likely to panic since he has to forge a new unity in the world. At this point he may begin a severe 'unfocused depression' interpreted as a 'state of mourning for the loss of the unity'. This profound depression and anxiety may become a generalized illness since 'a delinquent character can only become normal through the experience of a neurosis'. The next stage depends on a deep attachment to an available adult with whom a primary bond is established so that the eventual separation of the 'self' can be achieved.

Dockar-Drysdale describes this process in the case of John, a severely delinquent nine-year-old. 'Interruption' was caused by her making him acknowledge his real responsibilities for such minor delinquencies as throwing a towel into the bath.

John, usually very cool and tough, became pale, trembled and screamed terrible obscenities at me. I carried him back to the bathroom kicking and shrieking. I assured him again that he really had put the towel in the bath. He continued to scream, and screwed up his eyes. I stayed with him, holding him solidly, re-affirming the facts and reassuring him ; till at last, dreadfully afraid and trembling, he took the towel out of the water. Even now he turned his face away so as to avoid seeing what he was doing, then quite suddenly he gave a great shuddering sigh, wrung out the towel and hung it on the side of the bath. After which he turned to me with a transfigured and radiant face and ran into my arms. I carried him upstairs, tucked him up in bed and he sank almost at once into a deep sleep, still holding my hand.... The child in becoming instantly unaware of having thrown the towel into the bath, was using the reality blindness which had become so much part of him that he unconsciously employed this defence in every aspect of his life. The therapist, by bringing the defence to a conscious level, made a gap, which produced panic which the therapist then relieved by offering steady support and help to face reality. Constant and consistent repetition of such interruption, and protection brought John to a point ... without panic. Finally, we see him at a stage at which he can allow himself to be aware of his motions ... he has changed from a bright hard young tough – a 'wild one' in the making – to an anxious little boy; stormy, difficult, but attached to a teacher, whose approval he values and whose disapproval causes him pain.[22]

Such an exacting approach to individual therapy raises special problems of organization in the school context within which Dockar-Drysdale, although essentially a therapist, has done most of her work. The structure of such a therapeutic 'agency' has to be sufficiently flexible to allow the necessary therapeutic role to be played by members of the staff regardless of their specific 'function'. Only in an organization largely free of timetable and with flexible staff functions is it possible to provide for that complete involvement which is necessary for the reliving of 'primary experience'. Since in any institution continuity of treatment with a single 'provider' is impossible, 'localized regression' in terms of partial co-operation between the child and a number of different adults is all that is available.[23] Nevertheless to provide as much continuity as possible, particularly at critical periods, between one particular adult and one child the staff has to accept considerable flexibility of role. Teachers, whether male or female, must be prepared to act as 'mothers', administrators must play supporting roles as 'teachers' and so on. Both children and staff may require regular support from a skilled therapist acting either as 'mother' or in the supporting role of 'father'. Dockar-Drysdale has been largely responsible in her school, the Mulberry Bush, for this function. The 'paternal' supporting role will also be derived from the structure of the society (although this will be subordinate to the 'mother's' role), and from supporters within the community.

Such a therapeutic community for very disturbed children will be subject to considerable strains and tensions. Staff members must thoroughly understand the nature of their task and the importance of others in its undertaking. They must be mature enough to accept the demands made without feeling guilty about their involvement and without entering into a 'collusive' relationship with the child within which they share its delinquent or neurotic attitude. Society, both inside the school and in contact with it from outside, must understand the essentially therapeutic approach to destruction and aggression. Damage to property for instance, at times very apparent at the Mulberry Bush, is seen as an essential working out of the child's aggression. The transfer of this aggression to people will eventually be welcomed since it will then be more accessible to therapy. Damage, theft, aggression will be followed by feelings of guilt which will be relieved, not by punishment or enforced restitution, but in a way appropriate to the child's inner need. Restitution may be direct or indirect, e.g. cleaning the room of someone from whom you have stolen, or, initially, may be some symbolic 'undoing'. Such a non-punitive approach may not be easily understood by people who are not thinking in therapeutic terms and—like the aggression itself—this may put a severe strain on structure. But 'to understand all is to forgive all'.

Inevitably such an approach has not always found easy acceptance and the life of the Mulberry Bush has frequently been strained and threatened. Dockar-Drysdale's approach now, however, commands considerable respect and the school's existence at Standlake, in Oxfordshire, seems assured by the support of the D.E.S. and the Gulbenkian Foundation.

Like so many other pioneer ventures the Mulberry Bush school originated in the war at which time Dockar-Drysdale began a nursery school for her own children and for evacuees and their mothers. Apart from running a small family play-group in 1935 she had no previous experience, having lived a largely 'society' and academic life as the daughter of a professor of surgery of Trinity College, Dublin. The latter's death when she was fifteen had been for her a traumatic experience.

Her wartime work with disturbed children and their mothers brought her in contact with Milan Morgenstern, a refugee psychotherapist and friend of Anna Freud and Susan Isaacs. Morgenstern encouraged her to read Freud in the original. Her work also attracted the attention of Dr Dingwell of the National Association for Mental Health and of Miss Lindsay, an inspector of special schools. The Board of Education suggested that she should run a school for maladjusted children for an experimental period of five years and with considerable support and interest from educationalists, psychiatrists and psychologists she did so.

Doubting her ability and skill she worked for about eighteen months in the children's department of the Maudesley Hospital, attending conferences and doing varied therapeutic work with children under supervision from psychiatrists. She also underwent a three-year personal analysis which she found not only assisted her insight with the children but greatly helped her work with both parents and staff. She has subsequently become a full member of the Association of Psychotherapists, working both with adults and with children. She is best known, however, for her work with the latter, particularly at the Mulberry Bush.

When her husband was demobilized in 1948 they became co-principals of the school at Standlake. For the next fifteen years the school was an intensive psychotherapy unit for about forty primary-age children and twenty adults. All the children were very deeply disturbed but the purpose behind the intensive treatment was to return them to normal conditions as soon as possible—usually in about two years. The children were arranged into four official and many unofficial groups, graded in their degree of structure but with a strong bond with a single teacher. There was a strong 'support team' not only of psychiatrists and psychiatric social workers but also of auxiliary staff. The unending demands on the emotional and physical energies of the staff, particularly as it was a principle of the school never to close, produced certain recurrent crises. Recognition by the Ministry in 1959 produced new problems in the management of the school, now brought into closer contact with the expectations of the outside world. Dockar-Drysdale was supported by many influential psychiatrists and London clinics in maintaining her therapeutic approach and although she and her husband retired from the direct management of the school she continued as its therapeutic adviser. The present headmaster, John Armstrong, continues her policy and, in her own words 'out of the difficulties has emerged a therapeutic organization, in every area of which the provision of primary experience for emotionally deprived children remains the basic task.'

Since it involves highly specialized techniques of psychotherapy her treatment policies cannot be easily generalized either to the majority of schools or for the majority of children. She has, however, pioneered a technique of treating very disturbed children suffering from the effects of extreme emotional deprivation. She is almost alone as a pioneer in attempting to deal with the intractable problem of the psychopathic child in an educational environment and it is significant that one of the most important developments of her work has been at the Cotswold Community, an approved school run by Richard Balbernie,[24] to which institution for disturbed delinquents she is consultant psychotherapist.

Her aim has always been to achieve an objective of 'experience, followed by realization followed by conceptualization'. Experience is then put into a form which can be communicated.

RUDOLPH STEINER

Although, as Rudolf Steiner realized, many people regarded his system of beliefs and of education as 'a kind of religious sectarianism only fit for some fanatical enthusiasts'[25] it deserves attention not only as the first and most complete conceptualization of a method of education appropriate for the handicapped and disturbed child but also because of its practical application. At the moment there are five Steiner schools for maladjusted children in Britain, a larger number than owe allegiance to any single philosophy other than the worthy but motley company which arrays itself under the capacious banner of 'planned environmental therapy'.

Steiner himself, a mystic with a powerful sense of identity which transcended physical space and recorded time, was no mere madman. He was trained as a scientist in the Technical College of Vienna, and by the age of twenty-two had achieved sufficient distinction to be asked to edit a new edition of Goethe's natural-scientific writings. He was distinguished in philosophy, in which subject he took his doctorate, and in his subsequent career achieved some importance and respect among eminent people in fields as diverse as theology, drama, architecture, mathematics, sculpture, agriculture, medicine and education.

Although his principles of education are embodied in lectures he gave in 1907[26] he was not actually engaged in the process of the education of children until 1919 (when he was fifty-eight). After the First World War his appeals addressed to the world's leaders for a peace based on a new spiritual social order were largely unheeded except by the manager and employees of the Waldorf Astoria cigarette factory in Stuttgart. With their support the Free Waldorf School was founded at Stuttgart and, from this, anthroposophist— or 'Waldorf'—schools spread rapidly throughout Europe.

Steiner himself instructed the first teachers both in the theory and practice of education although it is important—in view of later criticism of anthroposophical educational methods—to realize that he himself stressed the error of the stereotyped application of pedagogic method. The teachers were, above all, to learn from the children what was necessary for their own spiritual development and the teachers also were to regard teaching as an art in which the highest form was to be achieved by individual application of sound principles.

These principles were to be based on Steiner's insights into the nature of spiritual growth. For Steiner, life was a well marked process of maturation from the physical to the spiritual. In infancy the child becomes gradually aware of, and moulded by, the environment provided by his guardians until his re-birth into an 'etheric' stage of existence at about the age of seven (the cutting of his 'own' teeth). At puberty, the 'astral' body is born and the adolescent becomes capable of independent judgement and it becomes possible for him to develop his own individual spiritual 'ego' separate from, but united with, all spiritual identities throughout creation and throughout time. Shorn of its spiritual content (which to Steiner would have meant without life) this organismic developmental outline is not dissimilar in form either from Piaget's model of cognitive development or from Freud's pattern of personality development.

Like Freud, Steiner stresses the importance in infancy of 'identification' with worthy adult models in an atmosphere of loving care. 'Within such an atmosphere of love the imitation of healthy models is possible, the child is in his right element'.[27] Since growth is through the senses, formal instruction is considered irrelevant at this period but much emphasis is put on environment and on experience. Physical surroundings must be carefully chosen in form and colour, toys must involve activity, feeding be correct, and the whole environment be so carefully structured that everything in it may be imitated so that the child need never be constrained.

At this stage writing may be copied and speech imitated but reading is considered too symbolic an activity to be undertaken. The rhythms of song and dance are especially important in the production

of balanced physical growth and harmony, and spontaneous drama-
tization of archetypal folk and fairy-tales are fundamentally
important.

In the 'etheric' stage, roughly from seven until adolescence
(Piaget's 'concrete-operational stage') the emphasis is on spiritually
concrete rather than 'abstract' experience. This Steiner considers to
be the age of 'authority' and hero-worship and these are combined in
studies of both living and historical heroes. Symbols and allegories
are considered spiritually 'concrete' and nature is a particularly
fruitful source. Agriculture, animal husbandry, building, craft-work
and a study of the seasons and nature are undertaken both as
valuable experience and as of great symbolic importance. 'It is very
important for a person to receive the secrets of Nature in allegories
before they appear to his soul in the form of natural laws'.[28] On the
other hand Steiner considers it necessary during this period to learn
and memorize things which are not fully understood so that they may
be available when understanding matures. 'Until the time of puberty
the youth should assimilate into the memory treasures over which
mankind has meditated; later on it is time to permeate with ideas
that which has been impressed on his memory. A man ought therefore not to retain merely what he has understood, but he ought now
to understand the things that he knows. . . .'[29] This storehouse for
eventual comprehension will include historical facts, geographical
data, basic movements and techniques of painting, all of which will
acquire their full meaning only with the birth of the 'astral' body at
puberty.

The role of 'authority' in the 'etheric' stage is of vital importance.
This authority rests solely with the adults in the community whose
task it is to control carefully the child's personal and intellectual
development so that he does not proceed too rapidly to 'astral' birth
before his 'etheric' development is complete, a task which is undertaken without the aid of corporal punishment, systems of competition
or reward, or even shared responsibility. The teacher, who is with the
same class throughout this period, relies on the discipline induced by
the basic philosophy of the school. 'The heart of the matter is a deep
sense of peace in heart and mind, in home and school, in these days
especially in the school.'[30]

At puberty, when the adolescent obtains full 'ego-consciousness'
and understanding of abstract forms, control is still exercised to
prevent too rapid development of 'spiritual scepticism' and immature

prejudice. 'No greater injury can be inflicted on anyone than by too soon awakening within him his own judgement'. The means of thought are now available but 'before being qualified to think, one must place before oneself as a warning what others have thought'.[31] All the powers of the soul are now free to develop and to guide the intellect towards the ultimate achievement of identity with God.

Some of the implications of this philosophy for the education of the maladjusted will be immediately apparent. A regime based on love, co-operation, security and essential harmony might well provide a therapeutic environment. Steiner, however, had much more to say that was specific about the education of the *Seelenflegebedürftige* — literally 'clownish souls', in need of special care. In this context Steiner himself was thinking primarily of mentally retarded children whose progress through the vital stages was limited by actual defects. Of this type of child he had had some personal experience in his youth when he had acted as tutor to a ten-year-old hydrocephalid. Deemed virtually ineducable this child was within two years attending high school and later became a doctor.

Between 1920 and 1924 Steiner laid the foundations of anthroposophical medicine and evolved the principles of curative eurythmy and curative education. These are based on the proposition that since the spiritual being cannot be ill it is the physical expression of the bodily vehicle which is hindering development. The basic treatment suggested is based on systematic exercises designed partly to correct difficulties of movement and posture and to achieve maximum potential. But to Steiner such exercises were not merely to strengthen the body or to acquire proficiency in movement and speech but to have a spiritual effect which would enable the handicapped child to face his special situation in life. He believed that 'the smallest step forward was of the greatest importance for the development of the child's individuality'.

As early as 1911 he had emphasised the importance of gymnastics and children's games through which the 'etheric' child experienced the feeling of its own expansion. 'Gymnastic exercises ought to be so carried out that with every movement, with every step, the feeling rises in the inner self of the boy or girl: "I feel increasing power within me". And this feeling should manifest itself within as a healthy delight, as a sensation of pleasure'. The educator should 'possess a close, intuitive and sympathetic knowledge of the relations of joy and comfort to the postures and movements of the human body. The formulator of such exercises ought himself to experience how one movement or posture of the limbs will produce a pleasant and comfortable sensation, but another a loss of strength, and so forth'.

Later, aided by his wife, Marie von Sivers (a Russian-trained actress), he evolved eurythmy. 'Eurythmy is neither dance nor mime, but a new form of art, which brings to appearance in controlled movements the sound-quality of music and speech. When the human being speaks or sings he forms with his breath the air around him. Unseen gestures and movements accompany in us each sound and note. These hidden movements are the source of the art of eurythmy. Thus it can be called "visible speech" and "visible song".'[32]

This close connection between speech and movement was the basis of 'curative eurythmy', which was based on the elements of speech, vowels and consonants. The practice of vowels and consonants, associated with movement, were thought to affect various parts of the body where dysfunction or disharmony existed, and on these were based the treatment of 'disturbances of the metabolic system and difficulties of movement and posture'. Thus Steiner produced a rationale for that therapeutic function of dance movements which many, of other persuasions, have observed.

The therapeutic function of art, craft, music and religious feeling (of a basically Christian persuasion) was also emphasised in 'curative education' and was conceptualized and systematized with a confidence founded on the acceptance of the basic philosophy. Today over a hundred 'curative homes' practice these methods.

Maladjustment, not specifically defined in Steiner's day, posed, to some extent, a special problem for those concerned with children 'in need of special soul-care'. It was inevitable, however, that many disturbed children were in curative homes and their response to the regime was observed.

Basically, Steiner considered his educational system as a blueprint for mental and spiritual health. If the instructions were carried out the child would develop as a balanced, harmonious and complete individual adjusted not necessarily to the world but to his own individuality and capable of achieving his high spiritual destiny. Although he considered that 'one cannot make amends in all the succeeding years for that which has been neglected by a guardian during the first seven years'[33] the damage is not as significant as it would be in Freudian terms, since Steiner sees the next—etheric— stage as the one of primary significance for the development of affections, habits, conscience, character, memory and temperament. It is at this point that his instructions are most specific for, in the succeeding 'astral' stage, the 'ego-conscious' adolescent is able to work individually to modify his own character and temperament. Before this he must be carefully guided. His physical environment must be carefully structured, he must identify with the right models, he must acquire a sense of harmony through art, music and movement. ('The joy of life, the love for existence, the strength to work—all these arise for the whole being out of the cultivation of the sense of beauty and art').[34] The child must, above all, be purified and ennobled by religious experiences. Steiner considered that 'the will, and along with it the character, of a person will never develop healthily if he cannot experience at this epoch in life profound religious impulses. The result of the uniform organization of the will is that the person feels himself to be an organic fragment of the whole world. If a man does not feel himself to be indissolubly connected with a Divine Spirit, then must the will and character remain unstable, discordant and unhealthy'.[35]

To Steiner, therefore, maladjustment was largely the product of faulty experience and education and was to be corrected by a rectification of these means. Basic metabolism might tend to make a child nervous and excitable or lethargic and inactive but these differences presented little difficulty in the right environment. Maladjustment is seen as a failure in the process of the growth and integration of the physical, etheric, astral and ego stages of development. Failure to move through the stages, or a lack of balance between them, produces a faulty personality.

A delinquent child, in these terms, is one who has been 'sucked too deeply into matter', and this leads to a lack of refinement in human feelings, a fascination for immorality, an impulsive irresponsible outlook. It is claimed that such a person will tend to be physically large and strong with a small head, be weak at music and mathematics, and will have agile limbs which, together with his physique and amoral outlook, will make him dangerous.

A child who is unbalanced in the direction of being too 'ego-involved' will on the other hand have too little contact with the real world and may be withdrawn, neurotic or obsessional. The extreme case will be of the autistic child who has withdrawn to the point where he has ceased to relate to the hard reality of the world at all.

Adjustment to the world therefore is adjustment to the self

through the right 'incarnation' (a balance of the inner and the outer selves) and this is what makes the widely varied physical and intellectual experiences within the school important.

The 'ego-involved' or autistic child may have to be helped to find himself in the physical world first through such exercises in orientation as walking and clapping, leading to combined words and movement so that space and rhythm become one 'thought experience'. Such a child may never achieve the complete 'incarnation', or even be able to manage what may seem to be rather stereotyped techniques of eurythmics and recitation, but some results are impressive. When I visited Peredur, the first Steiner school for the maladjusted, three autistic boys were sitting on the floor with an Indian teacher knitting and were able to communicate both with another teacher and myself by giving their names, ages and the date — which basic information they had formulated into words after having associated them with movement exercises. Two very severely autistic boys had become excellent potters and another was responsible for much of the work done in the bakery. Another, who had been taught to use the cello as a means by which he might discover himself through basic movement and rhythm, had become an excellent musician.

It is interesting to note that, contrary to the usual treatment of autistic children, a one-to-one relationship is not sought for since, for autistic as for other unbalanced children, the community is seen as an essential part of the therapeutic process. Delinquent and neurotic children, it is thought, should be put together so that they can help one another to achieve the correct balance.

Less severely disturbed children are educated largely according to the lines laid down for ordinary children although emphasis is varied to suit the particular needs of the over-physical (who must be given greater etheric experience) or the over-spiritual who must be encouraged to make greater contact with the physical world.

For the latter, in particular, there is a wealth of practical experience opportunities in a community like Peredur—which I will use as an example, although it is stressed that all Steiner schools, although sharing a common philosophy, are independent of one another and may vary considerably in emphasis.

Peredur was founded in 1951 by Mr and Mrs Siegfried Rudel. Joan Rudel had, while working at Camphill school for the mentally handicapped, attended a conference in 1948 at which the problems of what were considered to be 'the new type of child' (the product, it was thought, of urban culture) were discussed. She was subsequently offered a legacy by the parents of one of her former pupils to found the first Steiner school to deal with this problem. The principles and practice of the school are basically Steinerian although the emphasis appears to be largely directed to the needs of the neurotic rather than the delinquent child. Apart from the formal school rooms based internally and externally, in education and in architecture, on approved Steiner models, the community also controls two farms, a pottery, a bakery, a laundry, various other craft rooms and a training centre to contain three hostels for those older pupils still in need of protective care.

The farms are run on 'bio-dynamic' principles originally evolved by Steiner in 1922 and the community makes stone-ground flour for bread from its own wheat, clothes from the wool of its own sheep which is dyed with natural dyes produced on the estate. The pottery uses largely Peredur clay and it is hoped that eventually the shoe-mending shop will use Peredur-produced and tanned leather. This emphasis on direct contact with the fruits of nature is not only an important part of Steiner's own mystical sense of communion but also of Mrs Rudel's own feeling for the importance of such communion in combating what is essentially seen as an urban and materialistic malaise.

It is difficult to evaluate the effect of such methods since the true Steinerian does not admit the possibility of failure. There is an implicit belief that the system, if properly applied, will release the maximum potential in the child — however limited that potential may be.

As I have suggested it is in the completeness of the conceptualization that anthroposophic education is unique. This has one very important corollary. It is a system that can be applied by anyone who has studied it and believes in it and this means that the continuity of the school or the transfer of its practice to another institution does not depend on the presence of any individual. In theory the trained and experienced adults in the community are of equal status and the ultimate responsibility rests with them all. No one is indispensable to the working of the system.

This also makes possible what is, perhaps, the only training course for workers with maladjusted children which is based on a complete and unitary set of concepts. This is a two or three-year practical and theoretical course concerned with a study of child development and care, with particular reference to maladjustment, and with practical experience for child-care staff in eurythmy, music (lyre and recorder playing and singing), story-telling and improvized dramatic work, play therapy (including singing games and folk-dancing), painting, drawing, modelling, puppetry, handicrafts and outdoor activities.

This common training should eventually increase that strength of community and unity of aim which is, perhaps, the most important therapeutic influence at work in Steiner schools.[36]

Writing of her own difficulties in the early days of the Mulberry Bush, Dockar-Drysdale says 'the establishment of the Association of Workers for Maladjusted Children . . . brought the Mulberry Bush into contact with other schools also doing experimental work; thus my isolation ended'.[37] Indeed, the formation of the A.W.M.C. in 1951 provided the first opportunity for the pioneers to discuss their practice and principles within the framework of a national organization. It thus had important implications for the development of conceptualization and the spread of communication. It contained among its earliest officials under Dr Portia Holman—its original chairman and current president—Otto Shaw, Dr Franklin, David Wills, W. G. Sharman, Barbara Dockar-Drysdale and Father Owen. Its aims were to provide a professional body which would develop treatment and educational techniques, support experiment and promote research and also strive to produce a better understanding of the work done in special schools both in the Ministry and by the general public.

It rapidly acquired wide support from the many 'disciplines' involved in the care and treatment of disturbed and deprived children and the evidence given by some of its more influential members to the Underwood Committee appears to have had considerable effect on that body's eventual conclusions. The A.W.M.C. was, after all, the only organization which could claim to represent the views of a majority of those who had had any direct experience of the 'special' education of maladjusted children.

Its work of communication included annual study conferences, regional meetings and reports on research projects. The opportunity for people engaged in experimental work to explain their theories and techniques to a wider audience has been a particularly valuable aid to conceptualization.

The growth of the A.W.M.C. was, however, another pointer to the end of the 'pioneer era.' Although the influence and prestige of the pioneer figures remained high, what had been an individual movement was by the early 1950s becoming a national concern—which fact was officially recognized by the publication of the Underwood Report in 1955.

State Intervention

The Minister shall make regulations defining the several categories of pupils requiring special educational treatment and making provision as to the special methods appropriate for the education of pupils in each category. — *Education Act* Section 33 (i) 1944.

The 1944 Act at least made local authorites, and others, aware of the problem of maladjustment. Postwar difficulties, problems of resettlement, the return of fathers to families which had adjusted themselves to life without them and, it is often claimed, the traumatic experience of the atom bomb, led to considerable emotional and social maladjustment and, what attracted public attention more, increased delinquency. 'The difficulties experienced in billeting maladjusted children in 1939 showed the need for residential accommodation',[38] but there was little available. Some hostels, like Chaigeley, were, converted into residential schools, others remained as hostels with the children attending local schools. Some of the pioneer schools I have mentioned survived into the postwar era (e.g. Red Hill, Hill Orchard School, Summerhill) although some were under new management or with their functions changed.

The tentative State recognition of the maladjusted child in the 1945 Regulations for Handicapped Pupils (in response to the 1944 Education Act) as one who had a special educational need was of great importance, although neither the nature of the condition nor of the need was very specifically defined. The local education authorities now had powers not, as under the 1921 Act, to support individual children at a few 'special', privately run, schools but to found, finance and control special schools of their own as well as to recognize, support and inspect existing schools.[39]

Provision was also made in the 1944 Act (Section 33) for handicapped children to be placed in schools not approved as special schools. This provision, slightly amended by the Education (Miscellaneous Provisions) Act, 1953, said that: 'The arrangements made by the local education authority for the special educational treatment of

K

pupils of any such category shall, so far as is practicable, provide for the education of pupils in whose case the disability is serious in special schools appropriate for that category, but where that is impracticable, or where the disability is not serious, the arrangements may provide for the giving of such education in any school maintained by a local authority or in any school not so maintained, other than one notified by the Minister to the local education authority to be, in his opinion, unsuitable for the purpose'.

Despite continued pressure by the Ministry on local education authorities urging them to make adequate provision for the handicapped in their own special schools, about half of the children ascertained as maladjusted continued to be placed in independent boarding schools. By December 1954, 1,077 maladjusted children were being maintained by authorities in independent schools compared with 1157 in boarding 'special' schools.[40] There were in existence in England, in that year, thirty-two boarding special schools, three day special schools and forty-five approved boarding homes. Provision was very uneven throughout the country and 681 maladjusted children in England and Wales were awaiting places in special schools — the 1944 Act (Section 34) having made the ascertainment of need a statutory obligation on local education authorities.

During the period 1945–55 there had been a considerable increase in child guidance clinics from seventy-nine to about 300, more than 200 of them being provided by L.E.A.s. These, although sometimes understaffed, normally had a full team of psychiatrist, psychologist and psychiatric social worker and were therefore more able than heretofore to give support both to schools and hostels and to parents.[41]

One of the major problems of the State's assumption of control was the difficulty of inspection. There had been, since the end of the nineteenth century, inspection of special schools for the blind and the deaf, but other special school inspection had been largely in the hands of the chief medical officer. In 1931 James Lumsden, a psychologist, had been appointed as the first inspector for special schools in England but it was his fellow Scot, Mary Lindsay, another psychologist, who was mainly faced with the enormous task of the registration of special schools for the maladjusted after the 1944 Act. Before this the School Medical Service had retained a primary interest in schools for the maladjusted since State support was dependent on the provision in the 1921 Act for children suffering from nervous conditions. Mental health was regarded, with physical health, as a province of the medical services, the last vestiges of which position, with regard to educational provision was removed by the Education (Handicapped Children) Act c 52 1970. This Act, as from April 1, 1971, transfers from local health authorities and regional hospital boards all responsibility for the ascertainment, training and education of all severely mentally handicapped children of school age to the local education authority. This means, as the D.E.S. Circular 15/70 (which amplifies the proposals of the Act) points out, that 'No child within the age limits for education . . . will be outside the scope of the educational system.'

Faced with this enormous task the inspectorate, seeing its function largely as a mediating one between the experimental school and the community at large, appears sometimes to have deferred too readily to public opinion—as in the cases of Chaigeley and Bodenham Manor[42] and in refusing recognition to Red Hill School until it ceased to be coeducational. The inspectorate's prejudice against coeducation, in particular, demonstrated a lack of sympathy with pioneer principles, but in other cases, as for instance in Mary Lindsay's support of the Mulberry Bush school, it was less swayed by the pressure of public and official fear and ignorance.

Five main types of school came under varying degrees of official supervision in post-war years.

1 The independent and the 'non-maintained' special schools.*
2 The L.E.A. special boarding school.
3 The private ordinary boarding school accepting a proportion of maladjusted children.
4 The L.E.A. ordinary boarding school accepting a proportion of maladjusted children.
5 The L.E.A. day special school.

*'Non-maintained' special schools (of which there are 113 of all types) are completely voluntary and independent of any local education authority. They are normally run by charitable bodies such as the N.A.M.H., or by boards of governors who are successors to the individual pioneers who founded the schools. However, the fees of the pupils are paid by the L.E.As and the schools are fully recognised by the D.E.S., from whom they can and do receive grants towards capital expenditure.

'Independent' schools are purely private schools which receive no grant. 'Maintained' schools are schools for which the L.E.A. has full financial responsibility.

Each of these either had to adapt themselves to new post-1944 conditions or to create new systems for dealing with old problems. There was still therefore much 'pioneering' to be done even though the period of the great individual pioneers was over.

BREDINGHURST

In what officials would call 'the private sector' schools of the old-fashioned paternalistic type continued to survive and to be founded — Shotton Hall is perhaps the best example.[43] Life in them was very demanding but the idea of being a father-figure to a fairly small group of maladjusted children, particularly if they were intelligent, remained attractive.

But the day of the professionals was at hand. The first school of the new type was Bredinghurst School, founded in 1948 as part of the London County Council's comprehensive and interlocking organization for the treatment of emotionally disturbed children.[44]

Bredinghurst 'incorporated into its structure a full psychiatric team', i.e. a full-time psychiatrist, psychotherapist and psychiatric social worker and a part-time psychologist — in addition, of course, to the headmaster and teaching and house staff. Dr D. W. Winnicott said of it: 'such a school may be called pioneer',[45] and the headmaster — Wilfred Kemp — who had had considerable experience in running evacuation hostels for the L.C.C. in Hertfordshire, wrote: 'Though we were enthusiastic, full of ideas, equipped with some knowledge and experience, it was nevertheless correctly called an experimental school'. With its emphasis on individual psychiatric treatment and psychotherapy it rapidly established a reputation as a treatment centre for the most disturbed boys who needed more than 'environmental therapy', and by 1962 two other schools had been established on the same pattern. Dr Shields, the school's psychotherapist, in whose book *A Cure of Delinquents* a full account of the experiment may be read, even goes so far as to suggest that the treatment he describes 'offers society one last chance to cure the anti-social child.'[46] This appears to be a rather summary dismissal of all the work which had been done, and was being done, with maladjusted children in other types of school. Dr Shields seems to have very little time for 're-educators'. Indeed, even within the school considerable inter-staff tensions were apparent as people found difficulty in confining themselves within their role or of accepting full responsibility for it. It could, perhaps, be said that the most important aspect of Bredinghurst's 'pioneering' is not in the use of a school-based psychiatric team, but in its recognition of the importance of clearly defined roles and functions. Another way in which Bredinghurst was significant was in the stress which was placed on maintaining direct and continuous contact with families. Many of the earlier pioneer foundations had failed in this respect partly because of their geographical remoteness and sometimes as a deliberate policy of isolating the children from the source of their disturbance. This inevitably made for problems of readjustment and also increased the probability of rivalry and jealousy developing between home and school. Bredinghurst profited by its situation in the urban area from which the children came, had an 'open door' policy towards parents, and maintained continuous contact through the psychiatric social worker, who was enabled to re-adjust the home to the child. The children also were progressively adjusted not only by frequent visits home but by considerable freedom to go outside the school and to join outside clubs. Almost half the boys attended local schools.[47]

Unfortunately the work done at Bredinghurst since 1948 cannot be easily assessed as, although it was set up as an experiment, no detailed report of results has been forthcoming since 1953, when Dr H. G. Williams reported a statistically significant improvement in those children who had received psychoanalytical treatment as compared with those who had not.[48] Dr Shields estimated however that of the 216 boys who were discharged between 1948 and 1959, 181 had made a normal adjustment, twenty-seven had been admitted to approved schools or Borstal and eight were having difficulties of adjustment. This, when one considers that there was an increasing tendency to send the most severely disturbed boys to Bredinghurst, is an impressive record.

MIDHURST

Despite Dr Shield's apparent lack of regard for 're-educators' it was still true that ten years after the 1944 Act a very large proportion of 'ascertained' children and an even larger proportion of the undiagnosed maladjusted—particularly from the middle classes—

were being re-educated at schools which were not special schools but ordinary schools with a special function. Sixteen, including Wennington, Dartington Hall, Carmel College (and several other Catholic colleges), appear in a list of independent schools published by the Association of Workers for Maladjusted Children in 1960, and others, for instance many Quaker schools, were well known for this function and were used by both L.E.A.s and anxious parents.

The success of private ordinary progressive boarding schools in dealing with disturbed children inevitably attracted official attention and some L.E.A.s began thinking of the provision of such schools for the education and care of deprived and disturbed children as well as for those normal children who had other needs for boarding education. There was some precedent in Rendcomb (see Chapter 8) for the establishment of county boarding schools, and it is interesting that in this second post-war period the most important experiment in this field was being conducted by N.B.C. Lucas, who had served under J. H. Simpson at Rendcomb between 1925 and 1927.

Since 1938 (and until he retired in 1967) Lucas pioneered an 'evolutionary' model of L.E.A. day boarding school which may well be the prototype for future development. Under his guidance Midhurst Grammar School in Sussex developed from a small and insignificant rural grammar school for boys into a large comprehensive, coeducational, day / boarding school serving the secondary needs of a wide and scattered area of West Sussex. These needs included those of maladjusted children, who were provided for in two large boarding houses which also contained all the children from the area who had need of boarding-school education for reasons other than maladjustment. This system evolved from a semi-autonomous boarding house for about eighty pupils which, during and after the war, accommodated, with the 'local' boys, a high proportion of highly intelligent maladjusted boys from all over England.

The form of 'treatment' given was largely 'environmental', within the framework of a normal local day grammar school, although some of the boys received individual psychiatric treatment by the child-guidance service. The key to Midhurst's success was partly in the tolerant and accepting attitude of the school (there were few rules and, at one time, no punishments), but particularly in the individual genius of the headmaster.

Mr Lucas himself had a very disturbed childhood—'I lived in about ten homes before the age of nine'—but despite his unhappiness and missing a year's school work between the age of fifteen and sixteen during which time he worked for his grandfather, he eventually secured a scholarship to Cambridge and achieved a first-class degree.

Although he 'drifted' into teaching mainly as 'a way of getting abroad' his childhood experiences had produced in him a humanist attitude which was in many ways very inconsistent with much current educational practice. After working with J. H. Simpson and afterwards at Highgate School (1927–30) he had a three-year period when, like Homer Lane at Buffalo, he reassessed his position and beliefs. He was much influenced by Georges Sorel, 'passed rapidly through Communism' and having lived in Italy for some time had a brief flirtation with Fascism, which 'helped me to cope with the problem of authority'. He was at this point greatly attracted by Catholic theology which, he says, 'taught me the importance of myth and reason based upon it. I came to the conclusion that the "myth of the Divine Child" might give me what I wanted and was more soundly rooted than Freud—who had also influenced me'.[49]

From these varying experiences and influences Lucas evolved a dynamic theory of education which makes clear why Midhust — although apparently doing little more than providing a congenially permissive environment—has had such remarkable success in enabling highly intelligent maladjusted boys to come to terms with themselves and the world. Maturing is regarded as a process of attaining inner freedom 'through interrelation of external attitudes to situations and people and getting one's own inner responses free'. Then follows freedom to external situations.

In defining maladjustment Mr Lucas says: 'Human animals have basic desires and impulses. If circumstances are favourable they work towards enlargement, sense of freedom, easy membership of others. Unfavourable circumstances cause the same desires to protect against fear, authority, tenderness, other people and therefore causes stiffening and hardening in the self. This can lead to an unadaptability and division in the self which maladjusts'.

This basic idea explains what was essential to the Midhurst 'therapeutic environment'—it constantly changed. Nothing was allowed to stiffen or harden. Everything had to be brought 'in and out of time and order' so that children were constantly faced with new situations to which they had to adapt until they achieved an inner integrity and organization which made rules only formally necessary. Rules existed, disappeared, changed. The syllabus, the structure of classes, the games played, the extent to which the community governed itself, even, as I have mentioned, the nature of the school itself, constantly changed (change was the only constant).

A disgruntled, and not unnaturally confused, member of the staff once said: 'Luke is like a scientist constantly poking at an anthill to see what happens'; he may not fully have appreciated the motive, and it was not intended as a perceptive tribute. The scientist does not disturb the anthill out of random curiosity, nor does he do it in a random way. There is method in his apparent madness.

Since Midhurst was, in essence, dynamic it is impossible to describe its structure except at a particular point of time. It is, however, possible to view its achievement and this is impressive both in terms of its therapeutic and its academic function. Being in structure a normal comprehensive school it could offer all those academic facilities and amenities which are not possible in the typical small special school of forty to fifty boys. It had a wide-ranging and well qualified academic staff (still unfortunately not true of most special schools).

As a grammar school of about 350 boys in the late 1940s and early 1950s it was seldom out of the 'top twenty' schools, winning major awards at Oxford and Cambridge (more than fifty during 1943–66), and it would, I think, be true to say that the majority of the award winners—at least in the 1950s—were boys who had been sent to Midhurst as maladjusted. Mr Lucas says with conviction: 'The two things are linked.' In 1966, as a comprehensive school of 1030 pupils, fifty-one got at least two Advanced Level passes, more than forty went to universities and ninety-two were already there.

I have spent some time on this remarkable school because it seems to me that it has many advantages which might make it the pattern for future education of maladjusted children if supplemented by more specialist provision for the very seriously disturbed.

1 It is dynamic and not, like so many special schools, wedded to a particular and unchanging theory.
2 It is part of the environment from which most of the pupils come and they are therefore kept in contact with their homes and with reality.
3 The mixture of well-adjusted and maladjusted children is of

benefit to both. The former learn tolerance, the latter some of the virtues of conformity.

4 Schools of this type can provide more and better facilities for maladjusted children than can small special schools.

5 They are a normal part of the national educational system, and can be regarded as normal both by educational administrators and by the general public.

All that is required is a supply of men of genius and vision to run them.

DAY SCHOOLS

One of the ways in which the effect of pioneer tradition had affected provision for the education of the maladjusted can be seen in the fact that in 1954 there were still only three day-schools for the maladjusted in England. Tradition dictated a closed community and a rural environment. The first break with this tradition was with the foundation of special day 'observation classes' for children suffering from severe behaviour difficulties, originally at Church School, Rose Lane, Oxford in 1930. The architect of the scheme was A. C. Cameron, (husband of Elizabeth Bowen, the novelist), the Secretary for Education to the Oxford City Education Committee. He argued that it was important to have a centre where 'difficult but not stupid children can have intense individual attention which will either fit them to take their place again in the ordinary school or prove them to need institutional care'. This then was conceived as an experimental observational situation designed specifically for disturbed children with behaviour disorders. Degrees of disturbance were recognized, and the necessity for a variety of provision. Above all it was felt to be valuable to keep children of primary school age in close contact with their homes and with normal schools (into which the majority were readmitted).

Since there was no child-guidance clinic until 1938 selection was originally largely the responsibility of the teacher-in-charge and the school medical officers (one of whom is now Lord Hill) and an 'educational clinic' team. The teacher-in-charge was Miss Gertrude Clarke, sister of Sir Fred Clarke. Her work rapidly achieved success and the confidence of the head-teachers and other classes were established. This raised problems of co-ordination and communication and in 1939 the classes were gathered together into one school—Northern House—the top floor of the building being occupied by the child-guidance clinic. In 1946 Northern House School was recognized by the Ministry as a day special school for maladjusted children of primary age.

Since its inception, Northern House School has been characterized by the close co-operation between the child-guidance clinic and the school and between the school and local teachers and parents. Although policy has varied with changes of staff in school and clinic the aim has usually been to provide as normal an environment as possible and 'to expect "normal" behaviour from the children, knowing full well that this would not be achieved, but not being worried or shocked by deviant behaviour.' Mr H. L. A. Pearce, who succeeded Miss Clarke as head-teacher in 1950, writes: 'For most of the children attending Northern House the school itself was a therapeutic situation and I would guess that about three-quarters of them received no other form of therapy. Of the remainder, some received regular help from the Psychiatrist and some from the Psychologist whilst a sizeable minority had regular sessions with a Play Therapist. My experience was that the shy, withdrawn children were most in need of this extra treatment and seemed to benefit most from it'.

The school has recently been expanded to allow about sixty children of primary age to be admitted.[50]

Although Oxford had a special class in 1930 the first actual day-school for nervous and difficult children with learning difficulties was Haddenham Road Experimental School, established by the Leicester Education Committee in January 1932.[51] Leicester had a long tradition of making special provision for those who could not cope with normal education. In 1894 it was the first authority to make 'educational provision suited to special needs of children of undeveloped or feeble intellect', in which 'the education of eye and hand is made an instrument to lead up to a small amount of book-learning'.[52] By 1900, when such provision became compulsory, Leicester had five special centres for 106 children in which 'Kinder-garten methods' were used and in which individual care and a brighter and happier environment produced 'such good results that after a year or two the child is fit to be classed with normal children.'[53] One comment of the school board in 1900 is interesting: 'This difficult work which is still in a state of development, promises, unless unduly hampered by impossible Government routine regulations, to become a very important branch of Education.'[54] Indeed so difficult did Leicester find it to comply with 'the restrictions and requirements of the Board of Education'[55] that four of the five classes were re-integrated into the normal primary schools.

Restrictions on the placement of normal but difficult and slow-learning children in 'special' classes may well have inhibited other attempts by local authorities to deal with a problem which became increasingly apparent in a compulsory but inflexible and unimaginative education system—the problem of those who did not fit in. In 1932, with the establishment of Haddenham Road School, Leicester tried again.

The 'experimental' school was specifically for 'nervous or difficult children and for those having special scholastic disabilities *not attributable to mental deficiency.*'[56] Children more suited to open-air schools, schools for the mentally defective or backward classes in ordinary schools were specifically excluded. Thus maladjustment was defined, as it were, by default and a fairly rigorous form of 'ascertainment' or assessment became necessary.

An effort is made to study the special needs of each child, whether the problem be one of temperament, habit formation or learning. When it seems advisable, children are allowed to work by themselves for a period, developing their own interest, until they are ready to join in a group. Children who have special difficulty in such subjects as reading and number work are given individual teaching or teaching in very small groups, with teachers who specialize in the work. The garden is freely used, and the domestic classes, under the care of a full-time teacher, have proved a very constructive outlet for both boys and girls.

While children are in attendance at the School, their homes are visited with a view to ensuring the co-operation of the parents which in the majority of cases is regularly given. (1932)[57]

In order to escape the 'regulations and restrictions' which had defeated their earlier enterprise it was necessary for the Leicester authorities to classify the 'experimental' school as a normal elementary school for 150 children 'of unfulfilled promise'. Despite its size and a higher ratio of children to staff than is normal in special schools, Haddenham Road School remained true to its designation as 'experimental' and much valuable pioneering work was done in which other authorities took an increasing interest, although, largely because of the advent of war, without result. Admission to the school was on the recommendation of the educational psychologist after consultation with parents, teachers and administrative officers.

The organization of work within the school was largely on an individual work-card system supplemented by a few class lessons and much specialized remedial instruction in the basic subjects. In number work no formal lessons were given until number concepts had been built up by play with bricks. Reading, which also was tackled in the spirit of play, was based on a six-stage programme worked through at the children's own speed with work-cards. Children could, if they wished, work with and consult one another and they recorded their own achievement—which was also tested termly by standardized tests. This continuation of individual work and systematic assessment was typical of all the activities in this consciously experimental school, which was 'organized round "the child's intention to learn" not "the teacher's intention to teach him" '. Nowhere was this more true than in the school's approach to emotional and social adjustment. Haddenham Road was the first school in which there was any systematic attempt not only to achieve but to measure 'social progress'. Children with behaviour problems usually had no formal lessons until play had led to social adjustment or the satisfaction of individual need to regress. 'The harmful effect of emotional disturbance on intellectual output is recognized', the headmaster, R. A. Dewhurst, wrote, 'and this play period relieves anxieties, modifies aggression and paves the way for ordinary lessons in the classroom'. This therapeutic use of play for infants is later followed by gardening, animal care, games and craft activities for the older children.

The principle was that 'There is something every child can do well . . . and we try to find what that something is. . . . When proficiency is found the child acquires a feeling of achievement and projects this feeling towards work of which he was previously afraid. Confidence in his work dispels the child's need of gaining compensation through obtrusive and difficult behaviour, so his energy is now directed into right channels and the behaviour problem clears up'. The sort of problem child treated in this experimental school and some of the methods with which it experimented appear in the case of

W.C. aged 7½ years, I.Q. 115. Problem: Nervousness, night terrors and enuresis, restlessness and excitability. The boy was average in school subjects, but his antagonism to authority was reflected in the quality of work produced. He was allowed to work freely in the garden, where he liked to take charge of others. This was encouraged. During the winter months he had a course of sun-ray treatment at the School Clinic. After a period of two years he was able to return to his old school and one year later he passed First Class in the Scholarship examination. . . .[58]

For measuring the social progress achieved, the two eminent psychologists to the education committee, R. B. Cattel and K. M. B. Bridges, used a 'Social progress rating chart' originally devised by Bridges in the McGill University nursery school.

The majority of the children returned to ordinary schools in less than two years or went to work: a few with very poor home circumstances, were sent to residential schools.

In 1948 Haddenham Road School became Manor House School for Maladjusted Children and, as such, continues to exist.

London, which now has approximately half the day-schools and day-units in England, was slow in the field. The first tutorial class (day unit) was opened in London, Division 9, in 1950 in charge of Miss Nancy Noel. Miss Noel subsequently moved to the Lilian Baylis School—London's first day-school for the maladjusted, in 1954. Children were drawn from all over London; many had been excluded from ordinary schools, some were extremely disturbed. Members of staff left every few weeks and there was no psychiatric team in support. Miss Noel, now teacher-in-charge of an Inner London Education Authority tutorial class and speech unit, writes: 'The children were supposed to feel suicidal or have their aggressive outbursts on the days they were supposed to attend the C.G.C.—and of course, they did not'. Although the teachers learnt rapidly from their mistakes, this could hardly be accounted a satisfactory way in which to begin an important experiment.

Although the war had put such a severe check on the establishment of day schools it had vastly accelerated the growth of hostels for disturbed children. In 1954 there were forty-five approved boarding homes, only one of which appears to have existed as a hostel for maladjusted children before 1939. This was Holyrood Hostel, Dallington, which was established by the trustees of an orphanage as a home for twenty-five maladjusted girls in 1932. The Board of Education, however, recognized L.E.A. expenditure in sending maladjusted girls to Holyrood as eligible for grant. This was an important precedent. Holyrood was inevitably used for evacuees during the war and in 1951 was reopened by the Northamptonshire

Education Committee as a hostel for twenty maladjusted boys. Although the boys are educated in local schools the hostel is run as a therapeutic unit using group methods and 'shared responsibility'.

Thus by the time that the committee on maladjusted children was conducting its investigation into existing facilities for the maladjusted (1950–5) there was already in existence a comprehensive although embryonic system of State provision on which it could suggest building.

17

The Scottish Scene

By the end of this year, if there is no improvement in special education in Scotland, a maladjusted child in London will have a chance of suitable education 17 times greater than a Scottish one.... Working from the number of children in special education in London, the proportionate figure for Scotland should be 3,180; the actual number is 191. – *The Guardian*. February 23, 1966

In 1955, the year in which the Underwood Report revealed forty-three special schools dealing with 2,234 maladjusted children in England and Wales, the annual report of the Secretary of State for Scotland, *Education in Scotland, 1955*,[59] mentioned maladjusted children as a separate category for the first time and showed that thirty-four pupils were receiving special education, although no separate classes or schools for the maladjusted were mentioned in the report. The Barns Hostel School, the first to be recognized by the Scottish Education Department, had been closed shortly before for want of suitable premises.

The Education (Scotland) Act 1962 made no specific provision for the ascertainment and treatment of maladjusted children, merely repeating Sections 53–55 of the Education Act (Scotland) 1946, relating to 'children requiring special educational treatment'.

These facts seem all the more extraordinary when one considers that as early as 1952 the Advisory Council on Education in Scotland had submitted a report entitled *Pupils who are Maladjusted because of Social Handicap* and in 1964 a working party appointed by the Secretary of State on the 'Ascertainment of Maladjusted Children in Scotland' subsequently stated: 'Of the 7,000 children up to the age of sixteen years (including about 800 children under the age of five) who were examined in education authority child guidance services for problems associated with maladjustment ... more than 400 were thought to require special educational treatment by reason of maladjustment in a residential school and about 500 in a day special school'; of the 1,500 children dealt with in hospitals by the child psychiatric services 'about 200 . . . were thought to require special educational treatment in a residential school' and a further 200 required 'day' treatment. Moreover both the child-guidance service and the hospital child psychiatric service had long waiting-lists of children to be examined (600 in Glasgow alone) and, as is generally accepted, many children in need of treatment for maladjustment were not referred since, as there was so little provision for them, the referral seemed pointless. (It had been shown in England that the number of children referred increased proportionately to the number of treatment places available).

This, as the report points out, 'compares with the actual number of some 150 residential places and eighty day places for maladjusted children of all levels of intelligence and of all ages in public and grant aided special schools in Scotland'. The report continued: 'We wish to emphasise that the existing facilities for adolescents are even less adequate than for younger children and are consequently in even more urgent need of improvement'.[60]

Education in Scotland, 1965, revealed 139 maladjusted children between the ages of four and eighteen receiving residential treatment and seventy-three receiving day treatment in a total number of twenty-four classes in public and grant-aided schools, out of a total of 863,899 school children, a population which, according to the lowest level of incidence reported in the Underwood Report—5 per cent, which is also the percentage accepted by the 1952 report[61]—would be expected to contain approximately 43,195 children maladjusted in some degree.

Nor can it reasonably be argued that the level of incidence is likely to be lower in Scotland than in England. Indeed, the 1964 report had distinguished twenty 'Descriptive characteristics of the developing personalities which in the *Scottish Cultural Environment* are frequently associated with maladaptive behaviour', including slow learning, high level distractibility, forgetfulness, stubbornness, lack or loss of spontaneity and initiative in talk and action, habitual rigid control of behaviour, unusual degrees of self-assertiveness or self-effacement, and 'talks and actions habitually highly coloured by imaginative ideas', many of which, it is implied, would be less frequently associated with maladaptive behaviour in other cultural environments.

The 1952 report (Section 31) had also been concerned about those aspects of school life such as over-pressure to achieve, harsh discipline, and 'harm done by the teachers' attitude to the early symptoms of maladjustment', which tended to foster maladjustment in Scottish schoolchildren. It will be remembered that in the figures quoted earlier (Chapter 2) the largest single category of reasons for referral to what was until very recently the only grant-aided residential secondary school for maladjusted children in Scotland— Lendrick Muir—was reluctance to go to school.

In the same year that the report *The Ascertainment of Maladjusted Children* appeared (1964), the Kilbrandon Report, *Children and Young Persons, Scotland,* made the same complaint of the inadequacy of residential provision for disturbed children (whether delinquent or maladjusted—Lord Kilbrandon does not accept the distinction)[62] and, while commending the activities of voluntary agencies stated, dogmatically, that: 'the lack of provision, however, is such that the major part must clearly fall to the education authorities.'

The response of L.E.A.s to this educational charge has been unimpressive. Of the 292 children currently being educated in special residential schools for the maladjusted only sixty-nine are the direct responsibility of local authorities, the remainder being cared for by voluntary bodies with some support from the Scottish Education Department. Eighty children are in local authority day schools (2) and special classes (1).[63] The proportion of Scottish schoolchildren, therefore, who are receiving special educational treatment as maladjusted (less than 0.05 per cent) is still less than one tenth of the proportion of London children receiving similar treatment.

The reason for this state of affairs appears to be partly geographical, partly cultural and partly historical. Largely rural areas inevitably have more difficulty in organizing and financing provision than do urban areas and greater use has been made in Scotland of L.E.A. child-guidance clinics operating largely through itinerant educational psychologists than has been the case in England. Some regional hospitals also maintain small therapeutic units. In 1966 however, the Scottish Campaign for Educational Advance noted not only the inadequacy of the psychological services to cope with the problems but also the almost complete absence of special school provision in the industrial region of central Scotland which suggests that some causes lie deeper than geography.

The S.C.E.A. memorandum suggested that part of the failure to recognize the problem arose from a tendency to regard maladjusted children in school as 'wilfully naughty', an attitude which led to a low incidence of maladjustment but a high incidence of juvenile delinquency. This, combined with a narrow concept of the teacher's role as that of an academic pedagogue and stern disciplinarian, may have resulted in a much greater use of punitive approved schools rather than of any therapeutic educational establishments. The Kilbrandon Committee suggested that 'in some cases children in approved schools appear to be there either because no more suitable forms of residential training exist, or because of the lack of adequate machinery for early detection of maladjustment and handicap'.[64] The consequent Social Work (Scotland) Act, 1968, apart from some general injunctions and some confusing rather than clarifying changes in nomenclature, appears to propose little specific change in approved schools or 'residential establishments where education is provided.'

Approved schools in Scotland in many ways shared a similar history to those in England. Pioneer work was done in the mid-nineteenth century by such people as Sheriff Watson of Aberdeen, whose work impressed and influenced Mary Carpenter, and by the Rev Dr Thomas Guthrie, who founded the original ragged school for boys in Edinburgh in 1847. Dr Guthrie, whose foundations have by a process of continuous evolution developed into two existing approved schools, was, like many contemporary philanthropists, an advocate of preventive measures with deprived children. The subsequent workings of reformatory schools tended, however, to belie their origins and the 1952 report noted that 'the change from punishment to treatment is still developing and its implications have not yet been fully appreciated'.[65]

In education the parallel with England is less exact since the Scots have for long prided themselves on their high academic standards, their traditional educational structure and their puritanical attitude to 'discipline'. This has led to a reluctance to experiment and to a degree of isolation from the changing educational scene in other countries. Scottish pioneer work has either had to be conducted outside her frontiers by iconoclasts such as A. S. Neill, who have failed to smash the system from within, or by a few brave but isolated individuals whose effect on the Scottish educational system has been, at best, marginal. The latter—such as John Aitkenhead, David Wills and, more recently, R. F. Mackenzie[66]—have discovered that 'therapeutic education' is not a concept readily accepted north of the Border.

NERSTON

The difference in attitude to the problems of maladjusted children in Scotland is well illustrated in accounts of the effects of evacuation. 'The majority of the householders dealt with evacuees troubles and difficulties on their own. There was varied help available in many districts from doctors, nurses, V.A.D.s and the W.R.I., but in no case, so far as our information goes, did the evacuation area give assistance either by sending doctors, nurses or child guidance experts.

'From time to time, one gathers, the suggestion was made that difficult children and their parents should be dealt with by some form of segregation. So far as can be judged, all that this amounted to in practice was the setting aside of empty houses for dirty families. Most districts, when confronted with any serious problem, seem to have been content with evasive action. They just sent the children home.'[67]

Other than the Barns Hostel School in which David Wills struggled to establish a therapeutic environment despite the Edinburgh education authorities[68] (see Chapter 12), only one of the dozen or so residential schools established was for maladjusted children. Even this one, Nerston Residential Clinic, was not under the aegis of the education committee but of Glasgow's Child Guidance Service.

This latter fact appeared to make little difference to the tone of the establishment. Despite the fact that the children who came to Nerston in September, 1940 were the most severely psychologically disturbed group of forty out of more than 200 difficult cases, it was 'decided from the beginning that discipline would be one of the features of Nerston despite the fact that some schools of thought postulate that complete self-expression is a necessity'[69] Rules were rigid and punishment included corporal punishment, loss of privilege, a day in bed without books or toys, loss of pocket money for one week or punishment tasks while others were at play.

It was considered that 'the teachers, in the nature of their work with such children, cannot allow defiance or impertinence', although it was recognized that 'these small personalities, groping

slowly towards stability, tend to be overwhelmed if they cannot re-
taliate overtly on the adults who control their lives'. A house-mother
was available for this purpose and to give affection if necessary.
When a child arrived at Nerston he was told: 'The teachers know
all about what you have been doing and what is wrong with you, but
none of the children know anything about you. They will not be told
unless you begin stealing here (in the case of theft), when they will be
told why you are here and that they will have to watch you.[70]

Of the children who experienced this regime 90 per cent were of
primary school age and the referral symptoms most often occurring
were 'anxiety and obsessional neurosis', 'soiling and enuresis' and
'emotional retardation and infantile behaviour'. One very aggressive
child had attempted to cut another child's throat, one seven-year-old
girl had completely bitten the lapels off two of her coats, a boy of
eight had eaten his own faeces and many had experienced rejection in
a number of billets. 'All were very unhappy individuals shut in a
world of their own and the big majority were either anti-social or
asocial. One visitor to the house in the second week remarked that
the children seldom smiled and the only laughter was hysterical
laughter'.[71]

During the first few weeks the children were often violently disturbed, group hysteria broke out and there were waves of delinquency, fear, anger and exhibitionism. 'There was no corporate life
and no tradition, and it was more necessary then to resort to corporal
punishment when all else had failed'!

Routine was eventually imposed and although it 'remained a house
of crises' there were some compensations. Work by the teacher-
psychologists was on an individual basis and the house and grounds
provided considerable scope for recreation. Even some of the recreational activities may, however, be regarded as somewhat strange.
'Original plans for recreational activities had to be abandoned before
Nerston was a week old. These neurotic children could not immediately form a cohesive group. They were all individuals out of
step with everyone else. This was admirably demonstrated in
ordinary marching. It took ten minutes practice for three weeks to
teach them to march to music'![72] It is also recorded that children
who threw mud at each other were punished by having to miss the
pictures in order to clean the soiled clothes.

It says little, perhaps, for the earlier experiences of many of these
children that it is claimed that: 'Little crippled personalities come

there, hating, fearing, distrusting, their whole view of life distorted by their unhappiness. They leave again in six, twelve or eighteen months, freer and happier individuals, grown whole again by self-knowledge, self-discipline, tolerance and sympathy for human weakness.'[73] The actual figures for the first two or three years are less reassuring. Out of 116 boys and girls only half had been discharged to camp, billets or homes. Of the remainder, thirty-nine were still receiving treatment, twelve left before the treatment was completed, four failed to respond to treatment and one had been certified.

It is particularly interesting that while this avowedly disciplinarian institution was being run and staffed by psychologists, the Barns Hostel School, which served a similar purpose for the highly disturbed evacuees of the Edinburgh area and which had a staff without psychologists, operated from what appears to be completely the opposite principle, but one which, it might be thought was more psychologically based:

Mother-love and father-love provide, as it were, a permanent sheet-anchor for the emotions, without which there is danger of drift and disaster. It has been necessary to stress this because, with this factor so often inadequate in the lives of children who come to Barns, we have regarded it as our first duty to supply that lack. They must be made to feel secure, not in the relatively superficial way in which a firm discipline provides security, but with the deeper and more permanent assurance which comes from the sense of being loved. The security arising from a firm discipline tends to disappear when the discipline is no longer present; the security provided by affection, once established, is more permanent in its effect. It tends to enhance the self-assurance which a firm discipline is apt to diminish, and to encourage the initiative which a firm discipline inhibits.[74]

KILQUHANITY

Another pioneer in Scotland who put forward this view is John Aitkenhead, headmaster of Kilquhanity House. 'The school which emphasises the importance of freedom, art and self-expression, and could at a glance seem undisciplined, is in actual fact encouraging those conditions required for the development of self-discipline by the individual.'[75] Aitkenhead is a pioneer in the sense that although his practice and principles are directly and consciously derived from the work of A. S. Neill he is working in a very different educational and cultural context.

Like Summerhill, Kilquhanity is not a school for maladjusted children but it inevitably attracts some children who are considered, at least by their parents, to have problems of adjustment to normal schools. It has a positive attitude to mental health based on a belief in freedom, association with nature, and fun. If, as Aitkenhead believes, 'Education is the generation of happiness' and if the maladjusted child is the unhappy child then the situation must in this sense be therapeutic.

Like Summerhill also, Kilquhanity is a small school of thirty to forty pupils and about ten members of staff which has struggled to survive against economic, educational and social pressures. It, also, has acquired an accepted position, and although its influence on the Scottish educational system is minimal, Aitkenhead is a prophet not without honour in his own country particularly among those who are dealing directly with maladjusted children.

Kilquhanity was founded in 1940 after the publication of an advertisement in which A. S. Neill gave the venture his blessing. It was an internationalist, pacifist school dedicated to an ideal of complete free-expression. 'We were against war, against violence, against corporal punishment, against uniforms, against authoritarianism, (and very likely against authority!) In fact largely "agin the government". We were for peace, for love, for life, for nature (and nature cure), and of course for freedom—and maybe for community.'[76]

This idealistic declaration of intent has been considerably modified in the light of both individual and community needs. Although children are free not to attend lessons they are not free to leave a course once they have started it. Although all children are part of the council they are not free to disregard its decisions. Freedom is seen as something relative to the needs of others. On matters such as the prohibition of drinking or smoking, Aitkenhead is prepared to exercise his authority as headmaster.

The therapeutic basis of the school, as I have indicated, lies in a close sense of identification with nature through the school farm and the use of the surrounding countryside. Aitkenhead's almost mystical sense of the importance of nature to education and mental health is not unlike that of Steiner. Close personal relationships within the community are also immensely important and the sense of community is intensified by a common, and much encouraged, interest in the arts. In this, as in general organization, Kilquhanity differs little from the normal English pattern of a small, all-age 'progressive' private school. It could, however, claim to be very exceptional in Scotland.

A Scot who preceded Aitkenhead as an educational innovator, who also acknowledged the influence of A. S. Neill, and whose work is of more direct relevance to a study of the treatment of maladjusted children is Mrs Janet Grieve, founder and co-principal until 1963 of Lendrick Muir School.[77] Lendrick Muir is the only residential special school in Scotland which caters exclusively and completely for the educational needs of intelligent, maladjusted adolescents.

It is ironic that Mrs Grieve might never have begun the work which led ultimately to the establishment of Lendrick Muir had she not been refused employment in State schools on the grounds that she was married. She was excluded despite the fact that she had no children of her own and was already well known in progressive educational circles for her work in Regent Road School, Edinburgh, where she had, in the late 1920s pioneered many new primary school methods. A special report to the Edinburgh Education Committee said of the Regent Road experiment: 'The work done in this school marks a milestone in Scottish education.' It was a milestone on a road along which few travelled.

Being compelled, therefore, to continue her pioneer work outside the State system, Mrs Grieve founded Riverview School, Alloa, in 1931, for children between the ages of three and thirteen. The children profited by a permissive atmosphere, by progressive methods and by Mrs Grieve's insight and psychological knowledge acquired both as a student and as a lecturer in the departments of psychology and education in the University of Edinburgh. The seventy-five children and four teachers worked together to follow the process of discovery and enquiry to its limits. Children could move where they liked, speak when they wished to, choose whatever area of activity they desired. Each pupil followed his own work plan for the basic subjects which were programmed. Enquiry ranged widely over all other subjects and much was done on a basis of individual and group projects. An American spelling in a programmed reading scheme would lead to exploration of American history, geography and society. The life of people of different ages and places was 'lived out' in terms of dress, cooking, eating etc., in their manner. Each week one group would entertain the school and their parents with the fruits of their week's exploration. The basic skills were acquired as the means of discovery and since the thirst for knowledge was unquenchable so was the desire to learn. No one was allowed to feel a failure, for the staff working with the children rejoiced in their success and treated moments of failure as ways to greater understanding.

Mrs Grieve soon had many influential supporters, including Arthur Woodbury—Secretary of State for Scotland—and Professor James Drever of Edinburgh University, and in 1946 the school was transferred to Naemoor, a large house with an extensive estate, at Rumbling Bridge. It became a coeducational boarding school, although some former Riverview pupils were collected daily from Alloa and the nearby Hillfoots villages. Boys and girls were originally housed in the same large mansion house.

The aim of the school will be to develop personalities. The classes will be small and pupils will be allowed to progress at their own rate of development. Individual attention and teaching will be given to all pupils who will be encouraged to discover their own potentialities both as individuals and as members of the community.

Discipline will be developed from within the pupils, who will be quite free from adult domination. (*Alloa Journal*).

The structure of the school was much like that of Chaigeley during the same period although, of course, originally Naemoor was not for maladjusted children but for private pupils whose parents thought that Naemoor had more to offer in the education of the individual child than the alternative State schools.

Regulations for day-to-day conduct were made through a weekly 'school meeting' and a permanent school council. Emergency meetings could be called and sometimes went on for several days. Committees were elected to run the shop, bank, library, sports, etc., and these tended to proliferate in response to new needs until they included such bodies as 'the brush and mop committee' and the 'old people's committee' (for distribution of gifts at Christmas time).

After breakfast each day committees would report on their activities and there would be an 'assembly' in which problems were discussed under the direction of Mr or Mrs Grieve or the house-masters.

The programme of academic work, like the importance attached to democratic processes, owed much to Dewey, being largely in the form of elaborate projects undertaken co-operatively and often closely associated with the immediate environment of Naemoor. 'Activity methods' involved the working of the school bank (on which Naemoor School cheques could be drawn), and the school shop, research work in the library, the writing and acting of plays and, of course, the procedure of the various school meetings. One of Mrs Grieve's characteristic remarks was 'There is something wrong with a roomful of silent children'.

Not unnaturally a school with such principles and prepared to take almost any child for whom the fees could be paid soon found, as its English equivalents had done, that it was considered by many people to have a special function in dealing with maladjusted adolescents for whom, in Scotland, there was no State provision other than in approved schools. This was particularly true in conditions of post-war tension, and Naemoor soon contained many children whose education had been broken in some way or other by the war.

It was then suggested, when in the early 1950s the school was in the considerable economic difficulties experienced by most private and progressive schools at this time, that Naemoor should in fact specialize in the treatment of highly intelligent maladjusted children with the support of the Scottish Education Department. Naemoor was then re-constituted as Lendrick Muir School(1961) and it was no longer open to ordinary private pupils.

During this transitional period several changes took place which are of the utmost importance when one considers such questions as the size and structure of schools for the maladjusted, the relative place of education and therapy, the relevance of progressive educational methods to maladjusted children, and the use and feasibility of 'shared responsibility'. Much may be learnt from the breakdown of this experiment although one must not underestimate personality factors. Mrs Grieve was happier with primary-age children, Mr Grieve, perhaps, less happy with maladjusted ones—the majority of whom were from deprived backgrounds quite unlike those of the former private pupils.

The school was very large, containing as it did eighty to a hundred boys and girls (twice the size recommended by Underwood). It was committed to preparing intelligent pupils for public examinations although there was a 'B stream' for children with severe learning difficulties. The children were, on the whole, expected to behave normally both in class and in school teams, which had considerable success against other Scottish grammar (senior secondary) and public schools.

Even before the school acquired its special function the individual work scheme was abandoned for normal class teaching under pressure from the public examination system. Discipline also was much modified and the executive and judicial functions were taken from the unwieldy 'school meeting' and given to a small committee.

With increasing numbers of maladjusted children the mood and structure of the school changed considerably. The atmosphere became distinctly authoritarian; indeed a member of staff who had moved from Riverside to Lendrick Muir said of the latter: 'I have never known a school with so many rules'. Although most of the structure of self-government nominally remained, the full 'school meeting' seldom met, the school council ceased to function, and the breakfast-time assemblies degenerated either into lengthy inquisitions about alleged thefts or the formal reporting of the non-activity of semi-defunct committees. Power was concentrated in the hands of a committee of three—the headmaster, a pupil secretary and the captain of the first eleven; the bank and most necessary committee functions were taken over by members of staff, and one final attempt to hold a full 'school meeting' ended, after a two-day session, in chaos.

Mrs Grieve, who was much concerned at the disappearance of the last vestiges of a democratic structure which she had laboured so hard and with such faith to build, explained this development largely in terms of the immaturity of emotionally disturbed children, their lack of persistence and their poor grasp of reality.[78] She saw the solution in terms of a return to the close child-staff relationships of Riverview, which were more satisfying to the maladjusted child's need for emotional security. Responsibility for decision making, other than at individual or class level, was handed to the staff and those senior pupils who were considered sufficiently mature to exercise it.

It is necessary to consider, however, not only the type of child involved but also the number of children. Although some normal 'progressive' schools have worked successfully through democratic systems of representative government there is no precedent for a system of 'shared responsibility' in a school for maladjusted children of this size (eighty to a hundred). It seems doubtful if one could be organized unless the adult 'share' was proportionately enlarged or the unit broken down into significant sections. Attempts were made at Lendrick Muir to transfer some of the responsibility to smaller 'house' divisions but since all the boys, in fact, lived in one house and the girls were, by this time, lodged about a mile away in another, these were really only nominal divisions largely for the convenience of sports organizers.

A more fundamental and successful part of the re-organization which Mr and Mrs Grieve established before they retired in 1963 was a school youth club under the direction of two trained youth leaders. 'The Clubs' not only divided the children into meaningful interest groups, and gave them areas of real responsibility within those groups, but also helped to solve most successfully one of the problems which beset almost all schools for maladjusted children. It is characteristic of the majority of maladjusted children that, while they are unable to persist at any activity for very long, it is essential, both for their good and that of the school, to keep them as fully occupied as possible in out-of-school hours. In most schools for the maladjusted this usually means that either the staff are on duty almost all the time—teaching, organizing activities, and 'putting to bed'—or else the teaching staff and the house staff are completely separate in their functions—which is in many ways undesirable.

At Lendrick Muir the presence of full-time youth leaders has meant that teaching staff may also, without undue strain, perform some of the functions of house parents at bedtimes as well as giving occasional help at 'the Clubs' according to their interests and without consuming an unreasonable amount of time.

Also, with the release from tension and the feeling of responsibility which 'the Clubs' with its many sporting, camping, recreational and other activities provides, it is possible to run the school, as at present, on fairly conventional—if tolerant and permissive—lines. It appears to cope very well with children who are 'socially maladjusted' rather than severely emotionally disturbed; children who are out of sympathy with their backgrounds, who have failed at school in large, over-disciplined classes and who can profit by a sympathetic and tolerant environment and occasionally a certain minimum of psychotherapy.[79] Much what the normal, English 'progressive' school of much the same size offers.

The chief disadvantage in Scotland is that there are scarcely any places for those adolescents who need more than this other than too few hospital units and too many untherapeutically orientated approved schools. This is particularly true for children of below the highest intelligence (Lendrick Muir does not normally take children with I.Q.s much below 120) and for children of secondary age.

Until the foundation of Lendrick Muir there was, in fact, no provision for any of the children leaving those few primary special schools which existed in the 1950s — such as Harmeny House, which was founded by the Save the Children Fund (and the first headmaster of which was Sidney Hill, who had worked both with Dr Fitch, and at Chaigeley), or Craigerne, established in 1957 by the Dr Barnardo's Society. This is still essentially true for those boys who do not meet Lendrick Muir's exacting educational requirements, since there are, as yet, only thirty to forty children of secondary age and of average or below-average ability in special schools for the maladjusted in the whole of Scotland.

It would be unrealistic, however, to think that increasing the number of places would solve the problem. The problem will only be solved if, as Dr Wolff has suggested,[80] there was a complete revolution in the teacher's concept of his role. Before Scotland can staff new schools it must have enough teachers who regard therapy as of at least equal importance to academic education. These are not at the moment forthcoming and a high proportion of teachers in existing special schools are English (including the present headmasters of Lendrick Muir, Harmeny House and Craigerne). The majority of the staff in what few Scottish schools there are have no specific training in dealing with maladjusted children. Nor, unlike their similarly unequipped English counterparts, have they much opportunity of acquiring any appropriate training in Scotland. There is no Scottish equivalent of diploma courses in the education of maladjusted children run by several English and Welsh universities, although 'maladjustment' does appear as one of the types of 'handicap' considered in a four-month theoretical six-month practical course at Moray House which leads to an endorsement of a teacher's certificate.

Perhaps the new concept of 'Social Education' introduced by the Kilbrandon Report and implemented, to some extent, in the Social

Work (Scotland) Act, 1968, will make people more conscious of the problem and more prepared to tackle it in a fundamental way. Scotland is still largely virgin territory for pioneers in therapeutic education.

REFERENCES

CHAPTER 15: Some Theories of Therapeutic Education

1   BARRON, A. T. What is Therapy—what is Training? in *Therapeutic Education. p* 35. Autumn 1969.
2   Some of the following material based on an interview with Dr Marjorie Franklin, 1969.
3   FRANKLIN, M. E. in *Studies in Environmental Therapy*, I *pp* 27-30. 1968.
4   TIMES EDUCATIONAL SUPPLEMENT. Correspondent, Arlesford Place Hostel School: Care and Cure of Maladjusted Youth. *p* 206. 16 March 1951.
5   Ibid.
6   FRANKLIN, M. E. Discussion Groups. *The AWMC Newsletter, p* 7. March 1968.
7   BARRON, A. T. The Inter-action of Psychotherapy and Environmental Therapy. (Unpublished—provisional title).
8   SUTTIE, I. D. *The Origins of Love and Hate.* Kegan Paul, Trench, Trubner, London, 1935.
9   WILLS, W. D. Eliminating Punishment in the Residential Treatment of Troublesome Boys and Young Men. *Studies in Environmental Therapy*, I. 1968.
10 —— Shared Responsibility, in *Problems of Child Development.* New Education Fellowship, London, 1948. *See also Evacuation in Scotland.* S.C.R.E. publication XXII. *p* 199. V.L.P. 1944.
11 NEILL, A. S. *The Free Child.* Herbert Jenkins, London, 1953.
12 FREUD, A. *The Psychoanalytical Treatment of Children.* Imago, London, 1946.
13 —— *Introduction to Psychoanalysis for Teachers, p* 93. Allen & Unwin, London, 1931.
14 Ibid., *p* 104.
15 FREUD, A. *The Ego Mechanisms of Defence.* Hogarth, London, 1936.
16 BURLINGHAM, D. and FREUD, A. *Young Children in Wartime, pp* 11-12. Allen & Unwin (for the *New Era*), London, 1942.
17 BOWLBY, J. *Maternal Care and Mental Health.* World Health Organization, Geneva. 1951.
18 BURLINGHAM, D. and FREUD, A. op. cit., *pp* 74-5.

REFERENCES

319

19 DOCKAR-DRYSDALE, B. based on interview and on her collected papers in *Therapy and Child Care*. Longmans, Green, London, 1968.

20 —— The provision of Primary Experience in a Therapeutic School. *J. of Cl. Psychology and Psychiatry* 7. *pp* 263-275. 1966: in *Therapy in Child Care* (above) *pp* 97-115.

21 DOCKAR-DRYSDALE, B. Residential Treatment of Frozen Children. in *Therapy in Child Care*, op. cit., *p* 18.

22 Ibid., *pp* 26-7.

23 DOCKAR-DRYSDALE, B. Role and Function in *Therapy and Child Care*, op. cit., *pp* 52–66.

24 BALBERNIE, R. *Residential Work with Children*. Pergamon, Oxford, 1966.

25 STEINER, R. *The Education of Children. p* 84. Theosophical Publishing Co., London, 1911.

26 Ibid.

27 Ibid. *pp* 50-51.

28 Ibid. *p* 58.

29 Ibid. *p* 68.

30 STEWART, W. A. C. *The Educational Innovators, p* 165. Macmillan, London, 1969.

31 STEINER, R. op. cit., *p* 80. CARLGREN, F. *Rudolf Steiner* Rudolf Steiner Pub. Co., Switzerland, 1964.

32 Ibid. *pp* 27-8.

33 STEINER, R. op. cit., *p* 41.

34 Ibid. *p* 75.

35 Ibid. *pp* 73-4.

36 See also STEINER, R. *Discussions with Teachers*, 1919; *The Story of My Life*, 1928; *Education and Modern Spiritual Life*, 1919; *The Kingdom of Childhood*, 1964. EDMUNDS, L. F. *Rudolf Steiner Education*, 1962. HARWOOD, A. C. *The Recovery of Man in Childhood*, 1958; *The Way of a Child*, 1940. SHEPHERD, A. P. *A Scientist of the Invisible*, 1954. HART, R. *The Inviolable Hills*. All published by the Rudolf Steiner Press, Switzerland.

37 DOCKAR-DRYSDALE, B. op. cit., *p* xiv.

CHAPTER 16: State Intervention

38 PRITCHARD, D. G. *Education and the Handicapped 1760–1960, p* 213. Routledge & Kegan Paul, London, 1963.

39 MINISTRY OF EDUCATION. *Handicapped Pupils and School Health Service Regulations*. H.M.S.O., London, 1945.

40 MINISTRY OF EDUCATION. *Report of the Committee on Maladjusted Children* (the Underwood Report) Section 50. H.M.S.O., London, 1955.

41 MINISTRY OF EDUCATION. *Education of the Handicapped Pupil, 1945–1955*. Pamphlet No. 30. *p* 15. H.M.S.O., London, 1956.

42 WILLS, W. D. *Throw Away Thy Rod*. Gollancz, London, 1960.

43 LENNHOFF, F. G. *Exceptional Children*. Allen & Unwin, London, 1960.

44 SHIELDS, R. W. *A Cure of Delinquents*. Heinemann, London, 1962.

45 Ibid. *p* 9.

46 Ibid. *p* 180.

47 KEMP, W. F., in *The Maladjusted Child—the Underwood Report and After, pp* 51-55. N.A.M.H. 1957.

48 SHIELDS, R. W. op. cit., *p* 152-3.

49 PERSONAL COMMUNICATION.

50 Information *re* Northern House, from personal communication with H. L. A. PEARCE AND J. GARNE. Chief Education Officer, City of Oxford.

51 GARNE, J. Article on Northern House School, in *Education*. **110.** (2850) 1957.

52 LEICESTER SCHOOL BOARD. *Eighth Triennial Report*, 1894.

53 ———— *Tenth Triennial Report*, 1900.

54 ———— *Eleventh Triennial Report*, 1903.

55 ELEMENTARY EDUCATION (Defective and Epileptic Children) Act, 1899.

56 CITY OF LEICESTER EDUCATION COMMITTEE. Annual Report, 1932.

57 Ibid.

58 CITY OF LEICESTER EDUCATION COMMITTEE. *The Education of Retarded and Difficult Children in the Leicester Schools*. Pamphlet *c* 1937.

CHAPTER 17: The Scottish Scene

59 SCOTTISH EDUCATION DEPARTMENT. *Education in Scotland* **1955,** H.M.S.O., Edinburgh, 1956.

60 ———— *Ascertainment of Maladjusted Children*, Sections 114-116. H.M.S.O., Edinburgh, 1964.

61 ———— *Pupils who are Maladjusted because of Social Handicap*. Section 38. H.M.S.O. Edinburgh, 1952.

62 SCOTTISH HOME and HEALTH DEPARTMENT. *Children and Young Persons, Scotland*. (The Kilbrandon Report) H.M.S.O., Edinburgh, Sections 187-9. 1964.

63 Figures provided by the Scottish Education Department, January 1970.

64 KILBRANDON REPORT. Section 179.

65 REPORT (Ref. 61) Section 181.

66 MACKENZIE, R. F. *A Question of Living*. Collins, London, 1963.

67 BOYD, W. (ed.) *Evacuation in Scotland*. Scottish Council for Research in Education. publication **XXII,** *p* 66. V.L.P. 1944.

68 WILLS, W. D. *The Barns Experiment.* Allen & Unwin, London, 1945.
69 BOYD, W. (ed.) op. cit., *p* 173.
70 Ibid. *p* 187.
71 Ibid. *p* 174.
72 Ibid. *p* 179.
73 Ibid. *p* 189.
74 Ibid. *p* 196.
75 AITKENHEAD, J. in *The Independent Progressive School,* H.A.T. Child (ed.) *p* 82. Hutchinson, London, 1962.
76 Ibid. *pp* 76-77.
77 GRIEVE, J. Some Experiences in Shared Responsibility with Normal and with Maladjusted Adolescents, in *Studies in Environmental Therapy* I, *pp* 83-91. The Planned Environmental Therapy Trust, 1968. (Based also on personal communication, conversations with colleagues and personal knowledge of Lendrick Muir School.)
78 Ibid. *p* 89.
79 MCNAIR, H. S. *A Survey of Children in Residential Schools for the Maladjusted in Scotland* (Moray House Publications). Oliver and Boyd. Edinburgh, 1968.
80 WOLFF, S. Two Recent Scottish Government Reports. *A.W.M.C. Newsletter* No. 4. *pp* 18-25. 1964.

PART EIGHT

Assessment and Evaluation

18

Assessment : Quantitative

He began by assaulting what he termed 'The Bible of Maladjustment', namely the 1955 Underwood Report on Maladjustment—Report of speech given by Mr J. E. Varley to the Association of Workers for Maladjusted Children (Midlands Branch), October 1966.

The Report of the Committee on Maladjusted Children, 1955, was, and remains, the most comprehensive consideration of the problems of the education of the maladjusted. In particular, the Underwood Report on this most neglected category of the handicapped revealed the immensity of the problem and the inadequacy of the provision. While acknowledging the work of independent pioneers[1] in the 1920s and the contribution of wartime hostels[2] it pointed out that not only was there no agreement about the definition of the term maladjusted, or the incidence of this condition among children, but also that by December, 1954, there were 681 children awaiting places in the thirty-two boarding special schools and three day schools available (the average size of which was about thirty pupils.) There were also more than a thousand children in independent schools, many of which were not recognized as efficient (even as ordinary schools) by the Ministry.

Nevertheless, the Underwood Committee considered that 'hostels and boarding schools should continue to be the main forms of residential provision for maladjusted children', and that they did so, and that even thirty-two boarding special schools should be available to maladjusted children, is a tribute to the small band of pre-1944 pioneers of 'therapeutic education', many of whose pioneer schools still existed and whose basic ideas were now generally acceptable—although often much modified. 'The broad lines on which existing hostels and special schools are run seem to us sound; we have, however, made a number of minor recommendations about their organization and functioning'.[3]

In recommending an increase in day-school provision, the

325

Underwood Committee had little pioneer evidence on which to base its suggestions. It was, however, sufficiently impressed by the examples of Oxford and Leicester and by the day special units in London to urge the advantages of keeping children in contact with their homes. The relative cheapness of day provision may also be an important factor which has influenced local authorities to make increasing provision of this type. The percentage increase of day schools maintained by local education authorities between 1955 and 1969 (three to thirty) has 'been ten times that of boarding schools both maintained and non-maintained (thirty-two to sixty-three). The number of L.E.A. hostels (thirty-seven) has remained constant while the numbers of day units and special classes of various sorts has increased so rapidly that no reliable figures are available. In 1965, 107 such classes existed[4] and in January, 1968, 1,692 children were in special classes and units associated with ordinary schools.[5] This would appear to represent an increase of over 50 per cent in those years.

Other recommendations of the Underwood Committee, based largely on pioneer precedent, have had varying effect. Although it was suggested that there was 'no *a priori* reason why, under favourable conditions, other schools should not have boys and girls over the age of eleven' and the committee considered that 'it is hard to see how maladjusted children can be prepared for life in the world and a healthy attitude to sex be developed if in adolescence they have no chance to mix with the other sex under good conditions',[6] L.E.A.s have yet to implement this suggestion. Of the sixty-three boarding schools wholly or partly supported by L.E.A.s only three — one with only six boarders and two for mixed handicaps — are coeducational at secondary level. Over half (thirty-two) are for senior boys only, seven are mixed junior schools and four have the peculiar structure, suggested in Section 298 of the Underwood Report, of junior boys and senior girls. In contrast, twenty-one of the thirty day schools are all-age mixed, although one would have thought that with children in daily contact with their homes the need for coeducation would have been less. Since eight of the thirty-seven hostels are also mixed at senior level one can only suppose that L.E.A.s doubt the capacity of teachers in boarding special schools to cope with any problems which may arise, although they appear to have more confidence in parents (however disturbed they may be) or in hostel wardens.

The committee's recommendations with regard to the size of special schools also reflected the practice established by small, patriarchal, pioneer establishments. A limit of between twenty and fifty pupils was suggested for both day and boarding establishments. Although fifty-three of the existing boarding schools in England and Wales fall within these limits they do, in fact, range between sixteen and 130 pupils and four day schools exceed the upper limit, the largest being 150).[7]

Although acknowledging the historical importance of independent schools the Underwood Committee suggested that 'the use of independent boarding schools should, in our opinion, be more strictly controlled and also reduced'. However, despite persistent attempts by the Ministry to implement this recommendation and frequent directives to L.E.A.s and the development of alternative L.E.A. provision, the independent boarding school—both special and ordinary—still plays an important part. Although according to Ministry figures in 1964 there were only sixteen non-maintained schools officially approved and financially supported for 'special education and treatment of maladjusted children' the A.W.M.C. list of schools which were then available for such treatment included seventy-two independent schools and hostels accepting maladjusted children. Of these, twenty-three had no psychiatric or psychological assistance and the majority of the rest depended on occasional visits from referring psychologists or contact with local child guidance clinics. Some claimed to be no more than 'orthodox boarding school; sympathetic handling', and many others specifically excluded the type of child most likely to be in need of boarding-school education, e.g. enuretics, truants, aggressives and 'those needing special care'. One school indeed claimed to have fifty maladjusted boys and girls between the ages of six and sixteen although refusing to accept those given to 'lying and stealing'.

With the continuing pressure for places for maladjusted children and the enormous difficulty of adequate inspection the present position is far from clear. In January 1968, however, the number of children placed, as maladjusted, in independent schools (2,592) was more than half the number in maintained and non-maintained special schools either day or boarding (4,315) and more than a quarter of those receiving any form of 'special educational treatment' (9,313).[8] Indeed, far from decreasing, the number of children sent by L.E.A.s to independent special schools increased from 2,125 in 1965 to 2,137 in 1967,[9] and during the same period the number in non-maintained schools increased from 904 to 919.* How many maladjusted children, not sent by L.E.A.s, there are in ordinary private schools, and what sort of education and therapy they are receiving, is not, of course, revealed by official statistics. One sometimes wonders, however, if in assessing the achievements of the pioneers one should not set against them the unintentional dissemination of the idea that anyone of good will can set up a school which will be of benefit to maladjusted children as long as they have a nice house available in a congenial part of the country. Such establishments may have been in Dr Oakeshott's mind when she wrote: 'For it [the school] to be merely a place where children are contained and not specifically treated is a travesty of special educational provision and a crime against the child and the community.'[10]

This stricture does not apply only to independent schools, many of which continue to have an important function in treating maladjusted children and in continuing experiment. Indeed the Ministry of Education in Circular 4/61, while in general disapproving of L.E.A.s who sent maladjusted children to schools which had not received official recognition, said: 'There will also be the continuing need for experiment in the educational provision for handicapped pupils, with the resulting possibility that an authority may wish to send a child to a new school before it has been recognised as efficient.' Thus even the Ministry acknowledged the value of that pioneer spirit without which even the present inadequate provision for maladjusted children would not exist.

It would, indeed, be easy to overlook the inadequacy of this provision by considering sum-total statistics. More than half of the day schools and units in Britain are, in fact, in London, as are more than 10 per cent of the boarding schools. The majority of small county boroughs with fewer than 40,000 school-age children have no special schools, either day or boarding, for maladjusted children and Weaver cites fourteen English counties which in 1966 lacked any such provision. Weaver's very thorough analysis of regional provisions[11] of any type for maladjusted children revealed variations ranging from 3.4 per 10,000 school children in the northern

*See footnote on page 291 for definitions of 'independent', 'maintained' and 'non-maintained'.

counties (Westmorland, Cumberland and Durham) compared with 28.3 per 10,000 in the London metropolitan area. The areas south of a line from Gloucester to the Wash all exceeded the provision of the most active area north of this line. In fact, provision in the southern area was almost exactly twice that in the combined northern area: i.e. 5,298 out of 3,100,000 compared with 2,235 out of 3,600,000. Moreover, the tendency since 1960 has been for the southern area to increase its provision twice as fast as the northern area and independent and non-maintained schools in the two regions have shown a similar tendency. Only in one respect, the provision in hospital schools and units, has this trend been reversed and one may speculate that this may be, to some extent, a byproduct of the absence of provision for mildly disturbed children. It would appear also that during the last five years the emphasis in the North has been on the provision of more boarding-school and child-guidance facilities on the traditional pre-Underwood pattern, while in the South there has been greater emphasis on experiment with day special schools and classes.

It is possible, therefore, that the legislation most likely to be of benefit to maladjusted children is not that directed specifically to their needs but the impending reorganization of local government into larger, more viable and, one hopes, more active units. It seems probable that London's achievement in this field is not so much a product of greater need, or of the stimulus which the presence of many eminent and concerned individuals provides, but of the size of the organization which allows for greater flexibility, experiment, integration and co-operation than is possible elsewhere.

Even in London, however, provision would have to be at least ten times greater than it is before all the maladjusted children within her bounds would be receiving the special educational and therapeutic help urged by the Underwood Report and reinforced by almost every other report directly or indirectly concerned with maladjusted children.[12] Dramatic increases in provision appear to make little difference to the numbers of children awaiting placement. In 1965 1,199 children ascertained as maladjusted were on the waiting list. In 1967, despite an addition of 1,494 places, the waiting list had, in fact, increased to 1,209. This phenomenon, that the number of maladjusted children appears to increase proportionally to the number of places, is hardly surprising. If, as is generally agreed, approximately 5 per cent. of schoolchildren require some attention as maladjusted, present special educational provision is available for only one maladjusted child in fifty.

A few pioneers may have pointed the way but we have, as yet, scarcely undertaken the journey.

19

Assessment : Qualitative

Professionals as well as laymen tend to offer services to the needy regardless of the known value of the services rendered. . . . On the basis of inching along, year by year, trying new methods and techniques, knowledge is built up which is both reliable and serviceable. Yet one limitation of previous methods of treating emotionally disturbed children has been the continuing absence of reasonable evidence that the methods used have been profitable ones.[13]

How far pioneer work is perpetuated by generalization depends not only on the conceptualization of the work but on how valid the concept is. Fortunately some of the pioneers have written books about their methods or have had books written about them, but these have tended to be either frankly propagandist, e.g. *Throw Away Thy Rod*,[14] or discursive and anecdotal, e.g. *Exceptional Children*.[15] Both types are singularly lacking in reliable evidence of achievement. Nor has anyone yet put forward an acceptable concept of what such evidence could consist.

The D.E.S. pamphlet No. 47 *The Education of Maladjusted Children* (1965)[16] devotes a chapter to 'The choice of the School for the Child and of the Child for the School', but apart from some general considerations about residential placement and educational provision it offers little guidance other than that 'each school should have some policy about the type and degree of disturbance they are best suited to deal with' and suggests that the headmaster will know what this is. Even if this were true, the placement of maladjusted children in schools is never the responsibility of the headmasters, and child guidance clinics are unlikely to have sufficient evidence about the relationship of provision to cure to be very specific. Indeed, as Pamphlet No. 47 suggests, placement may sometimes 'be left in the hands of an administrator who does not happen to know the schools'. Research has shown that both the procedure for assessment and the criteria for ascertainment and placement differ widely from area to area and depend largely on existing facilities. Of 108 authorities investigated by Weaver[17] only in twenty-three was ascertainment based on 'team' assessment and in thirty-three the psychiatrist alone was responsible. Even more surprising, in view of the essentially educational nature of provision, was that in eighteen authorities the school medical officer was considered the relevant person and in thirty-four others the psychiatrist, educational psychologist or school medical officer acted separately. If, as Pamphlet No. 47 suggests, schools were able to specify educational and treatment policies it would appear to follow that the value of ascertainment would depend on the appropriateness of placement, and vice versa. However, although in some cases the ascertaining authority, usually through the C.G.C., carefully matches child and school, in some areas children (particularly if requiring residential placement) are 'put on a general waiting list for a vacancy in any special school'.

There is, moreover, little agreement on the criteria for placement. Authorities disagree widely, for instance, on the appropriateness of residential placement for 'brain-damaged' children and for children suffering from stress caused by the psychosis of a parent. Many of the reasons for such placement are negative in that they are either the result of inadequate day provision or the operation of the principle that 'the more the child offends the community the more likely it is that residential care will be needed'.

This apparent confusion, and the haphazard nature of present provision, is largely the result of uncritical acceptance of the value of pioneer work with maladjusted children, and the absence of serious research evidence on the relationship between the needs of maladjusted children and the provision made in educational and treatment agencies. Because of the inherent difficulties of research into the working of any dynamic institution, with its multiplicity of constantly changing variables, greater attention has been paid to the more manageable problems of the symptoms and causes of maladjustment. This is not entirely irrelevant in that the usefulness of any agency must be seen in relation to the nature of the task. However, as F. J. Schonell points out in reviewing research into maladjustment before 1952, the definition of causes and symptoms is made difficult by the 'psychological relativity' of the condition. And scientific method would depend not only on some clearly established connection between cause and effect but also on some accurate measure of normality.

Most such studies which have been undertaken tend either to be categorizations seen in terms of the individual's own discipline[18] or have been based on arguing backwards from the symptoms actually exhibited by children who have already been ascertained or placed in special schools.[19] There is no shortage of such lists of symptoms and causes, which vary in their scope and emphasis, but they are of doubtful value since they differ widely according to the different disciplines from which they derive and the different purposes for which they are being used. The most comprehensive is probably that given by Jenkins and Glickman in 1946[20] based on 5,000 child guidance cases, but very few studies relate the symptoms observed in the clinical situation to the educational needs of the child. An exception is Cruickshank and Johnson's[21] classification of maladjusted children in terms of appropriate treatment agencies: (i) those requiring treatment in normal schools, (ii) those requiring school-centred guidance services, (iii) those requiring treatment services, and (iv) those needing residential facilities.[22]

One of the most significant findings in research related to causal factors is that of Burt and Howard[23] who in 1952 discovered, after a study involving 631 children, that 'in many cases the main, if not the sole, cause of maladjustment arises out of current conditions in the child's school', conditions such as inappropriateness of school or class, uncongeniality of teachers or fellow pupils, or absence from, or changes in, school. This would suggest that a concentration of interest and research on alternative provision may be misplaced and we ought to be looking at what changes are desirable in ordinary schools in order to prevent maladjustment rather than at appropriate provision in special schools for those children who have failed to withstand the stress of life in ordinary schools.

As far as the purposes of this study are concerned one can only make any critical assessment of the work of the pioneers largely from analogy with existing schools which embody their principles. Research into the nature of such provision and the principles and organisation of such schools has been sparse. Kellmer Pringle's study of the *Differences between Schools for the Maladjusted and Ordinary Boarding Schools*[24] revealed, in fact, surprisingly little difference betwen the two categories either in organization, in the range of symptoms of maladjustment exhibited or in the training and general attitudes of the staff, although staff ratios were usually more favourable in maladjusted schools, which tended also to be much smaller units. Educational provision was similar in nature and structure although there was more remedial work done in the special schools since a much higher proportion of the children referred to them was educationally retarded. Methods of discipline, whether therapeutic or retributive, were very similar, the most surprising difference being that while only 8 per cent of the ordinary schools used corporal punishment, 25 per cent of the special schools did so. Although maladjusted children in special schools exhibited much the same symptoms as those in ordinary schools these tended to be more severe in the former and, of course, affected a greater proportion of the school population. It is not surprising, therefore, that special schools put a greater emphasis on therapy and were much more likely to have the services of both a psychiatrist and a regular psychotherapist.

Since it is generally assumed that existing independent or non-maintained special schools embody pioneer principles more so than L.E.A. special schools, and since what little work has been done in research on the effectiveness of different forms of provision has been done in L.E.A. schools, Weaver's work is of particular relevance if one is to attempt any assessment of the effectiveness of pioneer schools by analogy.[25] Weaver examined Jones's assertion that there was a distinction between voluntary and L.E.A. schools.[26] The former, Jones considered, were characterized by 'the twin principles of affection and a permissive institutional environment' the latter by a training approach by which habits of obedience, order, regularity, cleanliness, etc. were instilled in a largely impersonal way within a highly structured regime. Weaver, after an intensive investigation of 95 schools and hostels, including some pioneer establishments rejected this hypothesis and found that 'local authority establishments, contrary to Howard Jones' contention, were not less therapeutically orientated than the voluntary ones'. Indeed local authority schools, in having greater access to clinical assistance, often had better provision for psychotherapeutic work. Such differences as appeared were largely in the realm of school work in which local authority schools laid greater emphasis on remedial work based on psychological assessment and were more flexible in timetabling and individual choice of work. Voluntary establishments also, perhaps partly because they lacked psychiatric and psychological assistance, laid greater stress on the therapeutic function of systems of 'shared responsibility'. Neither type of establishment was punitive in its attitude to discipline and punishment, although the voluntary establishments made significantly greater use of 'consequential' sanctions (e.g. fining and referral to the school meeting).

The few research studies that have been undertaken to assess the efficiency of therapeutic educational methods in special schools have, therefore, some relevance to assessing the work of pioneer establishments whether these studies were undertaken in L.E.A. schools or not.

The first such investigation, reported by Petrie in 1962,[27] was based on a sample of only twenty-three children in a residential special school of traditional form, the main treatment consisting of 'environmental therapy'. The study covered a period of eighteen months and standard tests were used to measure progress in I.Q., academic attainment, social adjustment, personality adjustment and modification in the children's attitudes to their families. Social workers, meanwhile, assessed any changes in the children's home circumstances. During the eighteen months there was significant progress in all areas, although it was noticeable that the rate of progress declined during the second half of the period, and that changes in attitudes and feelings (as assessed by projective tests) changed less than did overt behaviour. Intelligent children appeared to respond better than did the less intelligent and there was greater improvement among those children whose home conditions improved during the trial period than among those children for whom this was not the case.

Roe's more extensive study (1965)[28] of 142 children in boarding schools, day schools and tutorial classes organized by the Inner London Education Authority covered a period of twenty-one months and measured educational, behavioural and relationship changes and symptom reduction by means of teachers' assessments and ratings, attainment tests, clinical interviews, projective tests, questionnaires and psychomotor and perceptual tests. The results of the survey showed substantial gains by an overall majority of the pupils but there were significant differences between those receiving different educational experiences. Day-school children not only showed less marked improvement in most areas but on measures related to behaviour and attitude actually increased the number of maladjustment pointers. This does not, however, prove the superiority of the residential treatment derived from traditional models, since not only was there also more marked improvement in children in tutorial classes but Roe's research indicates clearly that the children placed in day schools were measurably more extremely disturbed than were the others.

A more intensive study of the effects of day special school provision has recently been completed by Critchley[29] over a two-year period, using as a control group boys of average or near-average intelligence suffering from extreme learning difficulties but not having been ascertained as maladjusted. The aims and methods of investigation were similar to those used by Roe although the experimental group was drawn from a single day school. There were thirty-two boys in each group. Critchley's results in his experimental group revealed an overall failure to make progress in academic attainment and although there was some general improvement in social adjustment almost a third of the sample (10:32) showed little or no improvement over the two-year period. This is perhaps the most significant result since it suggests that such children, characterized by extreme hostility to adults, are not well placed in day schools and may benefit from that chance of establishing more secure adult relationships which residential schools may provide.

None of these studies gives conclusive evidence of the usefulness of any form of special school provision since even where a control group existed it was not drawn from the same sample, and it is impossible to say if similar progress might not have been achieved by the experimental groups if they had been subjected to other forms of treatment or, indeed, had had no special treatment at all. Moreover, since the form of treatment offered has never been scientifically analysed and varies from school to school, changing even during the course of research, it tells us little about those factors which are important in producing change. Studies in the organizational structure of special schools,[30] where they exist, tend only to confirm that there is little common ground and, as has been pointed out of residential special schools, 'a large number of children are sent to these schools not primarily for any benefit that they may receive therefrom, but in order to remove them from an unsatisfactory environment. The great English public schools have handled maladjusted children, in the upper classes, along with ordinary members of the schools and we have no evidence to show that their methods of selection and treatment are better or worse than those of boarding special schools'.[31] Lunzer[32] also observes the apparent spontaneous remission of symptoms of maladjusted children in ordinary schools and Levitt,[33] Powers and Witmer[34] and Eysenck[35] all demonstrate similar phenomena in disturbed individuals untreated by any therapeutic methods.[36]

One is, therefore, thrown back on largely subjective assessment, on the results recorded by such pioneers as Shaw (see Chapter 11), and on the pioneers' own descriptions of their methods. The pioneers' own evaluation of their success varies both in objectivity and scope. Shaw's systematic analysis of his results based on clearly established criteria is unusual and represents one end of a continuum, with at the other end the Steiner schools which, for largely metaphysical reasons, do not admit to failure. Even when figures for results are given they are almost impossible to evaluate or equate since no exact comparison of the original samples is possible, methods of obtaining results vary widely, and no two sets of criteria for 'adjustment' are the same. One cannot equate Shaw's meticulous accumulation of data with the incomplete figures and largely subjective assessments of the 'results' of the Hawkspur Camp experiment any more than one can compare Shaw's highly intelligent neurotic adolescents with the Hawkspur team's much older delinquents.

One could generalize that where results are stated in any form, whether specific or not, it is usual to claim a success rate in the region of 70 per cent to 80 per cent but, as has been pointed out, this may differ little from the figures given by Eysenck[37] and others for the spontaneous remission of neurotic symptoms. The argument is not a good one in that not only is it impossible to compare the neurotic states of the children in each group but it is likely that the children who responded to treatment and non-treatment differed within the groups although representing the same percentage. Clearly what is required is a more detailed knowledge of those specific conditions which do, or do not, respond to particular forms of treatment.

COMMON PRINCIPLES

In specifying the essentials of their various forms of treatment the pioneers have frequently been scarcely more explicit than in reporting their results. Such conceptualizations as exist, as has been pointed out, are frequently couched in very general terms, and although they have certain common ground there are wide differences and some apparent inconsistencies.[38] Almost all pioneers adopted a pragmatic approach. 'They were not helped or hindered by custom or tradition because they were outside all existing systems and had no traditions. They approached their task, as it were, from first principles saying, in effect, 'This is the problem, how shall we tackle it?'[39] The 'first principles' consisted, on the whole, of a belief in therapy rather than punishment or constraint and in love as the necessary prophylactic and panacea.

I know of none who would not consider unconditional love and acceptance of the child (although not always of his actions) as of primary importance. This is not always easy since being loved and being loveable are, to some extent, cause and effect and many children who attend schools for the maladjusted are not naturally either. Marjorie Franklin, talking of the central importance of love, said: 'All writers on the subject seem agreed ... that love is an ingredient that is universally essential. Most of us would add some other almost equally important ingredients, but would probably disagree as to what they are and more particularly how they are to be used.'[40]

One such ingredient was 'free expression'. How far all actions were accepted, if not acceptable, depended on the individual pioneer's attitude to 'permissivism'. Some like Homer Lane or A. S. Neill saw this as fundamentally important therapeutically in allowing for the 'acting out' of repressions which were the basic causes of disturbance. Others with less conviction of the innate goodness of children (e.g. Dr Fitch and Dr Dodd) at least saw a reasonably permissive atmosphere as necessary if symptoms which required treatment were to reveal themselves.[41] The Underwood Report[42] gives a rather more general reason for permissivism: 'Anti-social behaviour must be tolerated, because maladjusted children need to work through their emotional problems for themselves. The staff's function is to help the child through the phase of love and hate, damage and restitution, until he attains some stability and feels safe in forming relationships with adults.' As the report points out, this may be followed by the expectation that, this phase having been worked through, the child can—and should—then learn to conform to more or less normal discipline.

The way in which this discipline is imposed is also one of the central questions, in answering which the pioneers reached considerable agreement. The necessary basis for most of them was self-discipline through self-governing (Lane, Wills, Shaw, Seel,

Grieve), the theory being that only in this way would the necessity of law in society become significant and acceptable to those who had previously rebelled against it.[43] Other equally positive advantages of 'self government' are advanced at length by Wills (see Chapter 12) and by J. H. Simpson.[44]

How far any maladjusted child is capable of exercising, responding to, and desiring self-government and how far such a system is opposite to, or consistent with, adult authority, paternalism — or what the Underwood Report calls 'benevolent dictatorship' — is another of the problems which the pioneers had to tackle with varying degrees of self-awareness. Some, like Dr Dodd, Lyward or Lennhoff, are frankly paternalistic, partly on the grounds that since most maladjusted children are emotionally immature they will be frightened of unbounded freedom and will prefer 'a regular pattern for their lives with an adult telling them what to do' (Underwood Report). A more reasoned argument against automatic 'self govern-ment' than that presented by the Underwood Report (which might, by the same token, advocate keeping drug addicts on drugs because they felt the need for them) is given by Lyward.

It is a step towards satisfying real needs to let children meet in session to make rules and pass judgements and to challenge them to run their communities with, or without, wages. But routine in such matters can become burdensome, and the secession of the adult can make for unreality: and anyhow living together is so much more than a business of producing law and order and anticipating the virtues and dangers inherent in political democracy. Children's committees and courts can be misleading. We mustn't imagine we are creating good democrats when we are merely training debaters and lawyers. Benevolent dictatorship and many other things not to be desired as final for the adult must all jostle each other in the Home as they do in any home. It is as recurring opportunities of breaking up the institutional soil that self-government should be chiefly welcomed and emulated.[45]

Although Lyward clearly recognizes his own guiding role, others like Lane and Neill attempted to deny that they exercised any control except through their single vote in the school assembly. This, as has often been pointed out, is self-deception. Such people retain direct control over some matters affecting the health, life and property of their pupils and over their relations with the outside world. Also within the form of government which — sometimes by inaction — they helped to create, their influence was necessarily more potent than that of a single vote. Such a notable experimenter in forms of 'shared responsibility' as J. H. Simpson says: 'Indeed, no form of government by discussion would be normally and healthily constituted in which the voice of experience did not find an adequate means of expression.'[46] Of Homer Lane's refusal to admit to any personal influence Simpson, who knew both Lane and the Little Commonwealth well, declared: 'To pretend that Lane's personal influence did not permeate the Little Commonwealth and determine the temper and spirit of the meetings would be the height of absurdity.... I find it difficult to reconcile the theory of "absolute freedom" with the exercise of an immense and potent influence.' The danger as Wills points out[47] is that such figures will progress from feeling that they are doing the will of God (or whatever Neill's alternative is), to believing that they are God—a being who controls everything while at the same time allowing the exercise of perfect free will. This might almost be diagnosed as 'pioneer's syndrome' and is frequently associated with strong feelings of persecution.

Others, like Wills himself, admit to certain areas of personal authority and to the effect of their personal prestige as father figures, while at the same time trying to minimize the scope of both. Thus, the idea of shared responsibility is not inconsistent with paternalism and in Wills's case the former is clearly an expression of the latter.

The persistence, however, of ideas both of self-government and of paternalism (whether acknowledged or not) is closely related to the size and nature of the schools we have been considering. Paternalism can clearly not operate effectively in a school which is too large for the headmaster to know every child personally and well (as reforming public school headmasters such as Howson had discovered earlier). Nor, on the other hand, can a system of self-government based on primitive democratic procedures operate successfully in a large school. Wennington found this difficulty at one point in its growth[48] and so, it will be remembered, did Lendrick Muir (see Chapter 17). Moreover, since the basis of self-government as an organizational and disciplinary system lies in conformity to group pressures and since there is a good deal of psychological evidence that neurotics are less conformist and susceptible to group pressures than those whose emotional adjustment is normal,[49] self-government does not seem a system ideally suited to maladjusted children.

Its exponents (among whom most of the pioneers are numbered) considered it of such therapeutic value that they were prepared to tolerate its inevitable inconvenience and inefficiency. Two factors assisted them. Their schools were sufficiently small (usually from ten to thirty children) to allow an effective balance of paternalism and shared responsibility. Secondly most of the pioneer schools and institutions were for adolescents—at an age when, as Redl points out, the child has moved from the dependency of infancy, through the 'gang' stage towards a 'growing preference for a more sublimated group formation'.[50] While remaining deeply dependent on the adult, the adolescent wishes to express his personal significance and assume some control of his own destinies.

Whatever the degree of self-government or of free expression two things remained true of all pioneer schools—a belief in the curative power of love and a recognition either from within or without, that ultimately 'the spirit of the place counts for most and this is the creation almost entirely of those who are in charge—those who represent the parental figure to the children'.[51]

EFFECT OF PIONEER WORK

How far the concepts of the pioneers are perpetuated in modern practice may not be a fair measure of their success, since the postwar situation is in many ways fundamentally different from that in which the pioneers sought an answer to their problems. The growth of psychological knowledge, the liberalization of discipline and method in ordinary schools, the dominance of the 'expert' and the growth of the control of the State have all had their effect. Even the emphasis which the pioneers put on unconditional love has been questioned both by those who see it as an unreliable (and rather amateurish) panacea and by those who consider that conditioning is more important than feeling. The tendency, particularly in America, has been away from paternalistic purveyors of environmental therapy towards an intensely clinical and psycho-analytical approach on the one hand[52] to a heavily structured re-educational programme, based largely on special classes in normal day schools, on the other.[53]

In England, the effect of pioneer tradition has been stronger and this has tended to inhibit experiment. Nevertheless, there have been attempts, as at Bredinghurst, to explore the possibilities of a more clinical approach, and the recently developed day classes and units, not yet having found a satisfactory rationale of their own, are open to experiment. The extent to which such experiment takes place is now largely in the hands of the State, which has traditionally been cautious in its approach to new methods. Conscious of their role as protectors of society against the discomfort of too rapid change, administrators have tended to wait until the results of experiments have been generally accepted before giving them their official support. This has usually meant that the real pioneers are always far in advance of actual provision and, with the decrease of genuinely independent ventures, there is danger that thought will become static and provision become stereotyped.

In the last analysis it will always remain impossible to devise any exact measure of what the pioneers achieved or of the validity of their concepts. One feels, however, through contact with them both in life and in literature, that they contributed something to individual human happiness and perhaps more to the relief of individual human misery. Ultimate evaluation of their work must use their own basic methods of intuition for it may indeed be that they provided a suitable environment in which children 'grew out of' their difficulties or that it was some unheeded aspect of institutional experience, other than those factors which the pioneers considered important, which effected the change.

Pioneers faced with an immediate and demanding problem could not wait for the eternity of certainty. They survived, and their influence survives, because they had faith in what they were doing however unscientific their procedures. As Wills says: 'If you have a boundless and invincible faith in what you are doing, and that faith is based on the unchanging and eternal verities, you will survive. But if your confidence in what you do is based on some pragmatic assessment of its value, measured against the yardstick of some human scientific concept, then I advise you to keep bees or become a business tycoon.'[54]

REFERENCES

CHAPTER 18: Assessment: Quantitative

1 MINISTRY OF EDUCATION. *Report of the Committee on Maladjusted Children*, Section 43. H.M.S.O., London, 1955.
2 Ibid. Section 47.
3 Ibid. Section 323.
4 D.E.S. *Health of the School Child. Chief Medical Officer's Report*, H.M.S.O., London, 1964–5.
5 HOWELL, D. Secretary of State for Education and Science, Parliamentary Answer, 6 Dec. 1968.
6 THE UNDERWOOD REPORT. Sections 296-298.
7 D.E.S. *List of Special Schools for Handicapped Pupils in England and Wales (List 42)* H.M.S.O., London, 1969.
8 HOWELL, D. op. cit.
9 D.E.S. Statistics in Education, H.M.S.O., London, 1967.
10 OAKESHOTT, E. *Times Educational Supplement.* 7 Feb. 1964.
11 WEAVER, A. F. A Survey of the Treatment of Maladjusted Children within the Educational System in England. Ph.D Thesis, (unpublished) Oxford University, 1968. *See*, in particular, *pp* 41-55 and very comprehensive tables.
12 *See* for instance. *The Kilbrandon Report.* Sections 172–177. H.M.S.O., Edinburgh, 1964, and *Report of the Committee on Local Authority and Allied Personal Social Services (the Seebohm Report)* Section 242. H.M.S.O., London, 1968.

CHAPTER 19: Assessment: Qualitative

13 HARING, N. G. and PHILLIPS, E. L. *Educating Emotionally Disturbed Children, p* 11. McGRAW-HILL, New York, 1962.
14 WILLS, W. D. *Throw Away Thy Rod.* Gollancz, London, 1960.
15 LENNHOFF, F. G. *Exceptional Children.* Allen & Unwin, London, 1960.
16 D.E.S. *The Education of Maladjusted Children.* Education Pamphlet No. 47 H.M.S.O., London, 1965.
17 WEAVER, A. F. op. cit.

18 BURT, C. *The Subnormal Mind, pp* 213–227, Oxford University Press, London, 1935. BARTON HALL, M. B. *Psychiatric Examination of the Child.* Arnold, 1947, *pp* 84–5, London.

19 MCNAIR, H. S. *A Survey of Children in Residential Schools for the Maladjusted in Scotland.* Oliver & Boyd, Edinburgh, 1968.

20 JENKINS, R. L. and GLICKMAN, S. Common Syndromes in Child Psychiatry Deviant Behaviour Traits. *Am. J. Orthopsychiatry* (16) *pp* 244-54.

21 CRUIKSHANK, W. M. and JOHNSON, G. V. *The Education of Exceptional Children and Youth.* Staples Press, London, 1958.

22 *See also* Chazan M. Maladjusted Pupils: Trends in Post-War Theory and Practice. *Educational Research.* VI (1) *pp* 30-33, 1963.

23 BURT, C. and HOWARD, M. The Nature and Causes of Maladjustment among Children of School Age. *Br. J. Psych (Stat)* V (1) *pp* 39-60, 1952.

24 PRINGLE, M. L. K. Differences between Boarding Schools for the Maladjusted and Ordinary Boarding Schools. *Br. J. Ed. Psych.* **XXVII** (1) *pp* 29-36. 1957.

25 WEAVER, A. F., op. cit.

26 JONES, H. *Reluctant Rebels.* Tavistock, London, *p* 217. 1960.

27 PETRIE, I. R. J. Residential Treatment of Maladjusted Children. A study of some factors related to progress in adjustment. *Br. J. Ed. Psych.* **XXXII** *pp* 29-37.

28 ROE, M. C. *Survey into Progress of Maladjusted Pupils.* I.L.E.A., London, 1965.

29 CRITCHLEY, C. An Experimental Study of Maladjusted Children. M.A. Thesis, (unpublished) Liverpool University. 1969.

30 ROYAL MEDICAL-PSYCHOLOGICAL ASSOCIATION, Report on Schools and Hostels for Maladjusted Children. *J. of Psychiatry*, March 1966.

31 Ibid.

32 LUNZER, E. A. Aggressive and Withdrawing Children in the Normal School—Patterns of Behaviour. *Br. J. Ed. Psych.* **XXX** *pp* 1-10, 1960.

33 LEVITT, E. E. The Results of Psychotherapy with Children: An Evaluation. *J. Cons. Psychol* (21) *pp* 189-196, 1957.

34 POWERS, E. and WITMER, H. *An Experiment in the Prevention of Delinquency.* Columbia University Press, New York, 1951.

35 EYSENCK, H. J. (ed.) *Handbook of Abnormal Psychology.* Pitman, London, 1960.

36 For general review of research on maladjustment *see also* THOULESS R. H. *Map of Educational Research*, Chapter 9, N.F.E.R. 1969.

37 EYSENCK, H. J. op. cit.

38 WILLIAMS, N. Criteria of Recovery of Maladjusted Children in Residential Schools. M.A. thesis (unpublished) Durham University 1961.

39 WILLS, W. D. *Throw Away Thy Rod. p* 29. Gollancz, London, 1960.

40 FRANKLIN, M. The Meaning of Planned Environmental Therapy. *A.W.M.C. Newsletter. p* 13. 7 June 1966.

41 SHIELDS, R. W. *A Cure of Delinquents. p* 20. Heinemann, London, 1962.

42 THE UNDERWOOD REPORT, Section 300 (ii-iv) 1955.

43 KERSHAW, J. D. *Handicapped Children. p* 174. Heinemann, London, 1961.

44 SIMPSON, J. H. *A Schoolmasters Harvest. p* 141-188. Faber & Faber, London, 1954.

45 LYWARD, C. A. In Conclusion, in *Problems of Child Development, p* 94. N.E.F. 1948.

46 SIMPSON, J. H. *An Adventure in Education.* Sidgwick & Jackson, London, 1917.

47 WILLS, W. D. *Homer Lane. pp* 213-214. Allen & Unwin, London, 1964.

48 CHILD, H. A. T. *The Independent Progressive School*, Hutchinson, London, 1962.

49 LEVINE, *et al.* Conforming Behaviour of Psychiatric and Mental Patients. *J. Abn. and Soc. Psych.* **49**, 1954; and JAHODA M. *Human Relations.* **12**, *pp* 99-117, 1959.

50 REDL, F. Group Emotions and Leadership, *Psychiatry* **5**. 1942.

51 BURNS, C. L. C. *Maladjusted Children.* Carter & Hollies, London, 1955.

52 BETTELHEIM, B. *Love is Not Enough.* Free Press of Glencoe, Illinois, 1950; *see also* PEARSON, G. H. J. *Emotional Disorders in Children.* Norton, New York, 1949; S. R. SLAVSON, *Re-educating the Delinquent Through Group and Community Participation.* Harper, New York, 1954.

53 For example, CRUICKSHANK, W. M. *Psychology of Exceptional Children and Youth*, Staples Press, London, 1958; *Teaching Methods for Brain Injured and Hyperactive Children.* Syracuse University Press, New York, 1961; with JOHNSON, G. V. *The Education of Exceptional Children and Youth*, Staples Press, London, 1958.

54 WILLS, W. D. Closing address to A.W.M.C. Conference 1968 on the occasion of his retirement.

PART NINE

Into The Future

20

The Future of Special Education

We believe there is need for an increase in special boarding school provision as well as day school places for maladjusted children in the local authority sector.... However attention should equally be paid to securing a greater range and flexibility of services.... — *Seebohm Report* (1968) Section 242.

However desirable it may be in theory, action cannot wait upon research. With such an immediate problem as the recovery of thousands of maladjusted children, who will have no second chance, one must proceed by acting not on academically pure principles — for there are none in this field — but on the basis of established precedent constantly made dynamic by enquiry and experiment. The pioneer period is over but, in some ways, it has had an unfortunate and unintentional effect. The authority of pioneer work, conducted under very different social circumstances and with little objective evaluation, has led too often to a mere repetition of antique models. It is particularly ironic that the great experimenters have, to this extent, discouraged experiment. Too often Local Authorities, embarrassed by their own inaction, have considered that the opening of a small residential school, with no particular educational or therapeutic policy, and as far out of touch as possible with the children's own environment, has solved the problem. There is too little evidence that either the magnitude of the variety of the need has been considered or has led to any over-all plan of action. Of all the maladjusted children in this country 98 per cent are receiving no special education.

If one accepts that, at least for administrative purposes, maladjusted children are 'pupils who show evidence of emotional instability or psychological disturbance and require special educational treatment to effect their personal, social and educational re-adjustment' the problem is clearly an educational one rather than one of mental health or social re-adjustment, although the three are obviously interrelated.

Children who are distinguished in the classroom by an apparent discrepancy between expectation and performance require remedial teaching based on accurate assessment. Children who are unable to adjust socially either to the teacher or to other children require classes which, in size, structure and discipline, are conducive to the development of healthy social relations. The majority of maladjusted children are distinguished by an unbalanced and immature emotional attitude which can be adjusted only if the emotional climate in the classroom is tolerant of aggression, encouraging to the withdrawn, and allows every child to be appreciated as an individual who may have need to regress emotionally and educationally to a point from which he can start his development again. The recognition and treatment of specific psychological disorders such as withdrawal, nervous mannerisms, aggressive behaviour, and excessive dependency readily produced by the classroom situation is also essential.

These are the minimum requirements for the effective education of maladjusted children and it is not unreasonable to suppose that most of them could be met within the context of the ordinary school. Indeed it is essential that they should be, since even the most optimistic idealist cannot anticipate a time when there will be adequate special educational provision for more than a small minority of maladjusted children.

The surveys carried out in Somerset (1952), Birmingham (1953) and Berkshire (1953) by the Ministry of Education as background to the Underwood Report revealed a 5.4 per cent to 11.8 per cent incidence of maladjustment among schoolchildren. Other studies based on assessment by teachers, psychologists and parents and the use of the Bristol Social Adjustment Guide vary in their estimates between 4 per cent and 13.4 per cent for serious maladjustment and range up to 46 per cent for children showing some symptoms of disturbance.[1] Even if one accepts an estimate of as little as 5 per cent for those children suffering from seriously handicapping maladjustment this would mean that an authority the size of Liverpool ought legally to make educational provision for 6,176 such children. This, if achieved only in terms of special schools, would require a total of 123 schools and, with as many as fifteen children per class, at least 410 teachers. The present provision in Liverpool, which is among the highest in the country, is five special schools for the maladjusted containing approximately 179 children and about thirty teachers.

ORDINARY SCHOOLS

It is clear, therefore, that, in the future, the problem must be tackled primarily in the ordinary schools, where the majority of maladjusted children are likely to remain, leaving the special schools to do a highly specialized job with children whose primary need is intensive therapy.

The general conditions necessary are clear. The first is the reduction of over-large classes which are not only productive of maladjustment but prevent it from being detected and treated. This is particularly true of primary schools, where preventive work can be done only in classes which are sufficiently small to allow effective individual contact between teacher and pupils. It seems unrealistic to expect this to happen unless classes are generally reduced to not more than thirty children. Earlier preventive work could be done by the establishment of more nursery schools, particularly in those areas known to be highly productive of maladjustment, and by the extension of 'at risk registers' to include families in which there are either children already recognizably disturbed or conditions likely to produce disturbance. There is also a need for educational and psychiatric social workers who can help and advise parents on the best ways of coping, educationally, with problems of abnormal development during the pre-school years. Much depends on the awareness of the problem by teachers in ordinary schools and more might be done at all levels to involve the teachers in the education of the whole child through 'in-service' and other courses, in initial training, and by direct assistance to staff by educational psychologists and other professional advisers.

More specifically there is need for an establishment of trained remedial teachers on the basis of not less than one per 250 children in ordinary schools. These teachers would be specialists, recognized as such, with a specific function which was seen as of vital importance to the welfare of the school. This would make possible the provision of small remedial classes in almost all schools and would be of greatest importance in primary schools where educational and emotional problems could be dealt with before they became chronic. This would also entail the recognition of maladjustment as a problem different from backwardness but equally requiring treatment in schools, not just as 'naughtiness', indiscipline or stupidity. Where a number of schools are too small to make individual remedial classes viable, a unit could be created in one of the schools. This would have the advantage of greater flexibility and more facilities while retaining the benefits of clear lines of communication with ordinary schools and with the neighbourhood from which the children are drawn. Ideally such units, whether used for short-term treatment, part-time attendance or as substitutes for special schools, should consist of at least two or three classes to avoid the disadvantages of limited facilities for the probable wide range of children, the isolation of the staff, or the dispersal of advice agencies. Although the use of such units is increasing rapidly, and for good reason, their greatest difficulty is frequently conflict with, or isolation from, the parent school of which they should be an integral part. This is caused partly by necessarily different objectives, expectations and patterns of discipline but should lessen as units become a more accepted part of the educational scene and as ordinary schools become more therapeutically orientated.

Treating maladjusted children should also be recognized by schools as being a social and psychological problem as well as an educational one. Recognition of the part played by tensions within the family in causing disturbance in the child should point the need for closer liaison between school and family. This would be achieved both directly and through the medium of Education Welfare officers, social workers and school counsellors. There seems to be a pressing need for more highly trained school counsellors particularly—but not solely—in large secondary schools where they can perform a vital preventive function. This would increase the provision of immediate 'first aid' to the emotionally disturbed child which would be expertly supplemented by trained psychologists working within the school. There is also scope for experiment in urban areas in the use of Social Education teams in which all the remedial education, psychological and social work skills are combined in one agency responsible for a particular, limited geographical area with which it is thoroughly acquainted. This should lessen the problem of interdisciplinary communication, which is often so hampering to effective action.

Much of the work done will be wasted unless there are effective counselling and support agencies which will continue work with disturbed children after they have left ordinary schools. Although after-care for children leaving special schools is inadequate it does exist, if only on a large informal basis. Other adolescents are not so fortunate and the maladjusted school-leaver from the ordinary school is one of the most serious and least regarded social problems of our time.

One thing which might possibly assist in solving this problem would be the provision of more hostels for those in need of a protective period of transition into adult life. The increase of hostel provision for children of school age would also have another important result. Many children who appear maladjusted in ordinary schools may only be suffering from the effect of very disturbed social or family environments. These conditions may, or may not, be permanent. In either case their problem is not an educational one and many such children are wasting places and receiving inappropriate help in special schools. They would be better off, both educationally and socially, in normal schools if there was adequate and good hostel accommodation.

These are by no means unrealistic objectives and some authorities have already seen the advantages, both educational and financial, of keeping maladjusted children within the normal school context while giving them expert help with their difficulties. In large authorities this makes for more flexible provision and conserves financial and other resources for necessary expenditure on the reduced number of special schools which are still required for those children who do not respond to more immediate provision. In small authorities, where previously no provision existed, it is possible by the use of skilled remedial teachers and special units to tackle the problem with very limited resources. One such authority, Chester, has within the space of three years moved by such means from being without provision to being the authority with the largest provision for maladjusted children in the country (one place for every 145 schoolchildren compared with the national average of less than one per thousand).

Although one would hope that with the growth of such provision and with the gradual change in the structure, methods and ethos of ordinary schools, the number of seriously disturbed children will be diminished, the need for special schools is likely to remain. We are not yet at the point where more than a minority of ordinary schools are likely to have enough staff trained to cope with, and to under-

M

stand, emotional disorders, or to have an attitude and structure conducive to mental health. The traditional school still retains aims of academic achievement and formal discipline in fundamental conflict with any therapeutic objectives.

SPECIAL SCHOOLS

If special schools are used for maladjusted children they must be 'special'. They must be doing a job which cannot be done in ordinary schools and have a clearly defined treatment policy and a structure designed to this end. This will involve therapeutic and educational facilities not normally available in the ordinary school. Both schools and classes will be of the optimum size for the task, and staff, both teaching and child-care, will be highly trained to fulfil their demanding roles adequately. Such special schools will use formal education as a tool in the therapeutic process and remedial teaching in all normal subjects should be available. They should be in close touch with the children's families and with the neighbourhood from which the majority of the children come and should have good lines of communication open to ordinary schools to allow easy placement and re-entry. Adequate psychological and psychiatric support and treatment should be readily and regularly available and this support should be extended to meet the individual needs of the staff if necessary.

Unless adequate and highly skilled advisory staff is available the school may have difficulty in assessing its function and functioning and may grow to lack any real purpose or policy and become a mere dumping ground for the 'scape goats' of ordinary schools. If this happens, and unless the majority of these conditions are fulfilled, no special school, either day or boarding, can justify its existence.

Day special schools, although more costly, have certain advantages over day units if adequately planned. They are probably easier to administer than a number of units and, being entities in themselves, will be more able to determine their own policies. Since they will normally be larger than units they should have more specialized and varied treatment facilities and their specialist staff will feel less isolated.

From the child's viewpoint they not only have the advantage of units in maintaining contact with the family but, possibly, also the advantage of not being too closely in contact with the school in which the child was unable to cope. Day schools are for 'children who need new schools and not new homes' — children, perhaps, who need a rest both from the pressures of home and the pressures of school in an environment which is acceptable to them just because it does not represent a situation of tension, competition or fear[2].

It is a common misconception that day special schools deal with children who are less deeply disturbed and need less expert help than those in residential schools. That the reverse appears to be more generally true is perhaps largely the result of day-school headmasters having less effective control over intake than have their residential colleagues. Also, day schools are often used for emergency placement of children in the midst of a crisis, children for whom residential places may be found subsequently.

Roe's investigations into I.L.E.A. day and boarding schools[3] revealed that, although boarding schools received more children who had difficulty in living with their families or who were rejected by society for their delinquent tendencies, day schools were more likely to contain children whose extreme behaviour disorders had led to difficulty in, and rejection by, ordinary schools. The latter were usually very aggressive children or very markedly withdrawn and over-timid. When tested on the Bristol Social Adjustment Guide they revealed more extremes of maladjustment and were less susceptible to psychotherapy.

If this is the case very careful thought and organization must clearly precede the establishment of more day schools. They must not be merely 'waste paper baskets to be filled up with all the vaguely diagnosed problems of the area'.[4] Laslett suggests that 'in some areas ... an Authority will set up a day school for maladjusted children with only the vaguest ideas of what the school is for, which children should go to it, what sort of staff is required, what is expected of the school and what sort of provisions must be made for it'.[5]

Apart from the criteria mentioned above, which apply to all special schools, there are clearly several specific requirements. The school should be designed to give the children the greatest feeling of security and intimacy. In this way it should be as unlike an ordinary school as possible. Although comprehensive remedial teaching is one of the fundamentals it is essential that this should be subservient to the child's psychological needs and should be conducted on an individual basis. It is doubtful if there is any place for the conventional classroom in such a school except possibly in the last stages of transition back to the ordinary school.

In order to make the best use of the day school's greatest asset—contact with families— things must be so structured, organizationally and in terms of staff provision, that the day school can be used, as Laslett suggests, as a treatment centre for 'a family with a maladjusted child'. Each school should have a psychiatric social worker maintaining contact with the family and the psychiatric and social work-team should be concerned with child, parent and school. The school psychological service will enhance the usefulness of the school as a diagnostic centre as well as giving support both to children and staff.

It is interesting that most of these conditions were fulfilled by the two pioneer day schools and deplorable that there are, at present, any special schools in which the provision is much less adequate. In the latter case day special schools will be distinguished from day units only by their disadvantages. There will normally be much greater stigma attached to attending a special school rather than a unit in an ordinary school. The former also may have much greater difficulty in maintaining adequate contact with families and neighbourhoods if their catchment area is too large (as was the case with the Lilian Baylis school), or if they are not carefully sited. Moreover their lines of communication with ordinary schools are not normally so flexible and direct as those of ordinary school units and they do not have the advantage of units of being in such close contact with ordinary schools that special staff and ordinary teachers are able to share their problems and interests in a way which is helpful to the understanding of both groups. If more teachers are to be encouraged to understand and work with maladjusted children a proliferation of isolated day schools is not likely to be helpful.

BOARDING SPECIAL SCHOOLS

The future provision and organization of boarding special schools is even more open to question. Their particular form and their prestige are largely historical artefacts and many existing schools lack the clarity of purpose which characterized most pioneer establishments.

There are two conditions which must exist before it is justifiable to send a child to a boarding special school. He must not only be suffering from his presence in a disturbed and disturbing family but from a form of maladjustment susceptible only to the conditions and treatment offered in a boarding special school. What such a form of maladjustment is is far from clear. Dr Roe's analysis of the reasons given by psychiatrists for recommending boarding-school treatment suggests that children are usually sent because their families cannot, for one reason or another, tolerate their presence, rather than that the children themselves are severely maladjusted or are maladjusted in any particular way. The removal of the child is not always even helpful to the family since 'out of sight' may mean 'out of mind' and the problem may become submerged only to reappear when the child returns. The situation may, in fact, have been aggravated by the jealousy directed by the parents towards the, often somewhat remote, school which may appear to be succeeding where they have failed. The placing of boarding special schools in the depths of the country may make effective and continuous contact with the parents almost impossible and once the child has been removed from a caseload by being placed in a school very little work may be done with the family itself. Unless these disadvantages can be overcome by siting residential schools near their main sources of supply, which is impossible in scattered rural areas or with schools having a national catchment area, a hostel structure plus appropriate day-school provision seems preferable.

In order to justify its existence a boarding school must have a therapeutic aim which cannot be fulfilled in any other way. Laslett suggests, for instance, that, for a variety of reasons, a day school cannot operate completely within the concept of 'planned environmental therapy'[6] and it seems unlikely that the sort of work done by Otto Shaw at Red Hill could be performed outside the context of a residential school. Hospital units also, in treating severe cases of school phobia, nocturnal and diurnal enuresis and encopresis, and psychosomatic illnesses may have a necessary special function. It is possible also that certain forms of delinquency impose such strain on society that the security provided by residential schools may be thought essential. Current experiments in treating highly disturbed delinquents in psychiatrically orientated residential units may also prove valuable.

As well as having a clearly defined special function, residential schools to be effective must have all the facilities, both educational and psychological, related to this aim. They must, for instance, have what so many of them lack, adequate educational provision so that emotionally and socially deprived children do not become educationally deprived. Few have the facilities which a child should have, particularly at secondary level, of following a broad course of study to the limits of his potential.

It is as a social experiment that residential schools are often thought to be most valuable and yet in many ways are often so inadequate. They frequently lack any wide and effective contact with the neighbourhood and become ingrown, concentrating all experience on a society which has few points of reference to life in the outside world. Moreover, by remaining single-sex at secondary level they deprive adolescents of the most important of all social experiences and may make them increasingly inadequate to deal with ordinary social intercourse even to the extent of fostering deviant behaviour.

Even on the mundane grounds of expense, but bearing in mind the disadvantages of much residential provision, it is clear that no child should be sent to a boarding special school if his disturbance is related only to his home or because of educational failure related to poor social conditions. Boarding placement either in hostels, ordinary boarding schools or 'county boarding schools' is desirable on educational, social and psychological grounds for many such children now taking expensive places in residential special schools which may be needed for genuinely and seriously emotionally disturbed children for whom intensive residential care is necessary.

The Government's policy with regard to future trends in the education of maladjusted children is not clear. There has been no major restatement of aims since the Underwood Report which, if no longer the holy writ for many workers in the field, still serves as the administrator's bible. There are signs, however, that this may no longer be so true in the highest levels of administration and that the impending Education Act may bring significant changes. One such change may be the rethinking of categories of handicap so that the present ten may be reduced to a single category of 'children with special needs'. This would give impetus to the present trend towards educating children with different forms of handicap together and towards closer integration with ordinary schools.

21

Teacher Training

Whatever the nature of the institution for maladjusted children little will be achieved other than a conscience-easing appearance of concern unless it has fully trained and highly skilled teaching, child care and advisory staff. The day of the inspired amateur is over: the age of the professional is at hand. At the moment there are too few of either. Most of the teachers in special schools and units for the maladjusted have no specific training and child-care staff in residential schools frequently lack even a basic qualification. Concerned but inexpert adults and willing but untrained girls cannot form a sound basis for a professional service directed to the solution of the problems of highly disturbed children. The right people for the job must be chosen and an appropriate training must be available.

Who the 'right' people are is a question which has occasioned a great deal of thought and very little research. Many of the people concerned with pioneer work have given answers from their experience although they are not always in agreement. This discrepancy is obviously the result of the individualistic ways in which they saw the task and the role of the person who was to carry it out. Indeed, the question cannot be answered except in terms not only of the perceived role but also of the actual role of the individual in terms of the function of the educational and treatment agency.

The worker in a school for maladjusted children may have an allotted role which allows for little variation. In some schools, for instance, the roles of the teacher, child-care staff and psychotherapist may be clearly delineated. This restriction may, however, be more apparent than real and in the majority of schools, particularly if residential, a member of staff will play more than one role either deliberately or unconsciously.

In residential schools, for example, all staff will normally share a parental role whether this is used therapeutically or expressed in practical, everyday care. Dockar-Drysdale, for instance, stresses the importance of all staff, whether male or female, being prepared to accept a maternal role, and Balbernie equally emphasises the importance of the paternal role particularly in work with delinquents. Balbernie, however, stresses the importance of undertaking this at a conscious, professional and therapeutic level and points to the often observed dangers of the reverse attitude. 'In unskilled hands this opportunity for healing is lost for the staff may then blindly fall into quasi-parental, possessive (mothering and fathering) roles, attempting to fill the gaps, or may attempt to minister to these wounds by covering them up with cotton-wool and bandages—responses which reflect only their own unconscious emotional needs.... Staff may provide new relationship experiences which supplement family experience or provide alternative forms of experience but can never provide a substitute for parental experience.'[7]

The teacher's therapeutic role will almost inevitably be imposed on him by his pupils and may be equally disastrously and unskilfully handled. He may have little professional psychotherapeutic help and may suffer severe stress by being at the centre of a psychodynamic process which he does not understand. Teachers and other workers with particular gifts and insight may do much to assist the disturbed child's understanding of himself, and may promote his mental health by sympathetic handling. They should be encouraged to do so. As Dockar-Drysdale points out, however: 'Insight can only be gained slowly, and one must not confuse insight with intuition. People can only do therapeutic work in terms of themselves as they really are. We cannot teach this kind of work; we can only give people permission to learn, and support them in meeting the child's needs when they realize what they really are.' It is significant, however, that few of the pioneers whose genius in this respect was recognized were in fact teachers, and many of the most eminent were either trained as psychotherapists, psychiatric social workers, psychiatrists or psychoanalysts (e.g. Dockar-Drysdale, Wills, Dodd, Shaw), or prepared themselves by a wide study of psychological literature, or by examining their own resources and motivation closely through personal psycho-analysis. Without either professional psychological training or intense self-awareness the teachers may do more harm than good. 'The worker cannot alleviate the sickness of others unless he has first attended to his own, and if he has not first washed his own hands he will contaminate others.'[8] The teacher may also, as Dr Wolff suggests, be too often hampered by a traditional authoritarian perception of his role to make a good therapist[9] although it is clear that many are not and develop considerable skill in this increasingly important part of their work.

It may be a reflection of the perceived function of pioneer establishments that very little attention has been paid to the teacher's role as an instructor. Maladjusted children not only have the same right as other children have to be taught well but often much greater need. Dr Franklin stresses not only the importance of remedial-teaching skills but also the need to recognize that success achieved by good teaching may be an important aid to psychological adjustment.[10] The teacher must therefore be a good instructor possessed not only of real skills but the ability to communicate them to children who have already experienced damaging failure in the hands of the less skilled. He must also understand the deeper underlying reasons for learning difficulties and be able to assess the child's needs accurately.

Of greatest significance in future therapeutic educational establishments, as in all pioneer ventures, is the role of the leader. This applies equally whether the school practises shared responsibility or is frankly paternalistic. It applies not only to the principal but to all those who exercise responsibility at any level. Carlebach describes the essential man as one 'who must know what he is doing, . . . must believe in what he is doing, and . . . must be able to formulate and communicate his aims, his motives and his methods'. He lays particular stress on the leader being an individual who wishes to guide and help 'from an inner conviction that he has the capacity to accept the unacceptable, to lead the uncertain, to inspire the defeated and to encourage the hopeless'.[11] David Wills puts the emphasis at the same point when, after describing himself as unapproachable, quick-tempered and sarcastic, he claims as his only virtue 'an invincible faith'.

Dr Wolff describes the pioneer leader in therapeutic education as 'an individual with exceptional gifts and a special and often highly individualistic philosophy of life which he is able to transmit to the rest of the staff. . . . Several experts from educational, medical and social-work fields have made contributions to the care of children by the exemplary running of their particular institutions and by combining dedicated care and love of children with high professional standards. All these individuals combined a high level of psychological insight with administrative abilities, with educational skills and with complete indentification with their own establishments'.

As facilities expand and diversify and become less personal creations we shall not however be able to rely on a supply of such people. Instead it is possible that less complete and sure leaders will depend increasingly on expert advisers, who will both help the leader and the led to make the best use of the organization and to see more clearly their own place in it and the nature of their relationships.[12]

In more general terms, most people who have written knowledgeably about the subject of personal qualifications have stressed the need for maturity. Peck and Havighurst write:

An adult who hopes to improve a child with immature character can only expect to do it by taking on the security-giving functions as well as the guiding functions ordinarily performed by parents. To do this effectively requires unusual wisdom, unusual personal maturity, and sometimes almost superhuman patience. It also requires a strong personal caring about the child albeit of an unsentimental kind. In short, in teaching character as in teaching intellectual knowledge, no one can teach what he does not know. In character education this includes much more than intellectual knowledge alone: it requires that the teacher of character personally possesses genuinely mature feelings, attitudes and ethical behaviour, or no success can be expected.[13]

Personal maturity is also necessary to accept a therapeutic role, and with it both the love and the hatred of the child, without becoming damagingly involved. As Shaw points out, many workers who are insufficiently mature project their own difficulties on to the child and become identified with him in a way which makes radical cure impossible.[14] Wills too, although probably accepting that one can never remain completely uninvolved with a person one is trying to love, says: 'In order to live with maladjusted children you have to be the kind of person who can live without them, and indeed without anyone. You have to be a whole, complete person, entirely sufficient unto yourself. Because if you *cannot* do without them, you are dependent on them. If you are dependent on them you and they have reversed roles to the ultimate damnation of both of you.[15]

Apart from these pragmatic judgements we have few guidelines for selecting and training future generations of workers with maladjusted children. A consensus of pioneer opinion is to be found in a report entitled *Qualities of Staff of Schools and Hostels for Maladjusted Children and Problems of Selection,* prepared by the A.W.M.C. committee. This considered all the functions which staff are asked to fulfil and also stressed the importance of questioning motivation and attitudes both to children and to maladjustment itself. It suggested that the characteristics to be avoided were those normally associated with a rigid training, long service in ordinary schools, or a tendency to form sado-masochistic relationships. Desirable qualities were: physical fitness, personal integrity, insight, a sense of vocation, humour, patience, consistency, a genuine love of children free from emotional dependency, objectivity towards one's own colleagues' emotional reactions, a non-condescending attitude to children, firm convictions about behaviour and moral standards, active outside interests, a capacity for detachment combined with a willingness to expend one's own emotional and spiritual resources, and the exercise of care in abiding by the rules of the community.

A much more detailed and thorough investigation of desirable 'teacher competences' conducted by the U.S. Department of Health, Education and Welfare in 1957[16] stressed many of the same points. It put a good deal more emphasis, however, on specific knowledge skills both educational and psychological. As the result of questionnaires sent to teachers of long experience and high repute, and to those who employed them, it eventually produced a check list of 157 'teacher competencies' under seven headings: Knowing the child (26); curriculum: materials and methods (46); testing and test information (18); guidance (19); the teacher as a professional team worker (20); parents and public relations (7); the teacher as a person (21). It would be valuable to examine these competencies in detail but even their scope and the emphasis indicated by the number of competencies in each group will suggest the extent to which the teacher of maladjusted children is regarded as a highly and widely skilled professional worker in a way which is not paralleled in England.

THE TRAINING

The American report suggests that the acquisition of these competencies should form the basis of a teacher-training programme extending over five years of higher education plus teaching experience. Training of teachers for work with maladjusted children in this country normally consists of a one-year course of theory and practice for those who already have a Certificate of Education and some relevant practical experience.

The first such course was started in 1953 when the London University Institute of Education planned a diploma course in the education of maladjusted children. By 1968, forty one-year training courses existed in England in universities (thirteen) colleges of education (seventeen) and Central Training Council centres (ten) (the last group including specialist training for house staff who would not normally, of course, have teaching qualifications). The total number of students was 757 of all types. Most of the teacher students (350) were on generic courses covering all types of handicap. Although this number of training places for teachers is double that set as a target by Underwood only a very small minority of these teachers would be specifically trained for work with maladjusted children and the target for house staff has not yet been met.[17]

Courses are very variously organized and have many different primary objectives, but it is difficult to see how any of them could give a thorough grounding in all the competences the American report regards as desirable, of which a knowledge of developmental psychology, social anthropology, sociology, psychological testing, criminology, psychopathology, curriculum method and evaluation, remedial techniques, organizational methods, counselling, vocational guidance, psychotherapy, social service organization, techniques of communication, work with parents, and the research evidence relevant to these topics are but a few.

Faced with this dilemma course organizers, who are as individualistic as any other body of pioneers, seek different partial solutions. Some concentrate on giving the student effective knowledge of himself, others on the acquisition of skills, others on understanding largely within the terms of a single psychological theory, some on covering as many bits and pieces as possible in the hope of making a significant pattern.

It seems desirable that, if the developing agencies for the education of maladjusted children are to be staffed by adequately trained workers in the future, the nature and organization of training courses (like those of the schools themselves), should be rigorously reassessed. We may need more courses or longer courses but neither of these is desirable unless the aims can be specified, the organization be adequate to the task, and the results be evaluated in terms of the effectiveness of the teachers in carrying out whatever multiple function research shows to be most necessary to the welfare of mal-adjusted children. As with schools, however, the need is immediate, the research evidence is not available, and the shortage of highly trained and experienced staff is acute. A valuable first step might be closer co-operation and greater communication between course organizers so that some sort of criteria might be evolved. Conferences of course tutors have been held under the aegis of the National Association of Mental Health for the past twelve years and by the D.E.S. for the past three years, but there seems to be a need for more direct communication between course organizers, perhaps at a regional level, and greater pooling of ideas rather than annual discussions of general problems. It is possible that more might be achieved by the establishment of a few larger centres for special education in which advanced courses could be given by a team representing many different areas of expertise. Much more effective work is also needed in initial training in colleges of education to ensure that teachers in ordinary schools are not so unprepared and ill-equipped to deal with the psychological difficulties of their pupils.

22

The Future of Child Care and Child Guidance

For our part we can only say this. If, as we have indicated, the problem of juvenile delinquency can with greatest hope of success be treated on the basis of an educational and preventive principle, the importance of early ascertainment of impaired intelligence and maladjustment, and appropriate special educational provision to meet such needs, is plain. — *Kilbrandon Report* (1964) Section 178

Although there have been no major changes in educational policy, projected developments in the allied fields of child care, child guidance and juvenile delinquency will inevitably affect provision for the maladjusted child. The probable effect of such changes is, however, difficult to estimate and may not be what their proponents expect. In Scotland the Kilbrandon Report (1964)[18] has already begun to have effect through the Social Work (Scotland) Act (1968) in the appointment of directors of social work under whose aegis most agencies concerned with the social care of the child will be combined. It is significant that the more comprehensive function and title, Director of Social Education, suggested by Kilbrandon, was rejected in the 1968 Act, thus preserving that distinction between education and other aspects of work with children which Kilbrandon deplored. The Act was, indeed, a very poor response to the Kilbrandon Committee's radical suggestions, being little more than a rationalization of normal child-care work and a reorganization of the legal procedures relating to young offenders. It is too early yet to assess its effect in terms of prevention of delinquency. Much depends on the early diagnosis and treatment of maladjustment, although this in itself would achieve little, hampered as Scotland is by the inadequacy of its educational provision for the disturbed. It is possible, however, that the experience already gained in Scottish approved schools in the handling of maladjusted children for whom there was no other educational provision will ultimately make their integration into a properly educational system easier.

366

In England the Seebohm Report (1968)[19] envisaged much the same unification of services for children in care and in need of special education, and urged a much greater range and flexibility of services for disturbed children. It was suggested that a social services department should be responsible both for child guidance and for reception centres, remand homes and approved schools. Responsibility for the supervision of special education would be shared betweeen the social services and education authorities.

These proposals are in general strongly resisted by the psychologists themselves on the grounds that education is the service most completely concerned with the welfare of all children and that it therefore remains the appropriate controlling agency.[20] It is considered that to concentrate on the family and on the needs of the maladjusted and, in particular, the delinquent, is to fragment rather than unify the service. To put the child-guidance service under the control of a social service department would be to give undue precedence to social factors as against educational and psychological factors, which are outside the competence of a social work agency. Also outside the competence of such an agency is control over children's change of schools and the appointment of child-care staff in special schools, both advocated by the Seebohm Report. To give powers of guidance at the moment possessed by Child-guidance clinics to a social work agency appears to reveal considerable ignorance of the extent of the activities of the child-guidance service and of the school psychological service at least since 1955. Because more family guidance is clearly necessary it does not follow that it should be only of a social-work type or that 'the guidance functions performed in child guidance clinics should become the responsibility of the social service department'. Because of a primary interest in delinquency it appears that the Seebohm Committee thought largely in terms of residential placement and, on the basis of a concern in this very minor part of educational and child-guidance provision for disturbed children, sought to acquire for the social services an unjustifiably large control in the general area of education. To isolate the child-guidance service from the school psychological service the school health service and the schools themselves would be to destroy necessary co-operation, to diminish the role of the C.G.C. itself, and to ignore the fact that the C.G.C. is primarily concerned with ordinary children in ordinary schools whose psychological and educational needs may not be the result of any social or family problem. It would appear therefore that the primary future need in this area of extreme importance to the maladjusted child—for no one doubts the importance of the family—is not the absorption of the C.G.C. into the social services but, as the Seebohm Report also suggests, an increase in the number of psychiatric social workers within the C.G.C. team.[21]

It is certainly to be hoped that work with families, and with pre-school children and school leavers, will be increased but it should be recognized that their needs are not necessarily primarily social ones nor, indeed, necessarily of social origin at all.

THE SUMMERFIELD REPORT

These points are well made in the Summerfield Report on Psychologists in Education Services (1968). This report is of great significance for the future treatment of maladjusted children. While recognizing the present shortage of educational psychologists and, in particular of psychiatrists and psychiatric social workers within the child-guidance service, it makes recommendations which it hopes will produce a ratio of 1 psychologist to 10,000 schoolchildren (1:6,000 in country districts) by 1990. It is hoped that this will be achieved largely in terms of increased facilities for training and the adoption of different modes of entry into the profession. This modest objective, it is suggested, can be reached only by the acceptance of one highly controversial principle. The committee recommends that it should no longer be necessary for psychology graduates to be trained and experienced teachers before appointment as educational psychologists. This, as the Association of Educational Psychologists points out[22] seems not only to limit the role and usefulness of the educational psychologist but also ignores the importance of the feelings of his chief 'consumer'—the teacher—towards him. Perhaps the chief difficulty which psychologists have at the moment is gaining acceptance by teachers. How much more will this be so if the teacher not only suspects, but knows, that the educational psychologist has little practical knowledge of the school environment in which the child's disturbance is expressing itself? How readily will the teacher, daily engaged in a task in which the practical application of psychological principles is essential, accept the advice of an academically trained 'expert' who has no experience of the practical problems? The more that the ordinary school adapts itself to deal with the education of all children, handicapped or not, the more essential will it be for the educational psychologist to work in the schools. Without a personal knowledge of school dynamics, of modern school practice and of the schoolchild in the learning situation he will find himself inadequately prepared for the fuller role which one hopes he will play not only as an assessor and diagnostician but as an adviser, supporter, therapist and counsellor both to staff and children.

While it remains necessary for the psychologist to appreciate the teacher's role through experience it will become increasingly important for the psychologist to define his own role more clearly. As the needs of all handicapped children of all ages and degrees of disturbance are more fully recognized and catered for it will not be possible for the psychologist to waste his time doing things which do not require a high degree of professional skill. School medical officers have for long been regarded as competent to give psychological tests for purpose of diagnosis and assessment after a course of training extending over less than four full weeks. It can no longer be realistically argued that experienced teachers, with their much more profound knowledge of children, cannot achieve equal competence after a longer period of intensive training. It will be essential, even if the target of one psychologist to ten thousand children is achieved, for teachers to do a major part of the initial diagnostic and attainment testing so that problems are discovered before they become chronic and so that the psychologist is able to devote his time to the more expert analysis and treatment of severe disorders. Such a development would increase the degree of understanding between teachers and psychologist, prevent the neglect of children with learning difficulties which exists at the moment in almost all schools, increase the teacher's understanding of his job, and free the psychologist from the shackles imposed on him by the present necessity of being primarily a tester.

It is not unrealistic to think at least in terms of one highly trained teacher who had done an appropriate supplementary course being appointed to every school even if all teachers cannot be given the necessary skill and experience.

N

One of the Seebohm Committee's proposals subsequently expanded in the White Paper—*Children in Trouble* (1968)[23] and incorporated in the Children and Young Persons Act, 1969[24] is for the establishment in every social service area of 'community homes'. What these homes will be and how they will differ in any significant way from existing children's homes and approved schools is never made clear. It seems likely, however, that they will either be aimless admixtures of existing places of care and detention or that they will be based primarily on the unproven concept that all that delinquent and maladjusted children lack is adequate substitute family care. The delinquent may suffer by being placed in an entirely mother-centred environment with too little opportunity for the masculine working-out of aggression or of ego-building through identification with masculine models. The severly maladjusted child in care may, however, be in danger of being sent to an existing but renamed approved school, which has the same staff, the same ethos and the same belief in training. Carlebach suggests that there is a possibility that if they 'operate as nearly as possible in the same way as a good family' they will only succeed in alienating the children further from their own families, to whom some may return after relatively short periods, and that a 'therapeutic approach to social education' may be taken to justify a neglect of any genuinely educational role. Carlebach also points out that the management and inspection of the new agencies is to be left in the hands of those who have proved so inadequate in the past, and that the problems of leadership and 'hierarchical asphyxiation' in existing approved schools are not considered. The most that can be hoped for is that the community homes will produce their own generation of 'pioneers', who will give effect to Carlebach's hope that a community home will be 'a unit run on community lines and established by, and closely intertwined with, the local community in which it is situated' —possibly, in fact, natural extensions of existing schools.[25]

THE COTSWOLD COMMUNITY

One of the Seebohm Report's chief individual critics, who regards community homes as 'a sentimental idea dreamt up by female child-care officers', is Richard Balbernie. He believes that such proposals ignore the reality of delinquency by pretending that it does not exist as a condition. Much as he hates approved schools he believes that they will always have to exist in one form or another to relieve the intolerable social pressure that delinquent aggression generates. Balbernie must be listened to with respect for he is a trained psychologist and psychotherapist, an experienced research worker, the former headmaster of a school for maladjusted children, the author of the best extant book on the residential treatment of disturbed children[26] and, as the principal of the Cotswold Community, is one of the few people who are at the moment doing interesting and experimental work in this field. He does not consider himself to be a pioneer; indeed, he thinks that we now know enough about the factors in the treatment of maladjustment and delinquency to consider that the pioneer period is over. His avowed aim is to use, in an efficient and professional way, the insights which the pioneers have handed on.

The Cotswold Community experiment is being expertly studied, controlled and evaluated with the intention of conceptualizing methods and communicating results, by Dr A. K. Rice, a member of the Centre of Applied Social Research at the Tavistock Institute[27]. Dr Rice's eventual report and Balbernie's own book, *Residential Work with Children*, make it unnecessary for me to do more than summarize briefly the general principles involved.

The work is with severely damaged and deprived $13\frac{1}{2}$- to 16-year-olds whose delinquency appears to be an integral part of their personality. They stay for a period of eighteen months. Work is in small groups of eight or nine boys and is often of a technically high standard. It is real work and the intention is to rechannel aggression into positive ego-building activities in genuine adult-work situations. This involves identification with masculine ideals directly, and also as they are expressed by carefully chosen and trained workers whose personal maturity and understanding is crucial. Although the adult-work situation and masculine identification is part of the tradition of approved schools the approach in the Cotswold Community is essentially non-punitive and it is accepted that delinquent aggression must express itself in order to be dealt with. This also gives the delinquent the chance to come to terms with his own delinquency by 'acting out' irresponsibilities and difficulties. This inevitably produces considerable disruption within the community but disintegration is prevented by a highly developed and sophisticated organization in which the roles and functions of the staff are clearly defined and everyone understands and accepts the purpose.

The ultimate aim is to encourage the delinquent adolescent to take more conscious and rational authority for his own decisions, a conclusion which cannot be reached in an institution in which any real decision making (e.g. whether to do right or wrong) is made impossible.

The Cotswold Community is described as a 'therapeutic unit' and indeed psychotherapeutic and psychiatric help is available, and regression—even to missed 'primary experience'—is given scope. Nevertheless the approach is a psychological rather than a mental-health one. Balbernie considers that few delinquents are primarily psychotic rather than primarily delinquent and that the medical approach characteristic of the new Home Office psychiatric units for 'highly disturbed' delinquents is unrealistic. He believes that such units, which represent another form of experimental approach, will become the dustbin of the dustbin at the end of a long line of 'scape-goating' from community homes downwards.

Balbernie sees his way as a middle way between the institutional-ized aggression in what he considers to be the typical, punitive, approved school (in which delinquency is given no chance to express itself and be changed by the possibility of ego-developing oppor-tunities), and institutionalized sentimentality in which the reality of delinquency is ignored and the pervading maternal ethos stifles real ego-development by perpetuating dependence[28].

It appears to me that what is most valuable is Balbernie's pro-fessionalism and his determination to make an experiment not only something which is different but something which is continuously and expertly assessed in terms of its aim, organization and achieve-ment. Much depends on an accurate diagnosis of the condition which is actually being worked upon. It is probable that 'delinquency' is too broad a term and that no one solution can be universally applied. If the variety of provision envisaged in the 1969 Children's Act were ever to be realized, and if there was sufficient expertise available to produce specific diagnoses and prescriptions for action, it seems likely that the general term 'delinquent' would be replaced by specific categories of need for which appropriate agencies would be created. In this unlikely event it might well be found that not only would there be need of more Cotswold Com-munities for what might be considered the delinquent delinquent but that the emotionally deprived (particularly if they had no actual families) might profit by more family-type community homes, and the estimated 3 per cent of delinquents whose main need is clinical treatment[29] would find it in medically orientated units. Within these broad general categories it might be possible to make further sub-divisions by an intensive examination of individual cases and it might be found, for instance, that Dockar-Drysdale's work with pre-psychopathic children might be capable of extension (in ways other than Balbernie's) to small groups of psychopathic adolescents.

Balbernie recognizes that there will never be a single appropriate solution to a problem which is concerned with individual adjustment, and it would be unfortunate if any apparent success of a particular method with one type of child should lead to its indiscriminate application to others. This is one of the fundamental dangers inherent in successful pioneer work.

[Note]—Since this chapter was written the Local Authority Social Services Act, 1970 has proposed changing the social service structure in England in much the same way as that effected in Scotland by the Social Work (Scotland) Act, 1968. The Act has given to the Social Services Committee and the Director of Social Services those powers which the Children's Department acquired under the Children and Young Persons Act, 1969 and has combined them with the powers of the Welfare Department and with responsibilities relating to mental health formerly held by the local health authority. The powers of the local education authority, including that over educational psychologists, are largely unimpaired although the position of education welfare officers is not clear. The orientation either towards education or towards child care will be determined largely by the local authorities and, in particular, by their choice of director of social services.

23

In Conclusion

Much the same approach as that suggested for delinquents might in future be applied to those children who at the moment are gathered under the wide umbrella of 'maladjustment'. Where the disturbance is severe it might be possible to distinguish specific conditions and to experiment with specific treatments. This is already being attempted with autistic children, who perhaps have an advantage in not previously having been considered 'maladjusted'. If, however, as current experiments suggest, this apparent psychosis may be caused by emotional trauma and may be curable, or at least modifiable, by largely educational means, autistic units would become part of special educational provision for maladjusted children. There are (February 1970) twenty-six such units—all but five in the south-east of England. There are estimated to be 5,000 autistic children[30] and it has been suggested that approximately 800 units are required[31]. Provision on this scale, unless preceded by much greater research into the nature of the condition and appropriate forms of treatment might well be unfortunate in introducing yet another wide general category of handicap.

An alternative solution to the proliferation of small and isolated units might be, as I have suggested, the provision of a wide variety of individually structured educational experiences within the framework of the ordinary school or in special schools for children suffering from many different forms of handicap. There is a great deal in common between the requirements of children with emotional, physical, social and educational handicaps. Individual attention, small-group work, a secure and, to some extent, protected environment, remedial education, psychological support, treatment and assessment, all within the context of an organization with a personal atmosphere and a high staffing ratio, all appear to be general desiderata. Such mixed-handicap schools would appear to have many social and educational advantages to the child. The non-communicating child could have greater opportunity to communicate, the physically handicapped might find a less limiting environment, the backward child would not be isolated from his more able peers, the disturbed child might be dealt with in a less disturbed setting. Moreover since the handicapped child tends to suffer from more than one condition e.g. P.H./E.S.N./maladjusted, there would be facilities for dealing with all facets of handicap and there would not be the present danger that, in dealing with one handicap in a highly specialized way, we may neglect one disorder while dealing with the dominant presenting symptoms of another.

There is some precedent for such practice in open-air schools such as Delamere Forest, Steiner schools such as Camphill in Scotland, and in day schools such as the Frank Merrifield School in Chester-field. The working and effectiveness of such schools should be studied and perhaps, in particular, the effect of their size. Camphill has 250 pupils of all ages and both sexes and the Frank Merrifield school 150. One of the most limiting factors on the extension of, and the work done in, special schools for the maladjusted has been the assumption, never thoroughly investigated, that they need to be limited to numbers customary in small, patriarchal pioneer establishments.

More attention also needs to be given to experiment in the methods used within special schools. The general psychoanalytical orientation of pioneer schools for the maladjusted has led to a neglect of alternative methods of approach. In particular there has been a resistance in this country to trying anything which is derived from behaviourist theory. In so far as the work with maladjusted children involves a process of 'relearning', this blinkered attitude may have prevented the development of useful new methods of approach. Work such as that directed by Haring and Phillips in America suggests that hyperactive children, in particular, may have much to gain from a carefully structured relearning experience.[32] Lowenstein[33] and Bandura and Walter[34] have produced research evidence to suggest that the principles of behaviourist learning theories may have application not only to the acquisition of basic skills but also to the child's ability to withstand stress. The restructuring of maladaptive behaviour by techniques such as 'selective reinforcement' and 'shaping' may, it is suggested, do more than remove socially unacceptable symptoms. It may also improve the child's concept of himself, increase his self-esteem, reduce anxiety and stress and promote mature behaviour which becomes habitual and no longer requires external reinforcement.[35]

Perhaps, also, although we may be antipathetic to Eysenck's

apparent advocacy of 'aversion therapy' as a basis for moral retraining,[36] we should pay more regard to his views on genetic determination of maladjustment.[37] Too little is known about the biochemical origins of neurotic behaviour to make the medical treatment of maladjustment feasible, at the moment, on a major scale but much more research is clearly called for if there is hope that such techniques might not only reduce anxiety producing symptoms (such as enuresis) but might produce permanent re-balancing which would not require the continuous support of drugs.

Before dramatic progress can be made in any of these directions we require reliable information and minds open enough to receive it. We require conceptualization based on further and more rigorous experiment by a new race of professional 'pioneers'. We require agencies based on specific aims and with organizations of demonstrable appropriateness to the task. A professional approach will not lessen the value of the individual worker of genius but rather increase the effectiveness of his work. We need to consider whether there is anything of educational value to be done for the maladjusted child which cannot be achieved in an ordinary school which pays due regard to the principles of the pioneers and the expertise of their successors. Perhaps the work of the pioneers will never be done until all homes and all schools are fit for all children to grow up in healthily and special schools cease to exist. Pioneers necessarily begin their work looking towards the millennium.

REFERENCES

CHAPTER 20: The Future of Special Education

1 *See* WALL, W. D. *Education and Mental Health.* Harrap (for UNESCO) 1955; CRITCHLEY, C. *An Experimental Study of Maladjusted Children.* M.A. thesis (unpublished) *pp* 11-22, Liverpool University, 1969; CHAZAN, M. *Maladjusted Children: Trends in Postwar Theory and Practice.* N.F.E.R. 1963.

2 LASLETT, R. The Place of the Day Special School in the Treatment of the Maladjusted Child. *A.W.M.C. Sixth Newsletter, pp* 6-12. November 1965.

3 ROE, M. C. Survey into Progress of Maladjusted Pupils. I.L.E.A. publication. 1965.

4 LASLETT, R. op. cit., *p* 12.

5 —— A consideration of some of the Principles of Planned Environmental Therapy and an enquiry as to whether these can be practised in a Day School for Maladjusted Children, in *Studies in Environmental Therapy.* I *pp* 62-66. P.E.T. Trust 1968.

6 —— Ibid.

CHAPTER 21: Teacher Training

7 BALBERNIE, R. *Residential work with Children.* Pergamon, Oxford, 1966. *p* 187.

8 DOCKAR-DRYSDALE, B. Possibility of Regression in a Structured Environment, in *Therapy in Child Care, pp* 78-9. Longmans, London, 1968.

9 WOLFF, S. Two Recent Scottish Government Reports. *A.W.M.C. Newsletter, pp* 18-25. December 1964.

10 FRANKLIN, M. The Meaning of Planned Environmental Therapy. *A.W.M.C. Newsletter, p* 16. June 1966.

11 CARLEBACH, J. *Caring for Children in Trouble, pp* 174-5. Routledge & Kegan Paul, London, 1969.

12 WOLFF, S. *Children Under Stress, pp* 191-2. Allen Lane Penguin Press, London, 1969.

13 PECK, R. F. and HAVIGHURST, R. J. *The Psychology of Character Development*. Wiley, New York, 1960.
14 SHAW, O. *Prisons of the Mind. p* 21. Allen & Unwin, London, 1969.
15 WILLS, W. D. closing address given at A.W.M.C. Conference, Cheltenham, May, 1968.
16 U.S. DEPARTMENT OF HEALTH, EDUCATION AND WELFARE. Teachers of Children who are Socially and Emotionally Maladjusted. Bulletin No. 11. 1957.

CHAPTER 22: The Future of Child Care and Child Guidance

17 WEAVER, A. F. *A Survey of the Treatment of Maladjusted Children within the Educational System in England. p* 181. Unpublished Ph.D. thesis. Oxford University, 1968.
18 SCOTTISH HOME and HEALTH DEPARTMENT. *Children and Young Persons. Scotland.* Cmnd 2306. H.M.S.O., Edinburgh, 1964.
19 HOME OFFICE and OTHERS. *Report of the Committee on Local Authority and Allied Personal Social Services.* Cmnd. 3703. H.M.S.O., London, 1968.
20 BRITISH PSYCHOLOGICAL SOCIETY, Memorandum on the Seebohm Report and the Summerfield Report. (unpublished). November 1968.
21 D.E.S. *Psychologists in the Education Services. (The Summerfield Report).* H.M.S.O., London, 1968.
22 ASSOCIATION OF EDUCATIONAL PSYCHOLOGISTS. Commentary on the Report Psychologists in the Education Services (unpublished). December 1968.
23 HOME DEPARTMENT. *Children in Trouble.* Cmnd. 3601. H.M.S.O., London, 1968.
24 CHILDREN AND YOUNG PERSONS ACT. 1969. Ch 54. H.M.S.O. (London).
25 CARLEBACH, J. *Caring for Children in Trouble, pp* 175-179. Routledge and Kegan Paul, London, 1970.
26 BALBERNIE, R. op. cit.
27 RICE, A. K. *Cotswold Community and School.* Working Note (1) (mimeographed). Tavistock Institute. February 1968.
28 PERSONAL COMMUNICATION, interview.

CHAPTER 23: In Conclusion

29 HOME DEPARTMENT. *Making Citizens. p* 29. H.M.S.O., London, 1946.
30 Figures given by the National Society for Autistic Children.
31 LADY ELLIOT OF HARWOOD, in House of Lords debate, 17 February 1970.

32 HARING, N. G. and PHILLIPS, E. L. *Educating Emotionally Disturbed Children*. McGraw-Hill, New York. 1962.

33 LOWENSTEIN, L. F. Group Operant Conditioning, 1966. Ph.D. Thesis., London University.

34 BANDURA, A. and WALTER, S. *Social Learning and Personality Development*. Holt, Rinehart and Winston, New York, 1963.

35 *See also*, for example, ULLMANN, L. P. and KRASNER, L. *Case Studies in Behaviour Modification*. Holt, Rinehart and Winston, New York, 1965.

36 EYSENCK, H. J. *Crime and Personality*. Routledge, London, 1964.

37 EYSENCK, H. J. and PRELL, D. B. The Inheritance on Neuroticism, an Experimental Study. *J. Ment. Sci.* **XCVII** *pp* 441-465. 1951.

Appendix

1834	4 & 5	Will. IV c.76	Poor Law Amendment Act
1840	3 & 4	Vict. c.90	Infant Felons Act
1854	17 & 18	Vict. c.86	Reformatory Schools (Youthful Offenders) Act
1857	20 & 21	Vict. c.48	Industrial Schools Act
1857	20 & 21	Vict. c.55	Reformatory Schools Act
1862	25 & 26	Vict. c.43	Poor Law (Certified Schools) Act
1868	31 & 32	Vict. c.122	Poor Law Amendment Act
1870	33 & 34	Vict. c.75	Elementary Education Act
1876	39 & 40	Vict. c.79	Elementary Education Act
1880	43 & 44	Vict. c.23	Elementary Education Act
1886	49 & 50	Vict. c.25	Idiots Act
1887	50 & 51	Vict. c.25	Probation and First Offenders Act
1899	62 & 63	Vict. c.32	Elementary Education (Defective and Epileptic Children) Act
1899	62 & 63	Vict. c.37	Poor Law Act
1901	64	Vict. c.20	Youthful Offenders Act
1902	2	Ed. VII c.42	Education Act
1903	3	Ed. VII c.13	Elementary Education (Defective and Epileptic Children) Amendment Act
1907	7	Ed. VII c.17	Probation of Offenders Act
1907	7	Ed. VII c.43	Education (Administrative Provisions) Act
1908	8	Ed. VII c.67	Children's Act
1913	3 & 4	Geo. V c.28	Mental Deficiency Act
1914	4 & 5	Geo. V c.45	Elementary Education (Defective and Epileptic Children) Act
1918	8 & 9	Geo. V c.39	Education Act
1921	11 & 12	Geo. V c.51	Education Act
1930	20	Geo. V c.17	Poor Law Act

1933	23 & 24	Geo. V c.12	Children and Young Persons Act
1937	1	Edw. VIII and 1 Geo. VI c.37	Children and Young Persons (Scotland) Act
1944	7 & 8	Geo. VI c.31	Education Act
1946	9 & 10	Geo. VI c.81	National Health Services Act
1948	11 & 12	Geo. VI c.40	Education (Miscellaneous Provisions) Act
1948	11 & 12	Geo. VI c.43	Children's Act
1958	6 & 7	Eliz. II c.65	Children's Act
1963	11 & 12	Eliz. II c.37	Children and Young Persons Act
1968	16 & 17	Eliz. II c.49	Social work (Scotland) Act
1969	17 & 18	Eliz. II c.54	Children and Young Persons Act
1970	19	Eliz. II c.42	Local Authority Social Services Act
1970	18 & 19	Eliz. II c.52	Education (Handicapped Children Act)

PARLIAMENTARY PAPERS, REGULATIONS and REPORTS

1851		Education and Training of Pauper Children. (Poor Law Inspectors)
1852-3		Criminal and Destitute Children. (Select Committee)
1876		Education of Pauper Children. (Local Government Board)
1904	Circular 432	Defective and Epileptic Children (Revised). Board of Education
1908	Cd. 4202	The Care and Control of the Feeble Minded
1908	Cd. 3899	Children under the Poor Law. (Macnamara Report)
1927	Cmd. 2831	Treatment of Young Offenders
1945	Cmd. 6636	The Boarding Out of Dennis and Terence O'Neill. (Monckton Report)

1945	S.R.O. 1076	The Handicapped Pupils and School Health Service Regulations. (Ministry of Education)
1945	Circular 241	Handicapped Pupils and Medical Service Regulations. (Ministry of Education)
1946		Making Citizens. (Home Department pamphlet)
1946	Cmd. 6911	Homeless Children. (Clyde Report)
1946	Cmd. 6922	Care of Children. (Curtis Report)
1952	Cmd. 8428	Pupils who are Maladjusted because of Social Handicaps. (Advisory Council on Education in Scotland. Scottish Education Department)
1953	Circular 269	The School Health and Handicapped Pupils Regulations. (Ministry of Education)
1954	Circular 276	Provision of Special Schools. (Ministry of Education)
1955		Maladjusted Children. (Underwood Report: Ministry of Education)
1956	Pamphlet No. 30	Education of the Handicapped Pupil, 1945-1955. (Ministry of Education)
1959	Circular 347	Child Guidance. (Ministry of Education)
1959	Circular 348	Special Educational Treatment for Maladjusted Children. (Ministry of Education)
1959	S.I. 365	The Handicapped Pupils and Special Schools Regulations. (Ministry of Education)
1960	Cmd. 1911	Children and Young Persons. (Ingleby Report)
1961	Circular 4/61	The Use of Independent Schools for Handicapped Pupils. (Department of Education and Science)
1964		Ascertainment of Maladjusted Children. (Scottish Education Department)
1964	Cmnd. 2306	Children and Young Persons. Scotland. (Kilbrandon Report)
1965	Pamphlet No. 47	The Education of Maladjusted Children. (Department of Education and Science)

1965	Cmnd. 2742	The Child, the Family and the Young Offender. (Home Department Report)
1968	Cmnd. 3601	Children in Trouble. (Home Department Report)
1968	Cmnd. 3703	Local Authority and Allied Personal Social Services. (Seebohm Report)
1968		Psychologists in the Education Service. (Summerfield Report) (Department of Education and Science)
1970	Circular 15/70	The Education (Handicapped Children) Act 1970. Responsibility for the Education of Mentally Handicapped Children

See also: Annual reports of the Poor Law Commissioners. Annual reports of the Inspectors of Reformatory and Industrial Schools.

Reports of the Children's Branch of the Home Office. The Chief Medical Officer's Reports.

List of Special Schools for Handicapped Pupils in England and Wales. (List 42) (Department of Education and Science).

Statistics in Education (Department of Education and Science).

Bibliography

ADAMS, Sir J. *Modern Developments in English Educational Practice*, 2nd edn. University of London Press, London, 1928.

AICHHORN, A. *Wayward Youth*. Imago Publishing Co. London, 1957.

ALLEN, Lady MARJORIE. *Whose Children?* Favill, London, 1945.

AUDEN, W. H. *Poems*. Faber & Faber, London, 1930.

—— and MACNEICE, L. *Letters from Iceland*. Faber & Faber, London, 1937.

BADLEY, J. H. *A Schoolmaster's Testament*. Blackwell, London, 1937.

BALBERNIE, R. *Residential Work with Children*. Pergamon, Oxford, 1966.

BANDURA, A. and WALTER, S. *Social learning and personality Development*. Holt, Rinehart and Winston, New York, 1963.

BARBE, W. B. *The Exceptional Child*. The Centre for Applied Research in Education, New York, 1963.

BARTON HALL, M. B. *Psychiatric Examination of the Child*. Arnold, London, 1947.

BAZELEY, E. T. *Homer Lane and the Little Commonwealth*. Allen and Unwin, London, 1928.

BERKOWITZ, P. H. and ROTHMAN, E. P. *The Disturbed Child. Recognition and psycho-educational therapy in the classroom*. New York University Press, N.Y., 1960.

BETTELHEIM, B. *Love is Not Enough*. Free Press of Glencoe, Illinois, 1950.

BLEWITT, T. *The Modern Schools' Handbook*, Gollancz, London, 1934.

BOWLBY, J. *Maternal Care and Mental Health*. World Health Organisation, Geneva, 1951.

BOYD, W., ed. *Evacuation in Scotland*. Publications of the Scottish Council for Research in Education, **XXII** University of London Press, London, 1944.

—— and RAWSON, W. *The Story of the New Education*. Heinemann, London, 1965.

BURLINGHAM, D. & FREUD, A. *Young Children in Wartime*. Allen and Unwin (for the *New Era*), London, 1942.

BURN, M. *Mr Lyward's Answer*. Hamish Hamilton, London, 1956.

BURNS, C. L. C. *Maladjusted Children*. Hollis & Carter, London, 1955.

BURT, C. *The Subnormal Mind.* Oxford University Press, London, 1935.
—— *The Young Delinquent* (4th edn.) University of London Press, London, 1944.
CAMERON, H. *The Nervous Child.* Oxford University Press, London, 1918.
CARLEBACH, J. *Caring for Children in Trouble.* Routledge and Kegan Paul, London, 1969.
CARLGREN, F. *Rudolph Steiner* 2nd edn. The Goetheanum School, Dornach, 1964.
CARPENTER, J. ESTLIN. *The Life and Work of Mary Carpenter*, Macmillan, London, 1879.
CARPENTER, M. *Reformatory Schools for the Children of the Perishing and Dangerous Classes and for Juvenile Offenders.* Gilpin, London, 1851.
—— *Juvenile Delinquents their Condition and Treatment.* W. & F. G. Cash, London, 1853.
CHAZAN, M. *Maladjusted Children: trends in post-war theory and practice.* N.F.E.R. 1963.
CHILD, H. A. T. (ed.) *The Independent Progressive School.* Hutchinson, London, 1962.
COLEMAN, J. *Childscourt.* Macdonald, London, 1967.
CRUICKSHANK, W. M. *Psychology of Exceptional Children and Youth.* Staples Press, London, 1958.
—— *Teaching Methods for Brain Injured and Hyperactive Children.* Syracuse University Press, New York, 1961.
—— and JOHNSON, G. V. *Education of Exceptional Children and Youth.* Staples Press, London, 1958.
D'EVELYN, K. *Meeting Children's Emotional Needs.* Prentice-Hall, Englewood Cliffs (New Jersey), 1957.
DOCKAR-DRYSDALE, B. *Therapy in Child Care.* Longmans, Green, London, 1968.
DODD, F. H. *Commonsense Psychology and the Home.* Allen and Unwin, London, 1933.
DUPONT, H. (ed.) *Educating Emotionally Disturbed children.* Holt, Rinehart & Winston, New York, 1969.
EDMUNDS, L. P. *Rudolph Steiner Education.* Rudolph Steiner Publications, London, 1962.
EYSENCK, H. J. (ed.) *Handbook of Abnormal Psychology.* Pitman Medical, London, 1960.

—— *Crime and Personality.* Routledge, London, 1964.

FLUGEL, J. C. *The Psychoanalytic Study of the Family.* Hogarth, London, 1948.

—— *A Hundred Years of Psychology.* Duckworth, London, 1951.

FRANKLIN, M. E. *Q Camp.* Planned Environmental Therapy Trust, London, 1966.

FREUD, A. *Introduction to Psychoanalysis for Teachers.* Allen and Unwin, London, 1931.

—— *The Ego Mechanisms of Defence.* Hogarth, London, 1936.

—— The *Psychoanalytical Treatment of Children.* Imago, London, 1946.

HARING, N. G. and PHILLIPS, E. L. *Educating Emotionally Disturbed Children.* McGraw-Hill, New York, 1962.

HART, R. *The Inviolable Hills.* Rudolph Steiner Press, London.

HARWOOD, A. C. *The Recovery of Man in Childhood.* Hodder & Stoughton, London, 1958.

—— *The Way of a Child.* Rudolph Steiner Press, London, 1940.

HEYWOOD, J. S. *Children in Care.* Routledge & Kegan Paul, London, 1965.

HINDE, R. S. E. *The British Penal System 1773-1950.* Duckworth, London, 1951.

HOLMES, E. *What Is and What Might Be.* Constable, London, 1911.

—— *The Tragedy of Education.* Constable, London, 1913.

—— *In Defence of What Might Be.* Constable, London, 1914.

—— *Give Me the Young.* Constable, London, 1921.

HOLMES, R. G. A. *The Idiot Teacher.* Faber & Faber, London, 1952.

HOVLAND, C. I., JANIS, I. L., KELLEY, H. H. *Communications and Persuasion,* Yale University Press, New Haven, Conn, 1953.

ISAACS, S. (ed.) *The Cambridge Evacuation Survey.* Methuen, London, 1941.

JONES, H. *Reluctant Rebels.* Tavistock, London, 1960.

KERSHAW, J. D. *Handicapped Children.* Heinemann, London, 1961.

LANE, H. *Talks to Parents and Teachers.* Allen & Unwin, London, 1928.

LENNHOFF, F. G. *Exceptional Children.* Allen & Unwin, London, 1960.

LEWIS, H. *Deprived Children.* Oxford University Press, London, 1954.

LORAND, S. (ed.) *Psychoanalysis Today.* Allen & Unwin, London, 1948.

LYTTON, Earl of. *New Treasure.* Allen & Unwin, London, 1934.

MACKENZIE, R. F. *A Question of Living.* Collins, London, 1963.

MCLUHAN, M. and FOIRE, Q. *The Medium is the Message.* Allen Lane, Penguin Press, London, 1967.

MACMUNN, N. *A Path to Freedom in the School.* Curwen & Sons, London, 1914.

MCNAIR, H. S. *A Survey of Children in Residential Schools for the Maladjusted in Scotland.* Oliver & Boyd, Edinburgh, 1968.

MAUDSLEY, H. *Mental Pathology.* London, 1879.

MAYS, J. B. *Crime and the Social Structure.* Faber & Faber, London, 1967.

MILLER, D. *Growth to Freedom.* Tavistock, London, 1946.

MORRIS, Van C. *Existensialism in Education.* Harper & Row, New York, 1966.

MUSSEN, P. H. (et al.) *Child Development and Personality.* Harper & Rowe, New York, 1963.

NEILL, A. S. *A Dominie's Log.* Herbert Jenkins, London, 1915.

—— *A Dominie Dismissed.* Herbert Jenkins, London, 1916.

—— *A Dominie Abroad.* Herbert Jenkins, London, 1922.

—— *The Problem Child.* Herbert Jenkins, London, 1926.

—— *The Problem Parents.* Herbert Jenkins, London, 1932.

—— *Is Scotland Educated.* Herbert Jenkins, London, 1936.

—— *That Dreadful School.* Herbert Jenkins, London, 1937.

—— *The Problem Family.* Routledge & Kegan Paul, London, 1948.

—— *The Free Child.* Herbert Jenkins, London, 1953.

—— *The Problem Teacher.* Herbert Jenkins, London, 1957.

—— *Summerhill,* Gollancz, London, 1967.

O'CONNOR, D. J. *An Introduction to the Philosophy of Education.* Routledge & Kegan Paul, London, 1958.

OLLENDORFF, I. *Wilhelm Reich.* Elek, London, 1969.

PADLEY, R. and COLE, M. *The Evacuation Survey* (Report to Fabian Society). Routledge, London, 1940.

PEARSON, G. H. J. *Emotional Disorders in Children.* Norton, New York, 1949.

PECK, R. F. and HAVIGHURST, R. J. *The Psychology of Character Development.* Wiley, New York, 1960.

PEDLEY, R. *Comprehensive Education—a New Appraisal.* Gollancz, London, 1956.

PEKIN, L. B. *Progressive Schools.* Hogarth, London, 1934.

PERRY, L. R. (ed.) *Bertrand Russell, A. S. Neill, Homer Lane, W. H. Kilpatrick, Four Progressive educators.* Collier-Macmillan, London, 1967.

POWERS, E. and WITMER, H. *An Experiment in the Prevention of Delinquency.* Columbia University Press, New York, 1951.

PRITCHARD, D. G. *Education and the Handicapped 1760-1960.* Routledge & Kegan Paul, London, 1963.

REICH, W. *The Function of Orgasm.* Penguin, London, 1965.

REID, J. H. and HAGAN, H. R. *Residential Treatment of Disturbed Children.* Child Welfare League of America Inc. New York, 1952.

ROE, M. C. *Survey into Progress of Maladjusted Pupils.* Inner London Education Authority, London, 1965.

ROSE, G. *Schools for Young Offenders.* Tavistock, London, 1967.

ROSWELL, F. and NATCHEZ, G. *Reading Disability.* Basic Books Inc., New York, 1964.

SAXBY, I. B. *Education of Behaviour.* University of London Press, London, 1921.

SCHAFFNER, B. (ed.) *Group Processes.* Josiah Macy Jnr. Foundation, New York, 1950.

SHAW, O. L. *Maladjusted Boys.* Allen and Unwin, London, 1965.
—— *Prisons of the Mind.* Allen & Unwin, London, 1969.

SHEPHERD, A. P. *A Scientist of the Invisible.* Hodder & Stoughton, London, 1954.

SHIELDS, R. W. *A Cure of Delinquency.* Heinemann, London, 1962.

SIMEY, T. S. *The Concept of Love in Child Care.* Oxford University Press, London, 1961.

SIMPSON, J. H. *An Adventure in Education.* Sidgwick & Jackson, London, 1917.
—— *A Schoolmaster's Harvest.* Faber & Faber, London, 1954.

SKIDELSKY, R. *English Progressive Schools.* Penguin, London, 1969.

SLAVSON, S. R. *Re-educating the Delinquent Through Group and Community Participation.* Harper, New York, 1954.

STEINER, S. R. *The Education of Children from the Standpoint of Theosophy.* Theosophical Publishing Co., London, 1911.
—— *Discussions with Teachers.* Rudolph Steiner Press, 1919.
—— *The Story of my Life.* (H. Collinson ed.) Anthroposophical Publishing Co. (London) 1928.
—— *Education and Modern Spiritual Life.* Rudolph Steiner Press, London, 1943.

—— *The Kingdom of Childhood*. Rudolph Steiner Press, London, 1964.

STEVENSON, G. and SMITH, G. *Child Guidance Clinics: a quarter century of development*. Commonwealth Fund, New York, 1934.

STEWART, W. A. C. *The Educational Innovators*. Macmillan, London, 1969.

STRAUSS, A. A. and KEPHART, N. C. *Psychopathology and the Education of Brain-Injured Children*. Grune & Stratton, New York, 1955.

SUTTIE, I. D. *The Origins of Love and Hate*. Kegan Paul, Trench, Trubner, London, 1935.

THOMSON, R. *The Pelican History of Psychology*. Penguin, London, 1968.

THOULESS, R. H. *Map of Educational Research*. N.F.E.R., 1969.

TREDGOLD, A. F. *A Text-book of Mental Deficiency*. Baillière, Tindall & Cox, London, 1952.

ULLMANN, L. P. and KRASNER, L. *Case Studies in Behaviour Modification*. Holt, Rinehart and Winston, New York, 1965.

WALL, W. D. *Education and Mental Health*. Harrap (for UNESCO), 1955.

—— *Psychological Services for Schools*. UNESCO Institute for Education, Hamburg, 1956.

WALMSLEY, J. *Neill and Summerhill*. Penguin, London, 1969.

WERTHAM, F. *The Circle of Guilt*. Dennis Dobson, London, 1958.

WHITBOURN, F. *Lex: Alexander Devine, Founder of Clayesmore School*. Longman Green, London, 1937.

WILLS, W. D. *The Barns Experiment*. Allen & Unwin, London, 1945.

—— *Throw Away Thy Rod*. Gollancz, London, 1960.

—— *Commonsense about Young offenders*. Gollancz, London, 1962.

—— *The Hawkspur Experiment* (2nd edn.) Allen & Unwin, London, 1969.

—— *Homer Lane*. Allen & Unwin, London, 1964.

WOLFF, S. *Children Under Stress*. Allen Lane Penguin Press, London, 1969.

WOODS, A. *Educational Experiments in England*. Methuen, London, 1920.

WOOTON, B. *Social Science and Social Pathology*, Allen & Unwin, London, 1959.

YOUNG, A. F. & ASHTON, H. T. *British Social Work in the 19th Century*. Routledge & Kegan Paul, London, 1956.

YOUNG, E. H. *The New Era in Education*. Phillips, London, 1920.

ARTICLES AND REPORTS

BARRON, A. T. Preparing a Child for Placement. *New Era* **43** (2) 1962.
—— What is therapy—what is training? *Therapeutic Education*, Autumn 1969.

BLOOM, L. Some Aspects of the Residential Psychotherapy of Maladjusted or Delinquent Children. *Br. J. Delinq.* **VI** (1), 1955.

BURLINGHAM, D. and BARRON, A. T. A Study of Identical Twins. *The Psycho-analytical Study of the Child*. **xxiii**. 1963.

BURT, C. and HOWARD, M. The Nature and Causes of Maladjustment among Children of School Age. *Br. J. Psych.* (*Stat*) **V** (1), 1952.

CHAZAN, M. Maladjusted Pupils: Trends in Post-War Theory and Practice. *Educational Research* **VI** (1), 1963.

CRITCHLEY, C. An Experimental Study of Maladjusted Children. Unpublished M.A. Thesis, Liverpool University, 1969.

CRUTCHFIELD, R. Conformity and Character. *Am. Psych.* **x**, 1955.

DANBY, J. F. About Finchden Manor. *New Era*, **37** (7), August 1956.

DOCKAR-DRYSDALE, B. The Residential Treatment of Frozen Children. *Br. J. Delinq.* **14** (2), 1958.
—— The Provision of Primary Experience in a Therapeutic School. *J. of Psychology and Psychiatry* **7**, 1966.

EYSENCK, H. J. and PRELL, D. B. The Inheritance of Neuroticism: an Experimental Study. *J. Ment. Sci.* **XCVII**, 1951.

FRANKLIN, M. B. The Meaning of Planned Environmental Therapy. *A.W.M.C. Newsletter*, June 1966.
—— Discussion Groups. *A.W.M.C. Newsletter*, March 1968.
—— The Work of David Wills. *A.W.M.C. Newsletter* (1), Autumn 1968.

FULTON, J. E. Factors influencing the growth and pattern of the child guidance services and school psychological services in Britain from 1900 to the present time. M.A. Thesis, (unpublished) Queen's University, Belfast, 1964.

GARNE, J. Article on Northern House School in *Education*. **110** (2850), 1957.

GRIEVE, J. Some experiences in Shared Responsibility with normal and with maladjusted adolescents in *Studies in Environmental Therapy* 1 (the Planned Environmental Therapy Trust), 1968.

HENSHAW, E. M. Some Psychological Difficulties of Evacuation, *Mental Health* (1), 1940.

HOARE, R. F. Principles of Discipline and Self-Government. An experiment at Riverside Village. Report of the Sixth Annual Conference of Educational Associations, 1918.

ISSACS, S. Some Notes in the Incidence of Neurotic Difficulties in Young Children. *Br. J. Ed. Psych.* 2 (Part 1), 1932.

—— Fatherless Children in *Problems of Child Development*, N.E.F., 1948.

JENKINS, R. L. and GLICKMAN, S. Common Syndromes in Child Psychiatry Deviant Behaviour Traits. *Am. J. Orthopsychiatry* 16.

KEIR, G. A History of Child Guidance in Symposium of Psychologists and Psychiatrists in the Child Guidance Service, *Brit. J. Ed. Psych.* xxii(1) 1952.

LASLETT, R. The Place of the Day Special School in the Treatment of the Maladjusted Child. *A.W.M.C. Sixth Newsletter*, November, 1965.

—— A consideration of some of the principles of Planned Environmental Therapy and an enquiry as to whether these can be practised in a Day School for Maladjusted Children in *Studies in Environmental Therapy* 1, P.E.T. Trust, 1968.

LEVINE, (et al.) Conforming Behaviour of Psychiatric and Mental Patients *J. Abn. and Soc. Psych.* 49, 1954.

LEVITT, E. E. The Results of Psychotherapy with Children: an Evaluation. *J. Cons. Psychol.* (21), 1957.

LUNZER, E. A. Aggressive and Withdrawing Children in the Normal School—Patterns of Behaviour. *Br. J. Ed. Psych.* xxx, 1960.

LYWARD, G. A. Feeling Their Way Through *New Era* 13 (7), 1938.

—— 'The Permanent Need for Discipline'. *Annual Conference Home & Schools Council*, 1938.

—— Loving Children. *New Era* 4 (12) 1940.

—— In Conclusion in 'Problems of Child Development', *New Education Fellowship*, London, 1948.

—— A comment on standards: particularly for parents. *New Era* 34 (7) 1953.

—— Loyalty to the Maladjusted Child. *New Era* 36 (3), 1954.

—— The Residential Care of Disturbed Children. *Proceedings of the 14th Inter-clinic Conference N.A.M.H.* 1958.

—— The School as a Therapeutic Community in *Psychiatry in a changing Society.* Tavistock, London, 1969.

NEILL, A. S. On Reich in 'William Reich and the sexual revolution'. *Anarchy* (105) 1969.

PETRIE, I. R. J. Residential treatment of Maladjusted Children: A study of some factors related to progress in adjustment. *Br. J. Ed. Psych.* **xxxii.**

PRINGLE, M. L. K. Differences between Boarding Schools for the Maladjusted and ordinary Boarding Schools. *Br. J. Ed. Psych.* **xxvii** (1) 1957).

—— and SUTCLIFFE, B. *Remedial Education—An Experiment* Published by the Caldecott Community and the Department of Child Study, University of Birmingham Institute of Education, 1960.

REDL, F. Group Emotions and Leadership. *Psychiatry* **5**, 1942.

RENDEL, L. *Child of Misfortune.* The Caldecott Community, 1952.

RICE, A. K. 'Cotswold Community and School', *Working note No. 1.* (mimeographed), Tavistock Institute, February, 1968.

RODWAY, S. Leila Rendel O.B.E. 1883-1969. *Therapeutic Education,* Autumn 1969.

ROYAL MEDICAL-PSYCHOLOGICAL ASSOCIATION REPORT. Schools and Hostels for Maladjusted Children. *J. of Psychiatry,* March 1966.

SLAVSON, S. R. Group therapy in Child Care and Child Guidance. *Jewish Social Services Quarterly* **XXV** (2), 1948.

SODDY, K. *Contribution Factors* in 'The Maladjusted Child—the Underwood Report & After'. Proceedings of N.A.H.M. Conference, 11-12 April, 1957.

TIMES EDUCATIONAL SUPPLEMENT: Correspondent, Arlesford Place Hostel School: care and cure of maladjusted youth. 16 March 1951.

U.S. DEPT. OF HEALTH, EDUCATION AND WELFARE. Teachers of Children who are socially and emotionally maladjusted. *Bulletin* No. 11, 1957.

WARNER, F. Mental and Physical Conditions Among Fifty Thousand Children. *J. Roy. Stat. Soc.* **LIX**, 1896.

WEAVER, A. F. A Survey of the Treatment of Maladjusted Children within the Educational System in England. Unpublished Ph.D. Thesis, Oxford University 1968.

WILLIAMS, N. Criteria of Recovery of Maladjusted Children in Residential School. Unpublished M.A. Thesis, Durham University 1961.

WILLS, W. D. Shared Responsibility in 'Problems of Child Development' *New Education Fellowship*, London, 1948.

—— Aftercare at Schools for Maladjusted Children. *A.W.M.C. Newsletter No.* 6, 1965.

—— Eliminating Punishment in the Residential Treatment of Troublesome Boys and Young Men in *Studies in Environmental Therapy* **1**, 1968.

WINNICOTT, D. W. and BRITTON, C. The Problem of Homeless Children in 'Problems of Child Development'. *New Education Fellowship*, London, 1948.

WOLFF, S. Two recent Scottish Government Reports. *A.W.M.C. Newsletter No.* **4**, 1964.

Name Index

Abbotsholme, 66, 123, 125
Adams, J. W. L., 17
Adler, A., 135, 144, 170, 179
Aichhorn, A., 179, 181, 249, 263
Aitkenhead, J., 306, 309, 310, 311
Allen, Lady, 220, 224
Anselm, Brother, 238
d'Arcampbell Association, 99, 105
d'Arcy Osborne, Lady, 255
Arlesford Place, 25, 94, 213, 214, 215, 216, 221, 264, 265, 266
Armstrong, J., 278
Arnold, T., 66
Arrowsmith, Mr, 140
Ashton, E. T., 55
Association of Workers for Maladjusted Children, 13, 37, 180, 194, 287, 288, 325, 327, 362
Auden, W. H., 101, 112
Baden-Powell, Lord, 248
Badley, J. H., 111, 132, 251, 255
Bain, A., 49
Balbernie, R., 13, 35, 53, 221, 279, 359, 360, 370, 371, 372, 373
Bandura, A., 375
Barbe, W. B., 32
Barnardo, Dr, 56, 58, 316
Barnes, K. C., 251, 252, 253
Barns Hostel, 35, 189, 191, 192, 193, 303, 307, 309
Barron, A. J., 13, 216, 217, 218, 219, 220, 221, 222, 223, 224, 252, 263, 264, 267, 268
Barton-Hall, S. and M., 149
Bateman, W. Hurst, 243
Bazeley, Miss E. T., 97, 101, 102, 108, 109, 111, 181
B.B.C., 214
Bedales School, 66, 111, 123, 251, 255
Beltane School, 249
Bettelheim, B., 169, 185
Birmingham Society for the Care of Invalid and Nervous Children, 243
Blackburn, Miss, 243
Bodenham Manor, 192, 193, 291
Booth, C., 150
Booth, W., 150
Borstal, 79, 182, 264, 293
Bowlby, J., 33, 61, 201
Boy Scouts, 248
Boyd, W., 110, 140

Brackenhill Theosophical Home School, 123
Breckenbrough, 151
Bredinghurst, 292, 293, 341
Bridges, K. M. B., 301
Bristol Working and Visiting Soc. 59
British Child Study Association, 51
Burgess Hill School, 249
Burlingham, D., 222
Burn, M., 163
Burns, C., 37, 209
Burt, C., 51, 52, 92, 93, 94, 147, 148, 149, 203, 208, 218, 333
Caldecott Community, 79, 80, 81, 82, 83, 85, 86, 87, 88, 89, 233, 236
Cambridge Evacuation Survey, 201,
Cameron, A. C., 297
Cameron, H., 144
Camphill, 375
Carlebach, J., 361, 370
Carmel College, 294
Carpenter, M., 56, 58, 59, 60, 61, 62, 63, 64, 65, 77, 228, 230, 306
Cattell, R. G., 49, 147, 148, 301
Central Training Council, 225, 364
Centre of Applied Social Research, 371
Chaigeley, 35, 94, 111, 192, 239, 244, 246, 289, 291, 312, 316
Child Guidance Clinics, 226, 367, 368
Child Guidance Council, 149
Child Welfare Association, 241
Children's Act 1908, 147
Children's Act 1948, 82, 201, 225,
Children's Act 1969, 63, 372
Children's Social Adjustment Society, 212, 264
Children's Village, 99
Children and Young Person's Act 1969, 14, 370, 373
Childscourt, 215
Chinn, Wilfred, 79
Church National Society, 234
Churchill, W., 194
Claparède, E., 142, 143, 155
Clarke, Sir F., 297
Clarke, Miss G., 297, 298
Clayesmore, 66, 68, 69
Clinical Therapeutic Institute, 124
Clyde Committee (Scotland), 224
Cole, M., 201

Topic Index